Clinical Dermatology

ed by the

be

at least

Libra

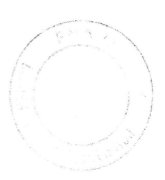

For Ruth, Patricia and Arlene

Clinical Dermatology

J.A.A. Hunter
OBE BA MD FRCP (Edin)
Professor Emeritus of Dermatology
University of Edinburgh
The Royal Infirmary
Edinburgh

J.A. Savin
MA MD ChB FRCP DIH
Former Consultant Dermatologist
The Royal Infirmary
Edinburgh

M.V. Dahl
BA MD
Professor and Chair
Department of Dermatology
Mayo Clinic Scottsdale
Scottsdale, USA, and
Professor Emeritus
University of Minnesota Medical School
Minneapolis, Minnesota, USA

THIRD EDITION

Blackwell
Science

© 1989, 1995, 2002 by Blackwell Science Ltd
a Blackwell Publishing company
Blackwell Science, Inc., 350 Main Street, Malden, Massachusetts 02148-5018, USA
Blackwell Science Ltd, Osney Mead, Oxford OX2 0EL, UK
Blackwell Science Asia Pty Ltd, 550 Swanston Street, Carlton, Victoria 3053, Australia
Blackwell Wissenschafts Verlag, Kurfürstendamm 57, 10707 Berlin, Germany

First published 1989
Reprinted 1990, 1992, 1994
Second edition 1995
Reprinted 1996, 1999
Third edition 2002

Library of Congress Cataloging-in-Publication Data

Hunter, J. A. A.
    Clinical dermatology / J.A.A. Hunter, J.A. Savin, M.V. Dahl.— 3rd ed.
      p. ; cm.
Includes index.
    ISBN 0-632-05916-8
    1. Skin—Diseases.   2. Dermatology.
    [DNLM: 1. Skin Diseases—diagnosis.   2. Skin Diseases—therapy. WR
140 H945c 2002]   I. Savin, John.   II. Dahl, Mark V.   III. Title.
    RL71 .H934 2002
    616.5—dc21

                                                              2002007252

ISBN 0-632-05916-8

A catalogue record for this title is available from the British Library

Set in 9/12 Sabon by Graphicraft Limited, Hong Kong
Printed and bound in Denmark by Narayana Press, Odder

Commissioning Editor: Stuart Taylor
Managing Editor: Rupal Malde
Editorial Assistant: Heather Johnson
Production Editor: Julie Elliott
Production Controller: Kate Wilson

For further information on Blackwell Science, visit our website:
www.blackwell-science.com

Contents

Preface to the third edition, vi
Preface to the first edition, viii
Introduction, ix

1   Skin disease in perspective, 1
2   The function and structure of the skin, 7
3   Diagnosis of skin disorders, 29
4   Disorders of keratinization, 41
5   Psoriasis, 48
6   Other papulosquamous disorders, 63
7   Eczema and dermatitis, 70
8   Reactive erythemas and vasculitis, 94
9   Bullous diseases, 107
10 Connective tissue disorders, 119
11 Disorders of blood vessels and lymphatics, 132
12 Sebaceous and sweat gland disorders, 148
13 Regional dermatology, 162
14 Infections, 189
15 Infestations, 224
16 Skin reactions to light, 233
17 Disorders of pigmentation, 242
18 Skin tumours, 253
19 The skin in systemic disease, 283
20 The skin and the psyche, 294
21 Other genetic disorders, 300
22 Drug eruptions, 307
23 Medical treatment, 314
24 Physical forms of treatment, 321

Formulary 1: Topical treatments, 328
Formulary 2: Systemic medication, 340

Index, 355

Preface to the third edition

Five years is a long time in modern medicine, and we feel that the moment has come for *Clinical Dermatology* to move into its third edition. As before, every chapter has been updated extensively, but our aim is still the same—to create an easily read text that will help family doctors to get to grips with a subject many still find confusing, despite the increasingly stodgy sets of guidelines that now land regularly on their desks.

We have selected the best elements of these guidelines for our new sections on treatment, which are therefore much more 'evidence based'. However, if we had to include only treatments based on flawless evidence, we would have to leave out too many old favourites that have stood the test of time, but have still not been evaluated properly. Next time perhaps.

We have also reacted to a survey of our readers, which showed that most of them spend little time on the chapters devoted only to the structure, function and immunology of the skin. We have pruned these back, but have put more physiology and pathology into the relevant clinical chapters where it should be of more use to a doctor struggling through a busy surgery.

Other changes too have been prompted by the helpful comments of our readers. They include a new chapter on regional dermatology, dealing with the special problems of areas such as the mouth and the genitalia; the replacement of several unloved clinical photographs; the insertion of a list of suggestions for further reading at the end of each chapter; more discussion of the ageing skin and of quality of life issues; and more emphasis on the types of surgery that can easily be undertaken by family doctors. More power to their elbows.

Finally, many important recent advances have entered every chapter on their own merits. Dermatoscopy, the expanding role of lasers, 'sun sense', and the drug treatment of AIDS are good examples of these. In addition, some new subjects, such as cutaneous anthrax, have been forced into the new edition by outside events.

We welcome you to our third edition.

Acknowledgements

Many of the clinical photographs come from the collection of the Department of Dermatology at the Royal Infirmary of Edinburgh and we wish to thank all those who presented them. We are most grateful to Graeme Chambers who has redrawn the previous line drawings as well as creating the new figures for the third edition, and to Geraldine Jeffers, Julie Elliott and Stuart Taylor of Blackwell Publishing for their help and encouragement in preparing this book.

We are also most grateful to the publishers for permission to use illustrations previously published in the following books:

Champion, R.H., Burton, J.L., Ebling, F.J.G. (1992) *Textbook of Dermatalogy*, 5th edn. Blackwell Scientific Publications, Oxford.

Edwards, C.R.W., Bouchier, I.A.D., Haslett, C., Chilvers, E.R. (1999) *Davidson's Principles and Practice of Medicine*, 17th edn. Churchill Livingstone, Edinburgh.

Gawkrodger, D.J. (1997) *An Illustrated Colour Text of Dermatology*. Churchill Livingstone, Edinburgh.

Kavanagh, G.M., Savin, J.A. (1998) *Self Assessment Picture Tests: Dermatology*. Mosby, London.

Munro, J., Campbell, I.W. (2000) *Macleod's Clinical Examination*, 10th edn. Churchill Livingstone, Edinburgh.

Percival, G.H., Montgomery, G.L., Dodds, T.C. (1962) *Atlas of Histopathology of the Skin*, 2nd edn. E.B. Livingstone, Edinburgh.

Savin, J.A., Hunter, J.A.A., Hepburn, N.C. (1997) *Skin Signs in Clinical Medicine: Diagnosis in Colour*. Mosby-Wolfe, London.

Sayer, H.P., *et al.* (2001) *Dermoscopy of Pigmented Skin Lesions*. EDRA Medical Publishing and New Media, Milan.

Disclaimer

Although every effort has been made to ensure that drug doses and other information are presented accurately in this publication, the ultimate responsibility rests with the prescribing physician. Neither the publishers nor the authors can be held responsible for any consequences arising from the use of information contained herein. Any product mentioned in this publication should be used in accordance with the prescribing information prepared by the manufacturers.

Preface to the first edition

Some 10% of those who go to their family doctors do so with skin problems. We have seen an improvement in the way these have been managed over the last few years, but the subject still baffles many medical students—on both sides of the Atlantic. They find it hard to get a grip on the soggy mass of facts served up by some textbooks. For them we have tried to create an easily-read text with enough detail to clarify the subject but not enough to obscure it.

There are many doctors too who are puzzled by dermatology, even after years in practice. They have still to learn how to look at the skin with a trained eye. Anyone who denies that clinical dermatology is a visual specialty can never have practised it. In this book we have marked out the route to diagnostic success with a simple scheme for recognizing primary skin lesions using many diagrams and coloured plates.

We hope that this book will help both groups—students and doctors, including some in general medicine and some starting to train as dermatologists —and of course their patients. We make no apologies for our emphasis on diagnosis and management, and accept that we cannot include every remedy. Here, we mention only those preparations we have found to be useful and, to avoid too many trade names, we have tabulated those used in the UK and the USA in a Formulary at the back of the book.

We have decided not to break up the text by quoting lists of references. For those who want to know more there are many large and excellent textbooks on the shelves of all medical libraries.

While every effort has been made to ensure that the doses mentioned here are correct, the authors and publishers cannot accept responsibility for any errors in dosage which may have inadvertently entered this book. The reader is advised to check dosages, adverse effects, drug interactions, and contraindications in the latest edition of the *British National Formulary* or *Drug Information* (American Society of Hospital Pharmacists).

Introduction

Our overall aim in this book has been to make dermatology easy to understand by the many busy doctors who glimpsed it only briefly, if at all, during their medical training. All too often the subject has been squeezed out of its proper place in the undergraduate curriculum, leaving growing numbers who quail before the skin and its reputed 2000 conditions, each with its own diverse presentations. They can see the eruptions clearly enough, but cannot describe or identify them. There are no machines to help them. Even official 'clinical guidelines' for treatment are no use if a diagnosis has not been made. Their patients quickly sense weakness and lose faith. We hope that this book will give them confidence in their ability to make the right diagnosis and then to prescribe safe and effective treatment.

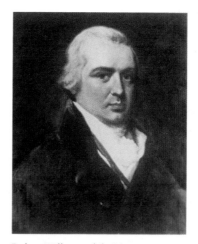

Robert Willan used the Linnaean system of botanical classification to divide skin diseases into eight orders.

To do so they will need some understanding of the anatomy, physiology and immunology of the skin (Chapter 2): but, as Robert Willan (1757–1812) (Figure) (recently elected as 'Dermatologist of the Millennium') showed long ago, the simple steps that lead to a sensible working diagnosis must start with the identification of primary skin lesions and the patterns these have taken up on the skin surface (Chapter 3). After this has been achieved, investigations can be directed along sensible lines (Chapter 3) until a firm diagnosis is reached. Then, and only then, will the correct line of treatment snap into place.

But another cloud of mystery has settled here, over the subject of topical treatment. We attempt to blow this away with a few simple rules governing the selection of the right active ingredient, and of the right vehicle in which it should be put up (Chapter 23). Correct choices here will be repaid by good results. Patients may be quick to complain if they are not doing well: equally they are delighted if their eruptions can be seen to melt rapidly away. Many of them are now joining in the quest for cosmetic perfection that is already well advanced in the USA and becoming more fashionable in the UK. Family doctors who are asked about this topic can find their answers in our new chapter on physical methods of treatment (Chapter 24).

We do not pretend that all of the problems in the classification of skin diseases have been solved in this book. Far from it: some will remain as long as their causes are still unknown, but we make no apology for trying to keep our terminology as simple as possible. Many doctors are put off by the cumbersome Latin names left behind by earlier pseudo-botanical classifications. Names like *painful nodule of the ear* or *ear corn* must now be allowed to take over from more traditional ones such as *chondrodermatitis nodularis helicis chronica*, and fist fights over the difference between dermatitis and eczema must now stop.

As well as simplifying the terminology, we have concentrated mainly on common conditions, which make up the bulk of dermatology in developed countries, though we do mention some others, which may be rare, but which illustrate important general principles. We have also tried to cut out as many synonyms and eponyms as possible. We have included some further reading at the end of each chapter for those wanting more information and, for the connoisseur, the names of some reference books at the end of this section.

We have, wherever possible, grouped together conditions that have the same cause, e.g. fungal infections (Chapter 14) and drug reactions (Chapter 22). Failing this, some chapters are based on a shared physiology, e.g. disorders of keratinization (Chapter 4) or on a shared anatomy, e.g. disorders of hair and nails (Chapter 13), of blood vessels (Chapter 11) or of the sweat glands (Chapter 12). In some chapters we have, reluctantly, been forced to group together conditions that share physical characteristics, e.g. the bullous diseases (Chapter 9) and the papulosquamous disorders (Chapter 6): but this is unsound, and brings together some strange bedfellows. Modern research will surely soon reallocate their positions in the dormitory of dermatology. Finally, we must mention, sooner rather than later, electronic communication and the help that it can offer both patients and doctors. Web sites are proliferating almost as rapidly as the epidermal cells in psoriasis; this section deserves its own heading.

Dermatology on the Internet

The best web sites are packed with useful information: others are less trustworthy. We rely heavily on those of the British Association of Dermatologists (www.bad.org.uk) and the American Academy of Dermatology (www.aad.org) for current guidelines on how to manage a variety of individual skin conditions. They also provide excellent patient information leaflets, and the addresses of patient support groups. The British Dermatologists Internet Site (www.bdis.org.uk) offers further guidelines for British general practitioners on the management of common skin diseases, including advice on when to refer them to a dermatologist.

Two other favourite sites are linked lists of dermatology websites (www.fammed.wisc.edu/education/presentation/derm/Dermcurriculum.html and www.medwebplus.com/subject/Dermatology). They provide many images of skin diseases, dermatology quizzes and lectures, interactive cases, and even an electronic textbook of dermatology. Finally, it is becoming easier to browse through dermatology journals online (www.mednets.com/dermatoljournals.htm). The full text of over half of the world's 200 most cited journals is now available on a web site (http//highwire.stanford.edu) that includes the famous 'Topic map': few pleasures exceed that of 'exploding' clinical medicine into its subcategories by a process of simple clicking and dragging.

Further reading

Braun-Falco, O., Plewig, G., Wolff, H.H. and Burgdorf, W.H.C. (eds). (1999) *Dermatology*, 2nd edn. Berlin & Heidelberg, Springer Verlag.

Champion, R.H., Burton, J.L., Burns, D.A. and Breathnach, S.M. (eds). (1998) *Textbook of Dermatology*, 6th edn. Oxford, Blackwell Science.

Crissey, J.T., Parish, L.C. and Holuber, K. (2001) *Historical Atlas of Dermatology and Dermatologists*. London, Parthenon.

Freedberg, I.M., Eisen, A.Z., Wolff, K., Goldsmith, L.A., Katz, S.I., Fitzpatrick, T.B. (eds). (1998) *Fitzpatrick's Dermatology in General Medicine*, 5th edn. New York, McGraw Hill.

Harper, J., Oranje, A. and Prose, N. (eds). (2000) *Textbook of Pediatric Dermatology*. Oxford, Blackwell Science.

Lebwohl, M., Heymann, W.R., Berth-Jones, J. and Coulson, I. (2002) *Treatment of Skin Diseases. Comprehensive Therapeutic Strategies*. New York, Mosby.

Shelley, W.B. and Shelley, E.D. (2001) *Advanced Dermatologic Therapy II*. Philadelphia, W.B. Saunders.

Sitaru, C. (1998) Dermatology resources on the Internet: a practical guide for dermatologists. *Int J Dermatol* 37: 641–7.

Skin disease in perspective

Dermatology is the study of the skin and its associated structures, including the hair and nails, and of their diseases. It is an immense subject, embracing some 2000 conditions, yet, paradoxically, some 70% of the dermatology work in the UK is caused by only nine types of skin disorder (Table 1.1). Similarly, in the USA, nearly half of all visits to dermatologists are for one of three diagnoses: acne, warts and skin tumours. Things are very different in developing countries where over-crowding and poor sanitation play a major part. There, skin disorders are even more common, particularly in the young, but are dominated by infections and infestations—the so-called 'dermatoses of poverty'—amplified by the presence of HIV infection.

A sense of perspective is important, and this chapter presents an overview of the causes, prevalence and impact of skin disease.

Causes

The skin is the boundary between ourselves and the world around us. It is an important sense organ, and controls heat and water loss. It reflects internal changes

Table 1.1 The most common categories of skin disorder in the UK.

Skin cancer
Acne
Atopic eczema
Psoriasis
Viral warts
Other infective skin disorders
Benign tumours and vascular lesions
Leg ulcers
Contact dermatitis and other eczemas

(Chapter 19) and reacts to external ones. Usually, it adapts easily and returns to a normal state, but some-times it fails to do so and a skin disorder appears. Some of the internal and external factors that are important causes of skin disease are shown in Fig. 1.1. Often several will be operating at the same time; just as often, no obvious cause for a skin abnormality can be found—and here lies much of the difficulty of dermatology. Nevertheless, when a cause is obvious, such as the washing of dishes and the appearance of irritant hand dermatitis, or sunburn and the develop-ment of melanoma, education and prevention are just as important as treatment.

Prevalence

No one who has worked in any branch of medicine will doubt the importance of diseases of the skin. A neurologist, for example, will know all about the Sturge–Weber syndrome, a gastroenterologist about the Peutz–Jeghers syndrome, and a cardiologist about the LEOPARD syndrome; but even in their own wards they will see far more of other common skin conditions such as drug eruptions, asteatotic eczema and scabies. They should know about these too.

In primary care, skin problems are even more important, and the prevalence of some common skin conditions, such as skin cancer and atopic eczema, is undoubtedly rising. Currently, skin disorders account for about 15% of all consultations in general practice in the UK, but this is only the tip of an iceberg of skin disease, the sunken part of which consists of problems that never get to doctors, being dealt with or ignored in the community.

How large is this problem? No one quite knows, as those who are not keen to see their doctors seldom star in the medical literature. The results of a study of

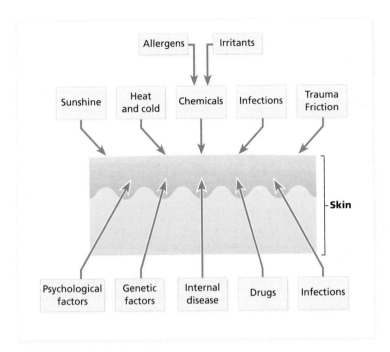

Fig. 1.1 Some internal and external factors causing skin diseases.

Table 1.2 Responses to minor ailments.

Did not use anything	45%
Used a home remedy	9%
Used an over-the-counter remedy	24%
Used a prescription remedy already in the house	13%
Saw a doctor	13%

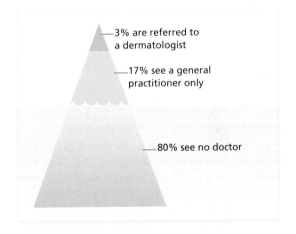

Fig. 1.2 The 'iceberg' of psoriasis in the UK during a single year.

the responses to minor ailments of all types are shown in Table 1.2; clearly a few sufferers took more than one course of action. These responses apply to skin disorders too, and form the basis for the 'iceberg' of psoriasis in the UK shown in Fig. 1.2. In the course of a single year most of those with psoriasis see no doctor, and only a few will see a dermatologist. Some may have fallen victim to fraudulent practices, such as 'herbal' preparations laced with steroids, and baseless advice on 'allergies'.

Several large studies have confirmed that this is the case with other skin diseases too.
• Of a large representative sample of the US population, 31.2% were found to have significant skin disease that deserved medical attention. Scaled up, these figures suggest that some 80 million of the US population may have significant skin diseases.

• A community study of adults in the UK found 22.5% to have a skin disease needing medical attention: only one in five of these had seen a doctor within the preceding 6 months. Self-medication was far more common than any treatment prescribed by doctors.
• In another UK study, 14% of adults and 19% of children had used a skin medication during the previous 2 weeks; only one-tenth of these were prescribed by

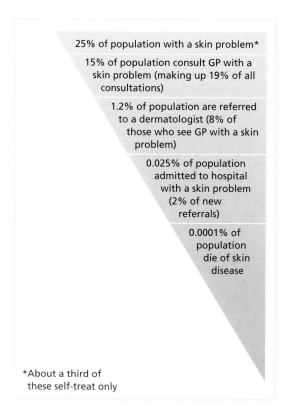

25% of population with a skin problem*

15% of population consult GP with a skin problem (making up 19% of all consultations)

1.2% of population are referred to a dermatologist (8% of those who see GP with a skin problem)

0.025% of population admitted to hospital with a skin problem (2% of new referrals)

0.0001% of population die of skin disease

*About a third of these self-treat only

Fig. 1.3 Skin problems in the UK and how they are dealt with in 1 year (derived from Williams 1996). Patients in the USA usually refer themselves to dermatologists.

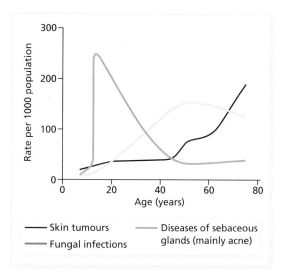

Fig. 1.4 The age-dependent prevalence of some skin conditions.

Table 1.3 Some factors influencing the prevalence of skin diseases in a community.

High level of	High incidence of
Ultraviolet radiation	Skin malignancy in Caucasians
Heat and humidity	Fungal and bacterial infections
Industrialization	Contact dermatitis
Underdevelopment	Infestations
	Bacterial and fungal infections

doctors. In a study of several tons of unused medicinal preparations, 7% by weight were manufactured for topical use on the skin.

• Preparations used to treat skin disease can be found in about half of all homes in the UK; the ratio of non-prescribed to prescribed remedies is about 6 : 1. Skin treatments come second only to painkillers in the list of non-prescription medicines. Even so, in the list of the most commonly prescribed groups of drugs in the UK, those for topical use in skin conditions still come second—behind diuretics.

Every 10 years or so we are given a snapshot of the way skin disorders are being dealt with in the UK, in a series of reports entitled *Morbidity Statistics from General Practice*. Some of the details from these, and from other studies, are given in Fig. 1.3. In addition, within each community, different age groups suffer from different skin conditions. In the USA, for example, diseases of the sebaceous glands (mainly acne) peak at the age of about 18 years and then decline, while the prevalence of skin tumours steadily mounts with age (Fig. 1.4).

The pattern of skin disease in a community depends on many other factors too, both genetic and environmental; some are listed in Table 1.3.

Impact

Much of this book is taken up with ways in which skin diseases can do harm. Most fit into the five Ds shown in Fig. 1.5; others are more subtle. Topical treatment, for example, can seem illogical to those who think that their skin disease is emotional in origin; it has been shown recently that psoriatics with great disability comply especially poorly with topical treatment.

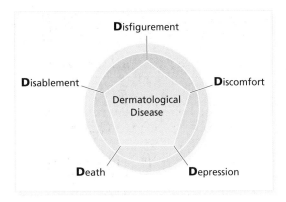

Fig. 1.5 The five Ds of dermatological disease.

In addition, the problems created by skin disease do not necessarily tally with the extent and severity of the eruption as judged by an outside observer. Quality-of-life studies give a different, patient-based, view of skin conditions. Questionnaires have been designed to compare the impact of skin diseases with those of other conditions; patients with bad psoriasis, for example, have at least as great a disability as those with angina. In the background lurk problems due to the costs of treatment and time lost from work.

Disfigurement

The possible reactions to disfiguring skin disease are described on p. 294. They range from a leper complex (e.g. some patients with psoriasis, p. 294), to embarrassment (e.g. port-wine stains, Fig. 1.6) or androgenetic alopecia in both men and women (p. 166). Disorders of body image can lead those who have no skin disease to think that they have, and even to commit suicide in this mistaken belief (dermatological non-disease, p. 295).

Discomfort

Some people prefer pain to itch; skin diseases can provide both. Itchy skin disorders include eczema (p. 70), lichen planus (p. 64), scabies (p. 227) and dermatitis herpetiformis (p. 113). Pain is marked in shingles (p. 206), leg ulcers (p. 139) and glomus tumours (p. 277).

Disability

Skin conditions are capable of ruining the quality of anyone's life. Each carries its own set of problems. At the most obvious level, dermatitis of the hands can quickly destroy a manual worker's earning capacity, as many hairdressers, nurses, cooks and mechanics know to their cost. In the USA, skin diseases account for almost half of all cases of occupational illness and cause more than 50 million days to be lost from work each year.

Disability and disfigurement can blend in a more subtle way, so that, for example, in times of unem-

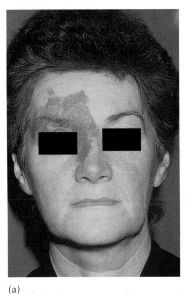

(a)

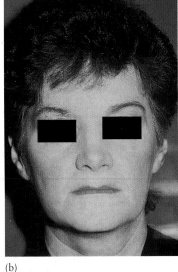

(b)

Fig. 1.6 (a) This patient has a port-wine stain. (b) Her life is transformed by her clever use of modern camouflage cosmetics, which take her less than a minute to apply.

ployment people with acne find it hard to get jobs. Psoriatics in the USA, already plagued by tactless hairdressers and messy treatments, have been shown to lose thousands of dollars in earnings by virtue of time taken off work. Even trivial psoriasis on the fingertips of blind people can have a huge effect on their lives by making it impossible to read Braille.

Depression

The physical, sensory and functional problems listed above often lead to depression and anxiety, even in the most stable people. Depression also seems to modulate the perception of itching, which becomes much worse. Feelings of stigmatization and rejection are common in patients with chronic skin diseases: up to 10% of patients with psoriasis that they think is bad have had suicidal thoughts. The risk of suicide in patients with severe acne is discussed on p. 155.

Death

Deaths from skin disease are fortunately rare, but they do occur (e.g. in pemphigus, toxic epidermal necrolysis and cutaneous malignancies). In addition, the stresses generated by a chronic skin disorder such as psoriasis predispose to heavy smoking and drinking, which carry their own risks.

In this context, the concept of skin failure is an important one. It may occur when any inflammatory skin disease becomes so widespread that it prevents normal functioning of the skin, with the results listed in Table 1.4. Its causes include erythroderma (p. 69), toxic epidermal necrolysis (p. 115), severe erythema multiforme (p. 99), pustular psoriasis (p. 53) and pemphigus (p. 108).

LEARNING POINTS

1 'Prevalence' and 'incidence rates' are not the same thing. Learn the difference and join a small select band.
(a) The **prevalence** of a disease is the proportion of a defined population affected by it at a particular point in time.
(b) The **incidence rate** is the proportion of a defined population developing the disease within a specified period of time.
2 A skin disease that seems trivial to a doctor can still wreck a patient's life.

Further reading

Black, M. (1999) Lessons from dermatology: implications for future provision of specialist services. *Journal of the Royal College of Physicians*, **33**, 208–211.

Table 1.4 The consequences of skin failure.

Function	Skin failure	Treatment
Temperature control	Cannot sweat when too hot: cannot vasoconstrict when too cold. Hence temperature swings dangerously up and down	Controlled environmental temperature
Barrier function	Raw skin surfaces lose much fluid and electrolytes Heavy protein loss Bacterial pathogens multiply on damaged skin	Monitor and replace High protein diet Antibiotic. Bathing/wet compresses
Cutaneous blood flow	Shunt through skin may lead to high output cardiac failure in those with poor cardiac reserve	Aggressively treat skin Support vital signs
Others	Erythroderma may lead to malabsorption Hair and nail loss later Nursing problems handling patients particularly with toxic epidermal necrolysis (p. 115) and pemphigus (p. 108)	Usually none needed Regrow spontaneously Nurse as for burns

Finlay, A.Y. (1997) Quality of life measurement in dermatology: a practical guide. *British Journal of Dermatology*, **136**, 305–314.

Grob, J.J., Stern, R.S., Mackie, R.M & Weinstock, W.A. eds. (1997) *Epidemiology, Causes and Prevention of Skin Diseases*. Blackwell Science, Oxford.

Royal College of General Practitioners (1995) *Morbidity Statistics from General Practice: Fourth National Study 1991–92*. HMSO, London.

Savin, J.A. (1993) The hidden face of dermatology. *Clinical and Experimental Dermatology*, **18**, 393–395.

Williams, H.C. (1997) Dermatology. In: Stevens, A., Raftery, J. (eds) *Health Care Needs Assessment*. Series 2. Radcliffe Medical Press, Oxford.

The function and structure of the skin

The skin—the interface between humans and their environment—is the largest organ in the body. It weighs an average of 4 kg and covers an area of 2 m^2. It acts as a barrier, protecting the body from harsh external conditions and preventing the loss of important body constituents, especially water. A death from destruction of skin, as in a burn, or in toxic epidermal necrolysis (p. 115), and the misery of unpleasant acne, remind us of its many important functions, which range from the vital to the cosmetic (Table 2.1).

The skin has two layers. The outer is epithelial, the *epidermis*, which is firmly attached to, and supported by connective tissue in the underlying *dermis*. Beneath the dermis is loose connective tissue, the *subcutis/hypodermis* which usually contains abundant fat (Fig. 2.1).

Epidermis

The epidermis is formed from many layers of closely packed cells, the most superficial of which are flattened and filled with keratins; it is therefore a stratified squamous epithelium. It adheres to the dermis partly by the interlocking of its downward projections (*epidermal ridges* or *pegs*) with upward projections of the dermis (*dermal papillae*) (Fig. 2.1).

Table 2.1 Functions of the skin.

Function	Structure/cell involved
Protection against:	
chemicals, particles	Horny layer
ultraviolet radiation	Melanocytes
antigens, haptens	Langerhans cells
microbes	Langerhans cells
Preservation of a balanced internal environment	Horny layer
Prevents loss of water, electrolytes and macromolecules	Horny layer
Shock absorber	Dermis and subcutaneous fat
Strong, yet elastic and compliant	
Temperature regulation	Blood vessels
	Eccrine sweat glands
Insulation	Subcutaneous fat
Sensation	Specialized nerve endings
Lubrication	Sebaceous glands
Protection and prising	Nails
Calorie reserve	Subcutaneous fat
Vitamin D synthesis	Keratinocytes
Body odour/pheromones	Apocrine sweat glands
Psychosocial, display	Skin, lips, hair and nails

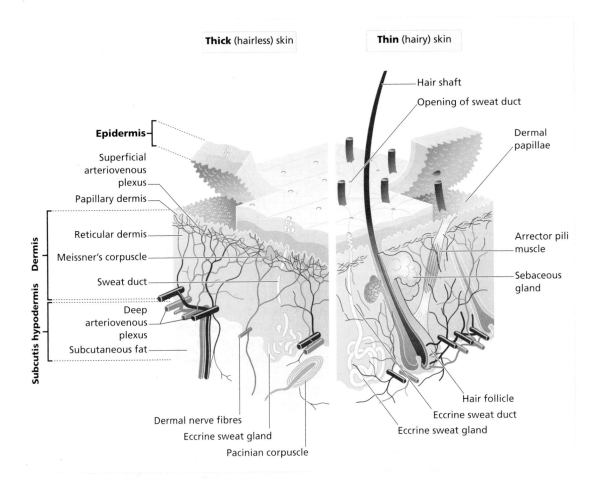

Fig. 2.1 Three-dimensional diagram of the skin, including a hair follicle.

The epidermis contains no blood vessels. It varies in thickness from less than 0.1 mm on the eyelids to nearly 1 mm on the palms and soles. As dead surface squames are shed (accounting for some of the dust in our houses), the thickness is kept constant by cells dividing in the deepest (*basal* or *germinative*) layer. A generated cell moves, or is pushed by underlying mitotic activity, to the surface, passing through the *prickle* and *granular cell layers* before dying in the *horny layer*. The journey from the basal layer to the surface (epidermal turnover or transit time) takes about 60 days. During this time the appearance of the cell changes. A vertical section through the epidermis summarizes the life history of a single epidermal cell (Fig. 2.2).

The *basal layer*, the deepest layer, rests on a basement membrane, which attaches it to the dermis. It is a single layer of columnar cells, whose basal surfaces sprout many fine processes and hemidesmosomes, anchoring them to the *lamina densa* of the basement membrane.

In normal skin some 30% of basal cells are preparing for division (growth fraction). Following mitosis, a cell enters the G_1 phase, synthesizes RNA and protein, and grows in size (Fig. 2.3). Later, when the cell is triggered to divide, DNA is synthesized (S phase) and chromosomal DNA is replicated. A short postsynthetic (G_2) phase of further growth occurs before mitosis (M). DNA synthesis continues through the S and G_2 phases, but not during mitosis. The G_1 phase is then repeated, and one of the daughter cells moves into the suprabasal layer. It then differentiates (Fig. 2.2), having lost the capacity to divide, and synthesizes keratins. Some basal cells remain inactive in a so-called G_0 phase but may re-enter the cycle and resume proliferation. The

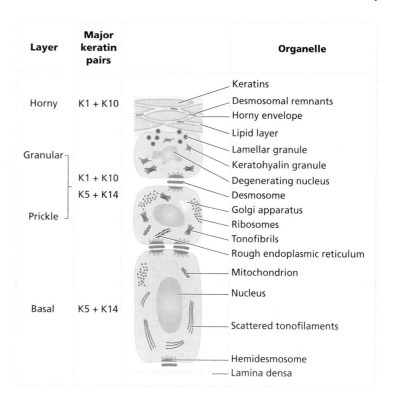

Layer	Major keratin pairs	Organelle
Horny	K1 + K10	Keratins
		Desmosomal remnants
		Horny envelope
		Lipid layer
Granular		Lamellar granule
	K1 + K10	Keratohyalin granule
	K5 + K14	Degenerating nucleus
		Desmosome
Prickle		Golgi apparatus
		Ribosomes
		Tonofibrils
		Rough endoplasmic reticulum
		Mitochondrion
		Nucleus
Basal	K5 + K14	Scattered tonofilaments
		Hemidesmosome
		Lamina densa

Fig. 2.2 Changes during keratinization.

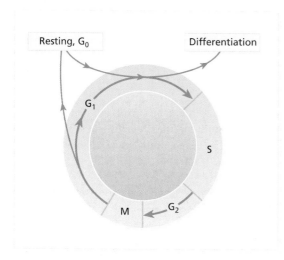

Fig. 2.3 The cell cycle.

cell cycle time in normal human skin is controversial; estimates of 50–200 h reflect differing views on the duration of the G_1 phase. Stem cells reside amongst these basal cells and amongst the cells of the external root sheath of the hair follicle at the level of attachment of the arrector pili muscle but cannot be identified by histology. These cells divide infrequently, but can generate new proliferative cells in the epidermis and hair follicle in response to damage.

Keratinocytes

The *spinous* or *prickle cell* layer (Fig. 2.4) is composed of *keratinocytes*. These differentiating cells, which synthesize keratins, are larger than basal cells. Keratinocytes are firmly attached to each other by small interlocking cytoplasmic processes, by abundant desmosomes and by an intercellular cement of glycoproteins and lipoproteins. Under the light microscope, the desmosomes look like 'prickles'. They are specialized attachment plaques that have been characterized biochemically. They contain desmoplakins, desmogleins and desmocollins. Autoantibodies to these proteins are found in pemphigus (p. 108), when they are responsible for the detachment of keratinocytes from one another and so for intraepidermal blister formation. Cytoplasmic continuity between keratinocytes occurs at *gap junctions*, specialized areas on opposing cell walls. Tonofilaments are small fibres running from the

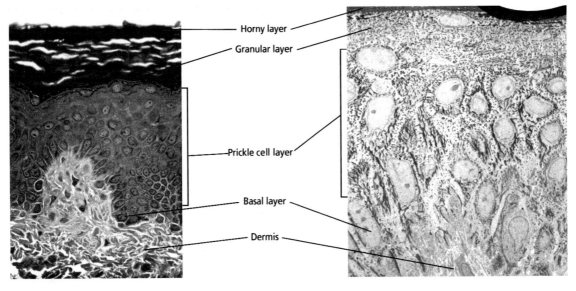

Fig. 2.4 Layers of the epidermis. (*left*) Light microscopy and (*right*) electron micrograph.

cytoplasm to the desmosomes. They are more numerous in cells of the spinous layer than of the basal layer, and are packed into bundles called *tonofibrils*. Many *lamellar granules* (otherwise known as membrane-coating granules, Odland bodies or keratinosomes), derived from the Golgi apparatus, appear in the superficial keratinocytes of this layer. They contain polysaccharides, hydrolytic enzymes and, more importantly, stacks of lipid lamellae composed of phospholipids, cholesterol and glucosylceramides. Their contents are discharged into the intercellular space of the granular cell layer to become precursors of the lipids in the intercellular space of the horny layer (see *Barrier function* below).

Cellular differentiation continues in the granular layer, which normally consists of two or three layers of cells that are flatter than those in the spinous layer, and have more tonofibrils. As the name of the layer implies, these cells contain large irregular basophilic granules of *keratohyalin*, which merge with tonofibrils. These keratohyalin granules contain proteins, including involucrin, loricrin and profilaggrin, which is cleaved into filaggrin by specific phosphatases as the granular cells move into the horny layer.

As keratinocytes migrate out through the outermost layers, their keratohyalin granules break up and their contents are dispersed throughout the cytoplasm,

leading to keratinization and the formation of a thick and tough peripheral protein coating called the *horny envelope*. Its structural proteins include loricrin and involucrin, the latter binding to ceramides in the surrounding intercellular space under the influence of transglutaminase. Filaggrin, involucrin and loricrin can all be detected histochemically and are useful as markers of epidermal differentiation.

The *horny layer* (stratum corneum) is made of piled-up layers of flattened dead cells (corneocytes)—the bricks—stuck together by lipids—the mortar—in the intercellular space. The corneocyte cytoplasm is packed with keratin filaments, embedded in a matrix and enclosed by an envelope derived from the keratohyalin granules. This envelope, along with the aggregated keratins that it encloses, gives the corneocyte its toughness, allowing the skin to withstand all sorts of chemical and mechanical insults. Horny cells normally have no nuclei or intracytoplasmic organelles, these having been destroyed by hydrolytic and degrading enzymes found in lamellar granules and the lysosomes of granular cells.

Keratinization

All cells have an internal skeleton made up of microfilaments (7 nm diameter; actin), microtubules (20–35 nm diameter; tubulin) and intermediate filaments (10 nm diameter). Keratins (from the Greek *keras* meaning 'horn') are the main intermediate filaments in epithelial cells and are comparable to vimentin in mesenchymal cells, neurofilaments in neurones and desmin in muscle cells. Keratins are not just a biochemical curiosity, as mutations in their genes cause a number of skin diseases including simple epidermolysis bullosa (p. 116) and bullous ichthyosiform erythroderma (p. 43).

The keratins are a family of more than 30 proteins, each produced by different genes. These separate into two gene families: one responsible for basic and the other for acidic keratins. The keratin polypeptide has a central helical portion with a non-helical N-terminal head and C-terminal tail. Individual keratins exist in pairs so that their double filament always consists of one acidic and one basic keratin polypeptide. The intertwining of adjacent filaments forms larger fibrils.

Different keratins are found at different levels of the epidermis depending on the stage of differentiation and disease; normal basal cells make keratins 5 and 14, but terminally differentiated suprabasal cells make keratins 1 and 10 (Fig. 2.2). Keratins 6 and 16 become prominent in hyperproliferative states such as psoriasis.

During differentiation, the keratin fibrils in the cells of the horny layer align and aggregate, under the influence of filaggrin. Cysetine, found in keratins of the horny layer, allows cross-linking of fibrils to give the epidermis strength to withstand injury.

Cell cohesion and desquamation

Firm cohesion in the spinous layer is ensured by 'stick and grip' mechanisms. A glycoprotein intercellular substance acts as a cement, sticking the cells together, and the intertwining of the small cytoplasmic processes of the prickle cells, together with their desmosomal attachments, accounts for the grip. The cytoskeleton of tonofibrils also maintains the cell shape rigidly.

The typical 'basket weave' appearance of the horny layer in routine histological sections is artefactual and deceptive. In fact, cells deep in the horny layer stick tightly together and only those at the surface flake off; this is in part caused by the activity of cholesterol sulphatase. This enzyme is deficient in X-linked recessive ichthyosis (p. 42), in which poor shedding leads to the piling up of corneocytes in the horny layer. Desquamation is normally responsible for the removal of harmful exogenous substances from the skin surface. The cells lost are replaced by newly formed corneocytes; regeneration and turnover of the horny layer is therefore continuous.

The epidermal barrier

The horny layer prevents the loss of interstitial fluid from within, and acts as a barrier to the penetration of potentially harmful substances from outside. Solvent extraction of the epidermis leads to an increased permeability to water, and it has been known for years that essential fatty acid deficiency causes poor cutaneous barrier function. These facts implicate ceramides, cholesterol, free fatty acids (from lamellar granules; p. 10), and smaller quantities of other lipids, in cutaneous barrier formation. Barrier function is also impaired when the horny layer is removed experimentally, by successive strippings with adhesive tape, or clinically, by injury or skin disease. It is also decreased by excessive hydration or dehydration of the horny layer and by detergents.

The rate of penetration of a substance through the epidermis is directly proportional to its concentration difference across the barrier layer, and indirectly proportional to the thickness of the horny layer. A rise in skin temperature aids penetration. A normal horny layer is slightly permeable to water, but relatively impermeable to ions such as sodium and potassium. Some other substances (e.g. glucose and urea) also penetrate poorly, whereas some aliphatic alcohols pass through easily. The penetration of a solute dissolved in an organic liquid depends mainly on the qualities of the solvent.

Epidermopoiesis and its regulation

Both the thickness of the normal epidermis, and the number of cells in it, remain constant, as cell loss at the surface is balanced by cell production in the basal layer. Locally produced polypeptides (cytokines), growth factors and hormones stimulate or inhibit epidermal proliferation, interacting in complex ways to ensure homeostasis. Cytokines and growth factors (Table 2.2) are produced by keratinocytes, Langerhans cells, fibroblasts and lymphocytes within the skin. After these bind to high affinity cell surface receptors, DNA synthesis is controlled by signal transduction,

Table 2.2 Some cytokines produced by keratinocytes.

Designation	Cytokine	Function
Interleukins		
IL-1	Interleukin 1	Lymphocyte activation
		Langerhans cell activation
		Acute phase reactions
IL-3	Interleukin 3	Colony-stimulating factor
IL-6	Interleukin 6	B-cell differentiation
IL-8	Interleukin 8	Chemotaxis
		Angiogenesis
IL-10	Interleukin 10	Inhibition of TH-1 T cells
IL-12	Interleukin 12	Induction of TH-2 T cells
Colony stimulating factors		
GM-CSF	Granulocyte–macrophage colony-stimulating factor	Proliferation of granulocytes and macrophages
G-CSF	Granulocyte colony-stimulating factor	Proliferation of granulocytes
M-CSF	Macrophage colony-stimulating factor	Proliferation of macrophages
Others		
TGF	Transforming growth factors	Inhibit inflammation
TNF	Tumour necrosis factors	Induce Class I antigens
		Antiviral states
IFN-α	Interferon-α	Antiviral state
IFN-γ	Interferon-γ	Amplification of type IV reactions

involving protein kinase C or inositol phosphate. Catecholamines, which do not penetrate the surface of cells, influence cell division via the adenosine 3′, 5′-cyclic monophosphate (cAMP) second messenger system. Steroid hormones bind to receptor proteins within the cytoplasm, and then pass to the nucleus where they influence transcription.

Vitamin D synthesis

The steroid 7-dehydrocholesterol, found in keratinocytes, is converted by sunlight to cholecalciferol. The vitamin becomes active after 25-hydroxylation in the kidney. Lack of sun and kidney disease can both cause vitamin D deficiency and rickets.

Other cells in the epidermis

Keratinocytes make up about 85% of cells in the epidermis, but three other types of cell are also found there: melanocytes, Langerhans cells and Merkel cells. (Fig. 2.5).

Melanocytes

Melanocytes are the only cells that can synthesize melanin. They migrate from the neural crest into the basal layer of the ectoderm where, in human embryos, they are seen as early as the eighth week of gestation. They are also found in hair bulbs, the retina and pia arachnoid. Each dendritic melanocyte associates with a number of keratinocytes, forming an 'epidermal melanin unit' (Fig. 2.5). The dendritic processes of melanocytes wind between the epidermal cells and end as discs in contact with them. Their cytoplasm contains discrete organelles, the *melanosomes*, containing varying amounts of the pigment melanin (Fig. 2.6).

Melanogenesis is described at the beginning of Chapter 17 on disorders of pigmentation.

Langerhans cells

The Langerhans cell is a dendritic cell (Figs 2.5 and 2.7) like the melanocyte. It also lacks desmosomes and tonofibrils, but has a lobulated nucleus. The specific

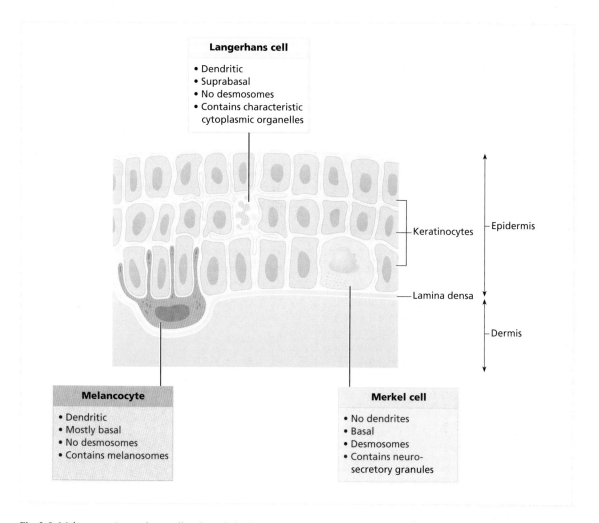

Langerhans cell

• Dendritic
• Suprabasal
• No desmosomes
• Contains characteristic
  cytoplasmic organelles

Keratinocytes — Epidermis

Lamina densa

Dermis

Melancocyte

• Dendritic
• Mostly basal
• No desmosomes
• Contains melanosomes

Merkel cell

• No dendrites
• Basal
• Desmosomes
• Contains neuro-
  secretory granules

Fig. 2.5 Melanocyte, Langerhans cell and Merkel cell.

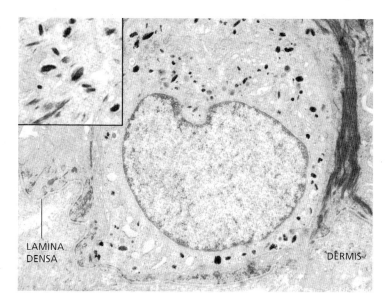

LAMINA
DENSA

DERMIS

Fig. 2.6 Melanocyte (electron micrograph), with melanosomes (inset).

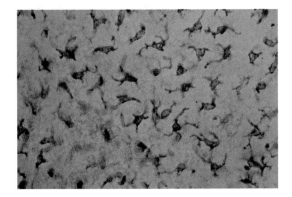

Fig. 2.7 Adenosine triphosphase-positive Langerhans cells in an epidermal sheet: the network provides a reticulo-epithelial trap for contact allergens.

granules within the cell look like a tennis racket when seen in two dimensions in an electron micrograph (Fig. 2.8), or like a sycamore seed when reconstructed in three dimensions. They are plate-like, with a rounded bleb protruding from the surface.

Langerhans cells come from a mobile pool of precursors originating in the bone marrow. There are approximately 800 Langerhans cells per mm^2 in human skin and their dendritic processes fan out to form a striking network seen best in epidermal sheets (Fig. 2.7). Langerhans cells are alone among epidermal cells in possessing surface receptors for C3b and the Fc portions of IgG and IgE, and in bearing major histocompatibility complex (MHC) Class II antigens (HLA-DR, -DP and -DQ). They are best thought of as highly specialized macrophages.

Langerhans cells have a key role in many immune reactions. They take up exogenous antigen, process it and present it to T lymphocytes either in the skin or in the local lymph nodes (p. 27). They probably play a part in immunosurveillance for viral and tumour antigens. In this way, ultraviolet radiation can induce skin tumours both by causing mutations in the epidermal cells, and by decreasing the number of epidermal Langerhans cells, so that cells bearing altered antigens are not recognized or destroyed by the immune system. Topical or systemic glucocorticoids also reduce the density of epidermal Langerhans cells. The Langerhans cell is the principal cell in skin allografts to which the T lymphocytes of the host react during rejection; allograft survival can be prolonged by depleting Langerhans cells.

Merkel cells

Merkel cells are found in normal epidermis (Fig. 2.5) and act as transducers for fine touch. They are non-dendritic cells, lying in or near the basal layer, and are of the same size as keratinocytes. They are concentrated in localized thickenings of the epidermis near hair follicles (hair discs), and contain membrane-bound spherical granules, 80–100 nm in diameter, which have a core of varying density, separated from the membrane by a clear halo. Sparse desmosomes connect these cells to neighbouring keratinocytes. Fine unmyelinated nerve endings are often associated with Merkel cells, which express immunoreactivity for various neuropeptides.

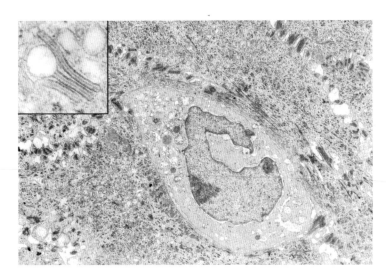

Fig. 2.8 Langerhans cell (electron micrograph), with characteristic granule (inset).

Epidermal appendages

The skin appendages are derived from epithelial germs during embryogenesis and, except for the nails, lie in the dermis. They include hair, nails and sweat and sebaceous glands. They are described, along with the diseases that affect them, in Chapters 12 and 13, respectively.

The dermo-epidermal junction

The basement membrane lies at the interface between the epidermis and dermis. With light microscopy it can be highlighted using a periodic acid–Schiff (PAS) stain, because of its abundance of neutral mucopolysaccharides. Electron microscopy (Fig. 2.9) shows that the *lamina densa* (rich in type IV collagen) is separated from the basal cells by an electron-lucent area, the *lamina lucida*. The plasma membrane of basal cells has *hemidesmosomes* (containing bullous pemphigoid antigens, collagen XVII and α6 β4 integrin). The lamina lucida contains the adhesive macromolecules, laminin-1, laminin-5 and entactin. Fine *anchoring filaments* (of laminin-5) cross the lamina lucida and connect the lamina densa to the plasma membrane of the basal cells. *Anchoring fibrils* (of type VII collagen), dermal microfibril bundles and single small collagen fibres (types I and III), extend from the papillary dermis to the deep part of the lamina densa.

Laminins, large non-collagen glycoproteins produced by keratinocytes, aided by entactin, promote adhesion between the basal cells above the lamina lucida and type IV collagen, the main constituent of the lamina densa, below it. The laminins act as a glue, helping to hold the epidermis onto the dermis. Bullous pemphigoid antigens (of molecular weights 230 and 180 kDa) are synthesized by basal cells and are found in close association with the hemidesmosomes and laminin. Their function is unknown but antibodies to them are found in pemphigoid (p. 111), a subcutaneous blistering condition.

The structures within the dermo-epidermal junction provide mechanical support, encouraging the adhesion, growth, differentiation and migration of the overlying basal cells, and also act as a semipermeable filter that regulates the transfer of nutrients and cells from dermis to epidermis.

Dermis

The dermis lies between the epidermis and the subcutaneous fat. It supports the epidermis structurally and nutritionally. Its thickness varies, being greatest in the palms and soles and least in the eyelids and penis. In old age, the dermis thins and loses its elasticity.

The dermis interdigitates with the epidermis (Fig. 2.1) so that upward projections of the dermis, the dermal papillae, interlock with downward ridges of the

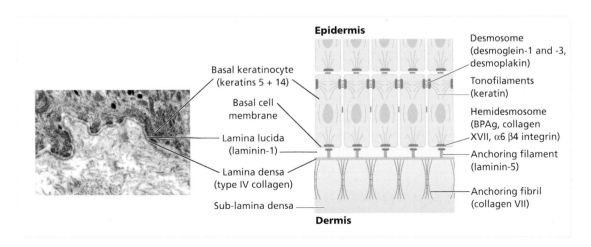

Fig. 2.9 Structure and molecular composition of the dermo-epidermal junction.

Table 2.3 Functions of some resident dermal cells.

Fibroblast	Synthesis of collagen, reticulin, elastin, fibronectin, glycosaminoglycans, collagenase
Mononuclear phagocyte	Mobile: phagocytose and destroy bacteria Secrete cytokines
Lymphocyte	Immunosurveillance
Langerhans cell and dermal dendritic cell	In transit between local lymph node and epidermis Antigen presentation
Mast cell	Stimulated by antigens, complement components, and other substances to release many inflammatory mediators including histamine, heparin, prostaglandins, leukotrienes, tryptase and chemotactic factors for eosinophils and neutrophils

epidermis, the rete pegs. This interdigitation is responsible for the ridges seen most readily on the fingertips (as fingerprints). It is important in the adhesion between epidermis and dermis as it increases the area of contact between them.

Like all connective tissues the dermis has three components: cells, fibres and amorphous ground substance.

Cells of the dermis

The main cells of the dermis are fibroblasts, but there are also small numbers of resident and transitory mononuclear phagocytes, lymphocytes, Langerhans cells and mast cells. Other blood cells, e.g. polymorphs, are seen during inflammation. The main functions of the resident dermal cells are listed in Table 2.3 and their role in immunological reactions is discussed later in this chapter.

Fibres of the dermis

The dermis is largely made up of interwoven fibres, principally of collagen, packed in bundles. Those in the papillary dermis are finer than those in the deeper reticular dermis. When the skin is stretched, collagen, with its high tensile strength, prevents tearing, and the elastic fibres, intermingled with the collagen, later return it to the unstretched state.

Collagen makes up 70–80% of the dry weight of the dermis. Its fibres are composed of thinner fibrils, which are in turn made up of microfibrils built from individual collagen molecules. These molecules consist of three polypeptide chains (molecular weight 150 kDa) forming a triple helix with a non-helical segment at both ends. The alignment of the chains is stabilized by covalent cross-links involving lysine and hydroxylysine. Collagen is an unusual protein as it contains a high proportion of proline and hydroxyproline and many glycine residues; the spacing of glycine as every third amino acid is a prerequisite for the formation of a triple helix. Defects in the enzymes needed for collagen synthesis are responsible for some skin diseases, including the Ehlers–Danlos syndrome (Chapter 21), and conditions involving other systems, including lathyrism (fragility of skin and other connective tissues) and osteogenesis imperfecta (fragility of bones).

There are many, genetically distinct, collagen proteins, all with triple helical molecules, and all rich in hydroxyproline and hydroxylysine. The distribution of some of them is summarized in Table 2.4.

Table 2.4 Distribution of some types of collagen.

Collagen type	Tissue distribution
I	Most connective tissues including tendon and bone Accounts for approximately 85% of skin collagen
II	Cartilage
III	Accounts for about 15% of skin collagen Blood vessels
IV	Skin (lamina densa) and basement membranes of other tissues
V	Ubiquitous, including placenta
VII	Skin (anchoring fibrils) Fetal membranes

Reticulin fibres are fine collagen fibres, seen in fetal skin and around the blood vessels and appendages of adult skin.

Elastic fibres account for about 2% of the dry weight of adult dermis. They have two distinct protein components: an amorphous elastin core and a surrounding 'elastic tissue microfibrillar component'. Elastin (molecular weight 72 kDa) is made up of polypeptides (rich in glycine, desmosine and valine) linked to the microfibrillar component through their desmosine residues. Abnormalities in the elastic tissue cause cutis laxa (sagging inelastic skin) and pseudoxanthoma elasticum (Chapter 21).

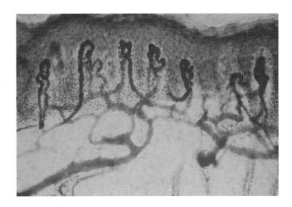

Fig. 2.10 Blood vessels of the skin (carmine stain).

Ground substance of the dermis

The amorphous ground substance of the dermis consists largely of two glycosaminoglycans (hyaluronic acid and dermatan sulphate) with smaller amounts of heparan sulphate and chondroitin sulphate. The glycosaminoglycans are complexed to core protein and exist as proteoglycans.

The ground substance has several important functions:
• it binds water, allowing nutrients, hormones and waste products to pass through the dermis;
• it acts as a lubricant between the collagen and elastic fibre networks during skin movement; and
• it provides bulk, allowing the dermis to act as a shock absorber.

Muscles

Both smooth and striated muscle are found in the skin. The smooth arrector pili muscles (see Fig. 13.1) are used by animals to raise their fur and so protect them from the cold. They are vestigial in humans, but may help to express sebum. Smooth muscle is also responsible for 'goose pimples' (bumps) from cold, nipple erection, and the raising of the scrotum by the dartos muscle. Striated fibres (e.g. the platysma) and some of the muscles of facial expression, are also found in the dermis.

Blood vessels

Although the skin consumes little oxygen, its abundant blood supply regulates body temperature. The blood vessels lie in two main horizontal layers (Fig. 2.10). The deep plexus is just above the subcutaneous fat,

and its arterioles supply the sweat glands and hair papillae. The superficial plexus is in the papillary dermis and arterioles from it become capillary loops in the dermal papillae. An arteriole arising in the deep dermis supplies an inverted cone of tissue, with its base at the epidermis.

The blood vessels in the skin are important in thermoregulation. Under sympathetic nervous control, arteriovenous anastamoses at the level of the deep plexus can shunt blood to the venous plexus at the expense of the capillary loops, thereby reducing surface heat loss by convection.

Cutaneous lymphatics

Afferent lymphatics begin as blind-ended capillaries in the dermal papilla and pass to a superficial lymphatic plexus in the papillary dermis. There are also two deeper horizontal plexuses, and collecting lymphatics from the deeper one run with the veins in the superficial fascia.

Nerves

The skin is liberally supplied with an estimated one million nerve fibres. Most are found in the face and extremities. Their cell bodies lie in the dorsal root ganglia. Both myelinated and non-myelinated fibres exist, with the latter making up an increasing proportion peripherally. Most free sensory nerves end in the dermis; however, a few non-myelinated nerve endings penetrate into the epidermis. Some of these are associated with Merkel cells (p. 14). Free nerve endings detect the potentially damaging stimuli of heat and pain (nocioceptors), while specialized end organs in the dermis, Pacinian and Meissner corpuscles, register deformation of the skin caused by pressure (mechanoreceptors) as well as vibration and touch. Autonomic nerves supply the blood vessels, sweat glands and arrector pili muscles.

Itching is an important feature of many skin diseases. It follows the stimulation of fine free nerve endings lying close to the dermo-epidermal junction. Areas with a high density of such endings (itch spots) are especially sensitive to itch-provoking stimuli. Impulses from these free endings pass centrally in two ways: quickly along myelinated A fibres, and more slowly along non-myelinated C fibres. As a result, itch has two components: a quick localized pricking sensation followed by a slow burning diffuse itching.

Many stimuli can induce itching (electrical, chemical and mechanical). In itchy skin diseases, pruritogenic chemicals such as histamine and proteolytic enzymes are liberated close to the dermoepidermal junction. The detailed pharmacology of individual diseases is still poorly understood but prostaglandins potentiate chemically induced itching in inflammatory skin diseases.

The skin immune system

The horny layer of the skin is able both to prevent the loss of fluid and electrolytes, and to stop the penetration of harmful substances (p. 11). It is a dry mechanical barrier from which contaminating organisms and chemicals are continually being removed by washing and desquamation. Only when these breach the horny layer do the cellular components, described below, come into play. The skin is involved in so many immunological reactions, seen regularly in the clinic

(e.g. urticaria, allergic contact dermatitis, psoriasis, vasculitis), that a special mention has to be made of the peripheral arm of the immune system based in the skin—the skin immune system (SIS).

The idea of an SIS as a functionally independent immunological unit is helpful. It includes the cutaneous blood vessels and lymphatics with their local lymph nodes and contains circulating lymphocytes and resident immune cells. Although it is beyond the scope of this book to cover general immunology, this section outlines some of the intricate ways in which antigens are recognized by specialized skin cells, mainly the Langerhans cells, and how antibodies, lymphocytes, macrophages and polymorphs elicit inflammation.

Some cellular components of the skin immune system

Keratinocytes (p. 9)

Their prime role is to make the protective horny layer (p. 11) and to support to the outermost epithelium of the body but they also have immunological functions in their own right. Keratinocytes produce large numbers of cytokines (see Table 2.2), and can be induced by γ-interferon to express HLA-DR. They can also produce α-melanocyte-stimulating hormone (p. 243), which is immunosuppressive. Keratinocytes play a central part in healing after epidermal injury (Fig. 2.11).

Langerhans cells (p. 12)

These dendritic cells come from the bone marrow and circulate through the epidermis, the dermis, lymphatics (as 'veiled cells'), and also through the T-cell area of the lymph nodes where they are called 'dendritic' or 'interdigitating' cells. They can be identified in tissue sections by demonstrating their characteristic surface markers (e.g. CD1a antigen, MHC Class II antigens, adenosine triphosphatase) or S-100 protein in their cytoplasm (also found in melanocytes). Langerhans cells have a key role in antigen presentation.

Dermal dendritic cells

These poorly characterized cells are found around the tiny blood vessels of the papillary dermis. They bear MHC Class II antigens on their surface and,

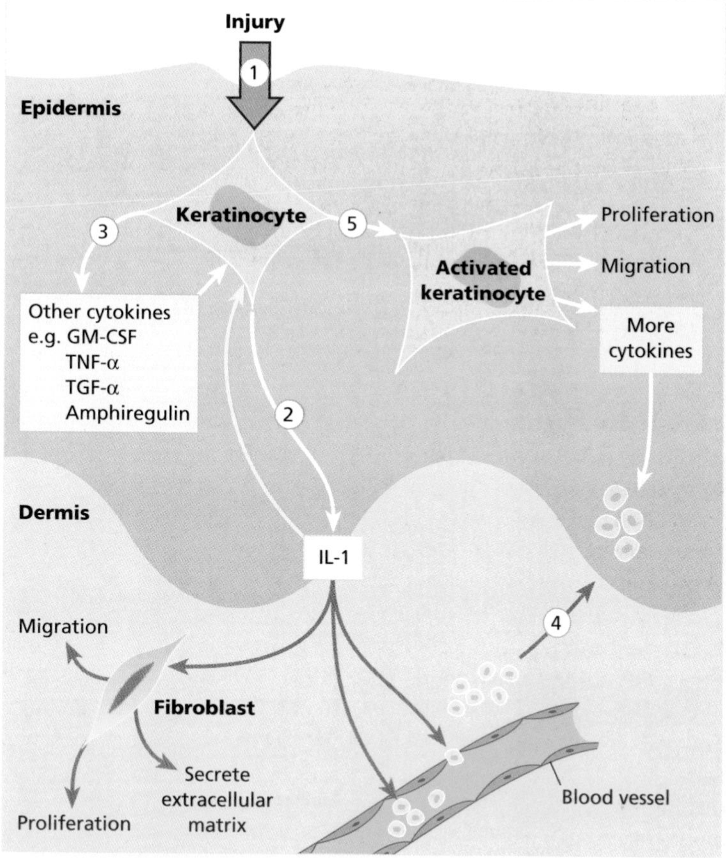

Fig. 2.11 The keratinocyte and wound healing. The injured keratinocyte turns on wound healing responses. When a keratinocyte is injured (1), it releases interleukin-1 (IL-1) (2). IL-1 activates endothelial cells causing them to express selectins that slow down lymphocytes passing over them. Once lymphocytes stop on the endothelial cells lining the vessels, IL-1 acts as a chemotactic factor to draw lymphocytes into the epidermis (4). At the same time, IL-1 activates keratinocytes by binding to their IL-1 receptors. Activated keratinocytes produce other cytokines (3). Among these is tumour necrosis factor α (TNF-α) that additionally activates keratinocytes and keeps them in an activated state (5). Activation of keratinocytes causes them to proliferate, migrate and secrete additional cytokines.

like Langerhans cells, probably function as antigen-presenting cells.

T lymphocytes

These develop and acquire their antigen receptors (T-cell receptors, TCR) in the thymus. They differentiate into subpopulations, recognizable by their different surface molecules (cluster of differentiation markers), which are functionally distinct.

T-helper (TH)/inducer cells

These help B cells to produce antibody and also induce cytotoxic T cells to recognize and kill virally infected cells and allogeneic grafts. TH cells recognize antigen in association with MHC Class II molecules (Fig. 2.12) and, when triggered by antigen, release cytokines that attract and activate other inflammatory cells (see Fig. 2.18). They are CD4+.

Helper T cells are divided into type 1 (TH-1) and type 2 lymphocytes (TH-2) according to the main cytokines that they produce (Fig. 2.13). Some skin diseases display a predominantly TH-1 response (e.g. psoriasis), others a mainly TH-2 response (e.g. atopic dermatitis).

T-cytotoxic (TC) cells

These lymphocytes are capable of destroying allogeneic and virally infected cells, which they recognize by the MHC Class I molecules on their surface. They are CD8+.

T-cell receptor and T-cell gene receptor rearrangements

Most T-cell receptors are composed of an α and β chain, each with a variable (antigen binding) and a constant domain, which are associated with the CD3 cell surface molecules (Fig. 2.12). Many different combinations of separate gene segments, termed V, D and

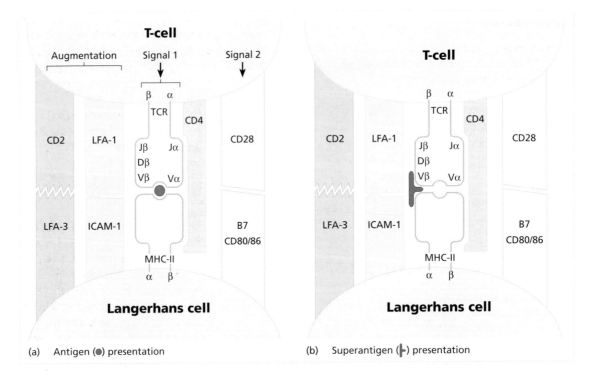

Fig. 2.12 T-lymphocyte activation by (a) antigen and (b) superantigen. When antigen has been processed it is presented on the surface of the Langerhans cell in association with major histocompatibility complex (MHC) Class II. The complex formation that takes place between the antigen, MHC Class II and T-cell receptor (TCR) provides signal 1, which is enhanced by the coupling of CD4 with the MHC molecule. A second signal for T-cell activation is provided by the interaction between the costimulatory molecules CD28 (T cell) and B7 (Langerhans cell). CD2/LFA-3 and LFA-1/ICAM-1 adhesion augment the response to signals 1 and 2. Superantigen interacts with the TCR Vβ and MHC Class II without processing, binding outside the normal antigen binding site. Activated T cells secrete many cytokines, including IL-1, IL-8 and interferon-γ, which promote inflammation (Fig. 2.13).

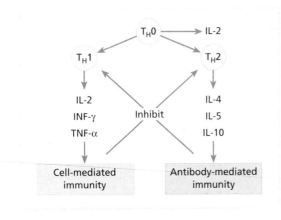

Fig. 2.13 Characteristics of TH-1 and TH-2 responses.

J, code for the variable domains of the receptor. An analysis of rearrangements of the gene for the receptor is used to determine whether a T-cell infiltrate is likely to be malignant or reactive. The identification of a specific band, on analysis of DNA from the lesion, which is not matched by the patient's DNA from other sites, indicates monoclonal T-cell proliferation, and suggests either malignancy or a T-cell response to a single antigen.

L cells/null (non-T, non-B) cells

These leucocytes have properties between those of T and myelomonocytic cells. Most have receptors for FcIgG. This subpopulation contains natural killer (NK) and killer (K) cells.

Natural killer cells

These are large granular leucocytes that can kill virally infected cells, or tumour cells that have not previously been sensitized with antibody.

Killer cells

These are not a separate cell type, but rather cytotoxic T cells, NK cells or monocytic leucocytes that can kill target cells sensitized with antibody. In antibody-mediated cellular cytotoxicity, antibody binds to antigen on the surface of the target cell: the K cell binds to the antibody at its other (Fc) end by its Fc receptor and the target cell is then lysed.

Mast cells

These are present in most connective tissues, predominantly around blood vessels. Their numerous granules contain inflammatory mediators (see Fig. 8.1). In rodents—and probably in humans—there are two distinct populations of mast cells, connective tissue and mucosal, which differ in their staining properties, content of inflammatory mediators and proteolytic enzymes. Skin mast cells play a central part in the pathogenesis of urticaria (p. 94).

Molecular components of the skin immune system

Antigens and haptens

Antigens are molecules that are recognized by the immune system thereby provoking an immune reaction, usually in the form of a humoral or cell-bound antibody response. Haptens, often chemicals of low molecular weight, cannot provoke an immune reaction themselves unless they combine with a protein. They are important sensitizers in allergic contact dermatitis (p. 80).

Superantigens

Some bacterial toxins (e.g. those released by *Staphylococcus aureus*) are prototypic superantigens. Sensitization to such superantigens is not necessary to prime the immune response. Superantigens align with

a variety of MHC Class II molecules outside their antigen presentation groove and, without any cellular processing, may directly signal to different classes of T cells within the large family carrying a Vβ type of T-cell receptor (Fig. 2.12). By these means, superantigens can induce massive T-cell proliferation and cytokine production leading to disorders such as the toxic shock syndrome (p. 192). Streptococcal toxins act as superantigens to activate T cells in the pathogenesis of guttate psoriasis.

Antibodies (immunoglobulins)

Immunoglobulin G (IgG) is responsible for most of the secondary response to most antigens. It can cross the placenta, and binds complement to activate the classical complement pathway. IgG can coat neutrophils and macrophages (by their FcIgG receptors), and acts as an opsonin by cross-bridging antigen. IgG can also sensitize target cells for destruction by K cells. IgM is the largest immunoglobulin molecule. It is responsible for much of the primary response and, like IgG, it can fix complement but it cannot cross the placenta. IgA is the most common immunoglobulin in secretions. It does not bind complement but can activate complement via the alternative pathway. IgE binds to Fc receptors on mast cells and basophils, where it sensitizes them to release inflammatory mediators in type I immediate hypersensitivity reactions (Fig. 2.14).

Cytokines

Cytokines are small proteins secreted by cells such as lymphocytes and macrophages, and also by keratinocytes (Table 2.2). They regulate the amplitude and duration of inflammation by acting locally on nearby cells (paracrine action), on those cells that secreted them (autocrine) and occasionally on distant target cells (endocrine) via the circulation. The term cytokine covers interleukins, interferons, colony-stimulating factors, cytotoxins and growth factors. Interleukins (IL) are produced predominantly by leucocytes, have a known amino acid sequence and are active in inflammation or immunity.

There are many cytokines (Table 2.2), and each may act on more than one type of cell causing many different effects. Cytokines frequently have overlapping actions. In any inflammatory reaction some cytokines

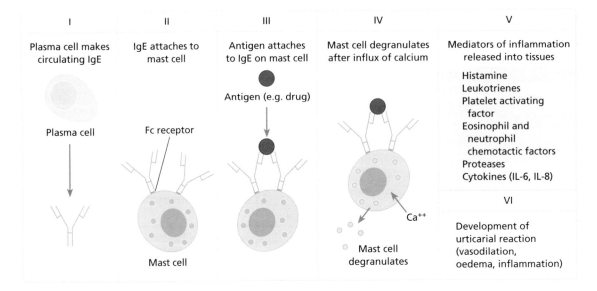

I	II	III	IV	V
Plasma cell makes circulating IgE	IgE attaches to mast cell	Antigen attaches to IgE on mast cell	Mast cell degranulates after influx of calcium	Mediators of inflammation released into tissues

Plasma cell

Fc receptor

Antigen (e.g. drug)

Mast cell

Ca^{++}

Mast cell degranulates

Histamine
Leukotrienes
Platelet activating factor
Eosinophil and neutrophil chemotactic factors
Proteases
Cytokines (IL-6, IL-8)

VI

Development of urticarial reaction (vasodilation, oedema, inflammation)

Fig. 2.14 Urticaria: an immediate (type I) hypersensitivity reaction.

are acting synergistically while others will antagonize these effects. This network of potent chemicals, each acting alone and in concert, moves the inflammatory response along in a controlled way. Cytokines bind to high affinity (but not usually specific) cell surface receptors, and elicit a biological response by regulating the transcription of genes in the target cell via signal transduction pathways involving, for example, the Janus protein tyrosine kinase or calcium influx systems. The biological response is a balance between the production of the cytokine, the expression of its receptors on the target cells, and the presence of inhibitors.

Adhesion molecules

Cellular adhesion molecules (CAMs) are surface glycoproteins that are expressed on many different types of cell; they are involved in cell–cell and cell–matrix adhesion and interactions. CAMs are fundamental in the interaction of lymphocytes with antigen-presenting cells (Fig. 2.12), keratinocytes and endothelial cells and are important in lymphocyte trafficking in the skin during inflammation (Fig. 2.11). CAMs have been classified into four families: cadherins, immunoglobulin superfamily, integrins and selectins. E-cadherins are found on the surface of keratinocytes between the desmosomes. γ-Interferon causes up-regulation of

Fas on epidermal lymphocytes. Interaction of these with Fas ligand on keratinocytes causes e-cadherins to 'disappear' leading to intercellular oedema (spongiosis) between desmosomes.

CAMs of special relevance in the skin are listed in Table 2.5.

Histocompatibility antigens

Like other cells, those in the skin express surface antigens directed by genes of the MHC. The human leucocyte antigen (HLA) region lies on chromosome 6. In particular, HLA-A, -B and -C antigens (the Class I antigens) are expressed on all nucleated cells including keratinocytes, Langerhans cells and cells of the dermis. HLA-DR, -DP, -DQ and -DZ antigens (the Class II antigens) are expressed only on some cells (e.g. Langerhans cells). They are poorly expressed on keratinocytes except during certain reactions (e.g. allergic contact dermatitis) or diseases (e.g. lichen planus). Helper T cells recognize antigens only in the presence of cells bearing Class II antigens. Class II antigens are also important for certain cell–cell interactions. On the other hand, Class I antigens mark target cells for cell-mediated cytotoxic reactions, such as the rejection of skin allografts and the destruction of cells infected by viruses.

Table 2.5 Cellular adhesion molecules important in the skin.

Family	Nature	Example	Site	Ligand
Cadherins	Glycoproteins Adherence dependent on calcium	Desmoglein	Desmosomes in epidermis	Other cadherins
Immunoglobulin	Numerous molecules which are structurally similar to immunoglobulins	Intercellular adhesion molecule-1 (ICAM-1)	Endothelial cells Keratinocytes Langerhans cells	LFA-1
		Cluster of differentiation antigen 2 (CD2)	T lymphocytes Some NK cells	LFA-3
		Vascular cell adhesion molecule 1 (VCAM-1)	Endothelial cells	VLA-4
Integrins	Surface proteins comprising two non-covalently bound α and β chains	Very late activation proteins (β1-VLA)	T lymphocyte	VCAM
		Leucocyte function antigen 1 (LFA-1)	T lymphocyte	ICAM-1
		Macrophage activation antigen 1 (Mac-1)	Macrophages Monocytes Granulocytes	C3b component of complement
Selectins	Adhesion molecules with lectin-like domain which binds carbohydrate	E selectin	Endothelial cells	Sle^x (CD15)

Hypersensitivity reactions in the skin

Hypersensitivity is the term given to an exaggerated or inappropriate immune reaction. It is still helpful, if rather artificial, to separate these into four main types using the original classification of Coombs and Gell. All of these types underlie reactions in the skin.

Type I: immediate hypersensitivity reactions

These are characterized by vasodilatation and an outpouring of fluid from blood vessels. Such reactions can be mimicked by drugs or toxins, which act directly, but immunological reactions are mediated by antibodies, and are manifestations of allergy. IgE and IgG4 antibodies, produced by plasma cells in organs other than the skin, attach themselves to mast cells in the dermis. These contain inflammatory mediators, either in granules or in their cytoplasm. The IgE antibody is attached to the mast cell by its Fc end, so that the antigen combining site dangles from the mast cell like a hand on an arm (Fig. 2.14). When specific antigen combines with the hand parts of the immunoglobulin (the antigen-binding site or Fab end), the mast cell liberates its mediators into the surrounding tissue. Of these mediators, histamine (from the granules) and leukotrienes (from the cell membrane) induce vasodilatation, and endothelial cells retract allowing transudation into the extravascular space. The vasodilatation causes a pink colour, and the transudation causes swelling. Urticaria and angioedema (p. 94) are examples of immediate hypersensitivity reactions occurring in the skin.

Antigen may be delivered to the skin from the outside (e.g. in a bee sting). This will induce a swelling in everyone by a direct pharmacological action. However, some people, with IgE antibodies against antigens in the venom, swell even more at the site of the sting as the result of a specific immunological reaction. If they are extremely sensitive, they may develop wheezing, wheals and anaphylactic shock (see Fig. 22.5), because of a massive release of histamine into the circulation.

Antigens can also reach mast cells from inside the body. Those who are allergic to shellfish, for example, may develop urticaria within seconds, minutes or hours of eating one. Antigenic material, absorbed from the gut, passes to tissue mast cells via the circulation, and elicits an urticarial reaction after binding to specific IgE on mast cells in the skin.

Type II: humoral cytotoxic reactions

In the main, these involve IgG and IgM antibodies, which, like IgE, are produced by plasma cells and are present in the interstitial fluid of the skin. When they meet an antigen, they fix and activate complement through a series of enzymatic reactions that generate mediator and cytotoxic proteins. If bacteria enter the skin, IgG and IgM antibodies bind to antigens on them. Complement is activated through the classical pathway, and a number of mediators are generated. Amongst these are the chemotactic factor, C5a, which attracts polymorphs to the area of bacterial invasion, and the opsonin, C3b, which coats the bacteria so that

they can be ingested and killed by polymorphs when these arrive (Fig. 2.15). Under certain circumstances, activation of complement can kill cells or organisms directly by the 'membrane attack complex' (C5b6789) in the terminal complement pathway. Complement can also be activated by bacteria directly through the alternative pathway; antibody is not required. The bacterial cell wall causes more C3b to be produced by the alternative pathway factors B, D and P (properdin). Aggregated IgA can also activate the alternative pathway.

Activation of either pathway produces C3b, the pivotal component of the complement system. Through the amplification loop, a single reaction can flood the area with C3b, C5a and other amplification loop and terminal pathway components. Complement is the mediator of humoral reactions.

Humoral cytotoxic reactions are typical of defence against infectious agents such as bacteria. However, they are also involved in certain autoimmune diseases such as pemphigoid (Chapter 9).

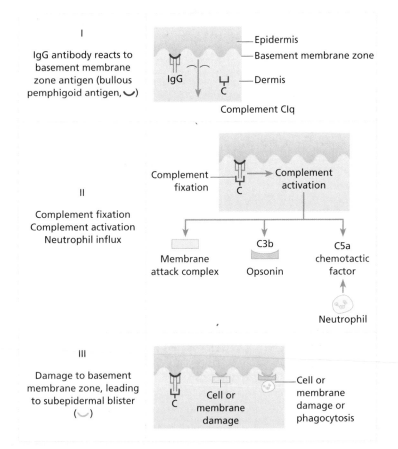

I
IgG antibody reacts to basement membrane zone antigen (bullous pemphigoid antigen, ⌣)

Epidermis
Basement membrane zone
IgG
Dermis
C
Complement Clq

II
Complement fixation
Complement activation
Neutrophil influx

Complement fixation
Complement activation
C

Membrane attack complex
C3b Opsonin
C5a chemotactic factor
Neutrophil

III
Damage to basement membrane zone, leading to subepidermal blister (⌣)

C
Cell or membrane damage

Cell or membrane damage or phagocytosis

Fig. 2.15 Bullous pemphigoid; a humoral cytotoxic (type II) reaction against a basement membrane zone antigen.

Occasionally, antibodies bind to the surface of a cell and activate it without causing its death or activating complement. Instead, the cell is stimulated to produce a hormone-like substance that may mediate disease. Pemphigus (Chapter 9) is a blistering disease of skin in which this type of reaction may be important.

Type III: immune complex-mediated reactions

Antigen may combine with antibodies near vital tissues so that the ensuing inflammatory response damages them. When an antigen is injected intradermally, it combines with appropriate antibodies on the walls of blood vessels, complement is activated, and polymorphonuclear leucocytes are brought to the area (an Arthus reaction). Degranulation of polymorphs liberates lysosomal enzymes that damage the vessel walls.

Antigen–antibody complexes can also be formed in the circulation, move to the small vessels in the skin and lodge there (Fig. 2.16). Complement will then be activated and inflammatory cells will injure the vessels as in the Arthus reaction. This causes oedema and the extravasation of red blood cells (e.g. the palpable purpura that characterizes vasculitis; Chapter 8).

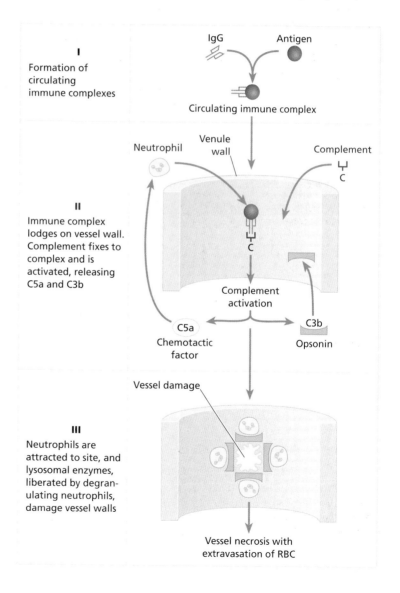

I
Formation of circulating immune complexes

II
Immune complex lodges on vessel wall. Complement fixes to complex and is activated, releasing C5a and C3b

III
Neutrophils are attracted to site, and lysosomal enzymes, liberated by degranulating neutrophils, damage vessel walls

IgG   Antigen

Circulating immune complex

Neutrophil   Venule wall   Complement

Complement activation

C5a
Chemotactic factor

C3b
Opsonin

Vessel damage

Vessel necrosis with extravasation of RBC

Fig. 2.16 Immune complex-mediated vasculitis (type III reaction).

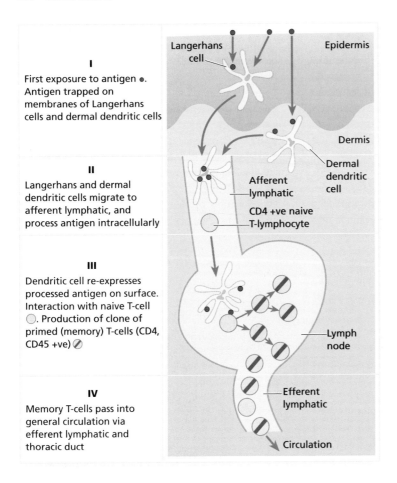

I

First exposure to antigen •. Antigen trapped on membranes of Langerhans cells and dermal dendritic cells

II

Langerhans and dermal dendritic cells migrate to afferent lymphatic, and process antigen intracellularly

III

Dendritic cell re-expresses processed antigen on surface. Interaction with naive T-cell ○. Production of clone of primed (memory) T-cells (CD4, CD45 +ve) ⊘

IV

Memory T-cells pass into general circulation via efferent lymphatic and thoracic duct

Fig. 2.17 Induction phase of allergic contact dermatitis (type IV) reaction.

Type IV: cell-mediated immune reactions

As the name implies, these are mediated by lymphocytes rather than by antibodies. Cell-mediated immune reactions are important in granulomas, delayed hypersensitivity reactions, and allergic contact dermatitis. They probably also play a part in some photosensitive disorders, in protecting against cancer, and in mediating reactions to insect bites.

Allergic contact dermatitis

There are two phases: during the induction phase naïve lymphocytes become sensitized to a specific antigen; during the elicitation phase antigens entering the skin are processed by antigen-presenting cells such as macrophages and Langerhans cells (Fig. 2.17) and then interact with sensitized lymphocytes. The lymphocytes are stimulated to enlarge, divide and to secrete

cytokines that can injure tissues directly and kill cells or microbes.

Induction (sensitization) phase (Fig. 2.17)

When the epidermal barrier is breached, the immune system provides the second line of defence. Among the keratinocytes are Langerhans cells, highly specialized intraepidermal macrophages with tentacles that intertwine among the keratinocytes, providing a net (Fig. 2.7) to 'catch' antigens falling down on them from the surface, such as chemicals or the antigens of microbes or tumours. During the initial induction phase, the antigen is trapped by a Langerhans cell which then migrates to the regional lymph node. To do this, it must retract its dendrites and 'swim upstream' from the prickle cell layer of the epidermis towards the basement membrane, against the 'flow' of keratinocytes generated by the epidermal basal cells. Once in the

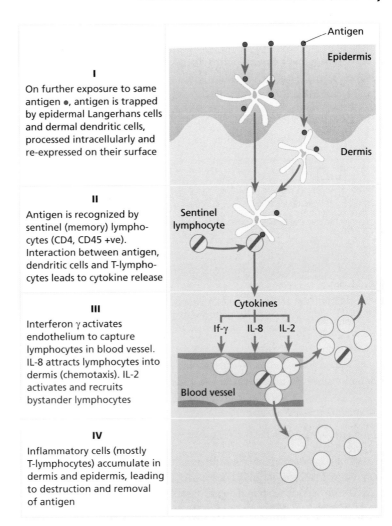

I

On further exposure to same antigen •, antigen is trapped by epidermal Langerhans cells and dermal dendritic cells, processed intracellularly and re-expressed on their surface

II

Antigen is recognized by sentinel (memory) lympho-cytes (CD4, CD45 +ve). Interaction between antigen, dendritic cells and T-lympho-cytes leads to cytokine release

III

Interferon γ activates endothelium to capture lymphocytes in blood vessel. IL-8 attracts lymphocytes into dermis (chemotaxis). IL-2 activates and recruits bystander lymphocytes

IV

Inflammatory cells (mostly T-lymphocytes) accumulate in dermis and epidermis, leading to destruction and removal of antigen

Fig. 2.18 Elicitation phase of allergic contact dermatitis (type IV) reaction.

dermis, the Langerhans cell enters the lymphatic system, and by the time it reaches the regional lymph node it will have processed the antigen, which is re-expressed on its surface in conjunction with MHC Class II molecules. In the node, the Langerhans cell mingles with crowds of lymphocytes, where it is most likely to find a T cell with just the right T-cell receptor to bind its now processed antigen. Helper (CD4+) T lymphocytes recognize antigen only in the presence of cells bearing MHC Class II antigens, such as the Langerhans cell. The interactions between surface molecules on a CD4+ T cell and a Langerhans cell are shown in Fig. 2.12. When a T cell interacts with an antigen-presenting cell carrying an antigen to which it can react, the T lymphocyte divides. This division depends upon the persistence of antigen (and the

antigen-presenting cells that contain it) and the T-cell growth factor interleukin-2 (IL-2). Eventually, a whole cadre of memory T cells is available to return to the skin to attack the antigen that stimulated their proliferation.

CD4+, CD45+ memory T lymphocytes circulate between nodes and tissues via lymphatic vessels, the thoracic duct, blood and interstitial fluid. They return to the skin aided by 'homing molecules' (cutaneous lymphocyte antigen, CLA) that guide their trip so that they preferentially enter the dermis. In the absence of antigen, they merely pass through it, and again enter the lymphatic vessels to return and recirculate. These cells are sentinel cells (Fig. 2.18), alert for their own special antigens. They accumulate in the skin if the host again encounters the antigen that initially stimulated their production. This preferential circulation of lymphocytes into the skin is a special part of the 'skin immune system' and reflects a selective advantage for the body to circulate lymphocytes that react to skin and skin surface-derived antigens.

Elicitation (challenge) phase (Fig. 2.18)

When a T lymphocyte again encounters the antigen to which it is sensitized, it is ready to react. If the antigen is extracellular, as on an invading bacterium, toxin or chemical allergen, the CD4+ T-helper cells do the work. The sequence of antigen processing by the Langerhans cell in the elicitation reaction is similar to the sequence of antigen processing during the induction phase, described above, that leads to the induction of immunity. The antigens get trapped by epidermal Langerhans cells or dermal dendritic cells, which process the antigen intracellularly before re-expressing the modified antigenic determinant on their surfaces. In the elicitation reaction, the Langerhans cells find appropriate T lymphocytes in the dermis, so most antigen presentation occurs there. The antigen is presented to CD4+ T cells which are activated and produce cytokines that cause lymphocytes, polymorphonuclear leucocytes and monocytes in blood vessels to slow as they pass through dermal blood vessels, to stop and emigrate into the dermis causing inflammation (Fig. 2.18). Helper or cytotoxic lymphocytes help to stem the infection or eliminate antigen and polymorphonuclear leucocytes engulf antigens and destroy them. The traffic of inflammatory cells in the epidermis and dermis is determined not only by cytokines produced by lymphocytes, but also by cytokines produced by injured keratinocytes (Fig. 2.11). For example, keratinocyte-derived cytokines can activate Langerhans cells and T cells, and IL-8, produced by keratinocytes, is a potent chemotactic factor for lymphocytes and polymorphs, and brings these up into the epidermis.

Response to intracellular antigens

Antigens coming from inside a cell, such as intracellular fungi or viruses and tumour antigens, are presented to cytotoxic T cells (CD8+) by the MHC Class I molecule. Presentation in this manner makes the infected cell liable to destruction by cytotoxic T lymphocytes or K cells. NK cells can also kill such

> **LEARNING POINTS**
>
> 1 Many skin disorders are good examples of an immune reaction at work. The more you know about the mechanisms, the more interesting the rashes become.
> 2 However, the immune system may not be the only culprit. If *Treponema pallidum* had not been discovered, syphilis might still be listed as an autoimmune disorder.

cells, even though they have not been sensitized with antibody.

Granulomas

Granulomas form when cell-mediated immunity fails to eliminate antigen. Foreign body granulomas occur because material remains undigested. Immunological granulomas require the persistence of antigen, but the response is augmented by a cell-mediated immune reaction. Lymphokines, released by lymphocytes sensitized to the antigen, cause macrophages to differentiate into epithelioid cells and giant cells. These secrete other cytokines, which influence inflammatory events. Immunological granulomas of the skin are characterized by Langhans giant cells (not to be confused with Langerhans cells; p. 12), epithelioid cells, and a surrounding mantle of lymphocytes.

Granulomatous reactions also occur when organisms cannot be destroyed (e.g. in tuberculosis, leprosy, leishmaniasis), or when a chemical cannot be eliminated (e.g. zirconium or beryllium). Similar reactions are seen in some persisting inflammations of undetermined cause (e.g. rosacea, granuloma annulare, sarcoidosis, and certain forms of panniculitis).

Further reading

Freinkel, R.K. & Woodley, D.T. (2001) *The Biology of the Skin*. Parthenon, London.

Uchi, T., Terao, H., Koga, T. & Furue, M. (2000) Cytokines and chemokines in the epidermis. *Journal of Dermatological Science*, **Suppl. 1**, S29–38.

Diagnosis of skin disorders

The key to successful treatment is an accurate diagnosis. You can look up treatments, but you cannot look up diagnoses. Without a proper diagnosis, you will be asking 'What's a good treatment for scaling feet?' instead of 'What's good for tinea pedis?' Would you ever ask yourself 'What's a good treatment for chest pain? Luckily, dermatology differs from other specialties as its diseases can easily be seen. Keen eyes and a magnifying glass are all that are needed for a complete examination of the skin. Sometimes it is best to examine the patient briefly before obtaining a full history: a quick look will often prompt the right questions. However, a careful history is important in every case, as is the intelligent use of the laboratory.

History

The key points to be covered in the history are listed in Table 3.1 and should include descriptions of the events surrounding the onset of the skin lesions, of the progression of individual lesions, and of the disease in general, including any responses to treatment. Many patients try a few salves before seeing a physician. Some try all the medications in their medicine cabinets, many of which can aggravate the problem. A careful inquiry into drugs taken for other conditions is often useful. Ask also about previous skin disorders, occupation, hobbies and disorders in the family.

Examination

To examine the skin properly, the lighting must be uniform and bright. Daylight is best. The patient should usually undress so that the whole skin can be examined, although sometimes this is neither desirable (e.g. hand warts) nor possible. The presence of a chaperone,

Table 3.1 Outline of dermatological history.

History of present skin condition
Duration
Site at onset, details of spread
Itch
Burning
Pain
Wet, dry, blisters
Exacerbating factors

General health at present
Ask about fever

Past history of skin disorders

Past general medical history
Inquire specifically about asthma and hay fever

Family history of skin disorders
If positive—inherited vs. infection/infestation

Family history of other medical disorders

Social and occupational history
Hobbies
Travels abroad
Relationship of rash to work and holidays
Alcohol intake

Drugs used to treat present skin condition
Topical
Systemic
Physician prescribed
Patient initiated

Drugs prescribed for other disorders (including those taken before onset of skin disorder)

ideally a nurse or a relative, is often sensible, and is essential if examination of the genitalia is necessary. Do not be put off this too easily by the elderly, the stubborn, the shy, or the surroundings. Sometimes

Table 3.2 Terminology of primary lesions.

	Small (< 0.5 cm)	Large (> 0.5 cm)
Elevated solid lesion	Papule	Nodule (> 0.5 cm in both width and depth) Plaque (> 2 cm in width but without substantial depth)
Flat area of altered colour or texture	Macule	Large macule (patch)
Fluid-filled blister	Vesicle	Bulla
Pus-filled lesion	Pustule	Abscess
Extravasation of blood into skin	Petechia (pinhead size) Purpura (up to 2 mm in diameter)	Ecchymosis Haematoma
Accumulation of dermal oedema	Wheal (can be any size)	Angioedema

make-up must be washed off or wigs removed. There is nothing more embarrassing than missing the right diagnosis because an important sign has been hidden.

Distribution

A dermatological diagnosis is based both on the distribution of lesions and on their morphology and configuration. For example, an area of seborrhoeic dermatitis may look very like an area of atopic dermatitis; but the key to diagnosis lies in the location. Seborrhoeic dermatitis affects the scalp, forehead, eyebrows, nasolabial folds and central chest; atopic dermatitis typically affects the antecubital and popliteal fossae.

See if the skin disease is localized, universal or symmetrical. Depending on the disease suggested by the morphology, you may want to check special areas, like the feet in a patient with hand eczema, or the gluteal cleft in a patient who might have psoriasis. Examine as much of the skin as possible. Look in the mouth and remember to check the hair and the nails (Chapter 13). Note negative as well as positive findings, e.g. the way the shielded areas are spared in a photosensitive dermatitis (see Fig. 16.7). Always keep your eyes open for incidental skin cancers which the patient may have ignored.

Morphology

After the distribution has been noted, next define the morphology of the primary lesions. Many skin diseases have a characteristic morphology, but scratching, ulceration and other events can change this. The rule is to find an early or 'primary' lesion and to inspect it closely. What is its shape? What is its size? What is its colour? What are its margins like? What are the surface characteristics? What does it feel like?

Most types of primary lesion have one name if small, and a different one if large. The scheme is summarized in Table 3.2.

There are many reasons why you should describe skin diseases properly.
• Skin disorders are often grouped by their morphology. Once the morphology is clear, a differential diagnosis comes easily to mind.
• If you have to describe a condition accurately, you will have to look at it carefully.
• You can paint a verbal picture if you have to refer the patient for another opinion.
• You will sound like a physician and not a homoeopath.
• You will be able to understand the terminology of this book.

Terminology of lesions (Fig. 3.1)

Primary lesions

Erythema is redness caused by vascular dilatation.

A *papule* is a small solid elevation of skin, less than 0.5 cm in diameter.

A *plaque* is an elevated area of skin greater than 2 cm in diameter but without substantial depth.

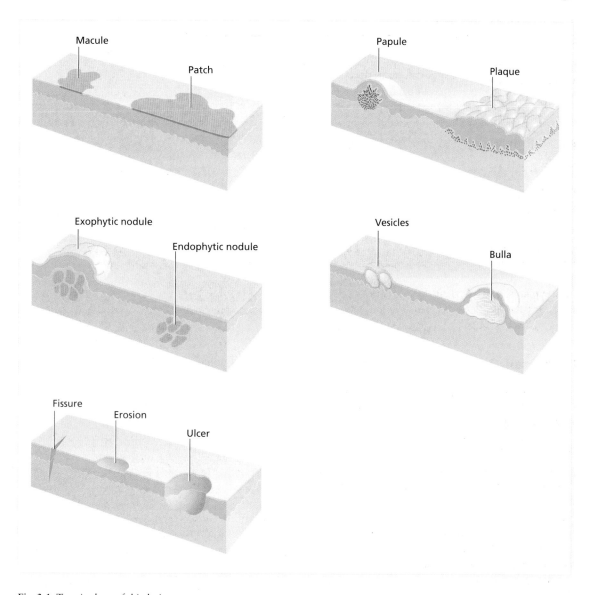

Fig. 3.1 Terminology of skin lesions.

A *macule* is a small flat area of altered colour or texture.

A *vesicle* is a circumscribed elevation of skin, less than 0.5 cm in diameter, and containing fluid.

A *bulla* is a circumscribed elevation of skin over 0.5 cm in diameter and containing fluid.

A *pustule* is a visible accumulation of pus in the skin.

An *abscess* is a localized collection of pus in a cavity, more than 1 cm in diameter. Abscesses are usually nodules, and the term 'purulent bulla' is sometimes used to describe a pus-filled blister that is situated on top of the skin rather than within it.

A *wheal* is an elevated white compressible evanescent area produced by dermal oedema. It is often surrounded by a red axon-mediated flare. Although usually less than 2 cm in diameter, some wheals are huge.

Angioedema is a diffuse swelling caused by oedema extending to the subcutaneous tissue.

A *nodule* is a solid mass in the skin, usually greater than 0.5 cm in diameter, in both width and depth, which can be seen to be elevated or can be palpated.

A *tumour* is harder to define as the term is based more correctly on microscopic pathology than on clinical morphology. We keep it here as a convenient term to describe an enlargement of the tissues by normal or pathological material or cells that form a mass, usually more than 1 cm in diameter. Because the word 'tumour' can scare patients, tumours may courteously be called 'large nodules', especially if they are not malignant.

A *papilloma* is a nipple-like projection from the skin.

Petechiae are pinhead-sized macules of blood in the skin.

The term *purpura* describes a larger macule or papule of blood in the skin. Such blood-filled lesions do not blanch if a glass lens is pushed against them (diascopy).

An *ecchymosis* is a larger extravasation of blood into the skin.

A *haematoma* is a swelling from gross bleeding.

A *burrow* is a linear or curvilinear papule, with some scaling, caused by a scabies mite.

A *comedo* is a plug of greasy keratin wedged in a dilated pilosebaceous orifice. Open comedones are blackheads. The follicle opening of a closed comedo is nearly covered over by skin so that it looks like a pinhead-sized, ivory-coloured papule.

Telangiectasia is the visible dilatation of small cutaneous blood vessels.

Poikiloderma is a combination of atrophy, reticulate hyperpigmentation and telangiectasia.

Secondary lesions

These evolve from primary lesions.

A *scale* is a flake arising from the horny layer.

A *keratosis* is a horn-like thickening of the stratum corneum.

A *crust* may look like a scale, but is composed of dried blood or tissue fluid.

An *ulcer* is an area of skin from which the whole of the epidermis and at least the upper part of the dermis has been lost. Ulcers may extend into subcutaneous fat, and heal with scarring.

An *erosion* is an area of skin denuded by a complete or partial loss of only the epidermis. Erosions heal without scarring.

An *excoriation* is an ulcer or erosion produced by scratching.

A *fissure* is a slit in the skin.

A *sinus* is a cavity or channel that permits the escape of pus or fluid.

A *scar* is a result of healing, where normal structures are permanently replaced by fibrous tissue.

Atrophy is a thinning of skin caused by diminution of the epidermis, dermis or subcutaneous fat. When the epidermis is atrophic it may crinkle like cigarette paper, appear thin and translucent, and lose normal surface markings. Blood vessels may be easy to see in both epidermal and dermal atrophy.

Lichenification is an area of thickened skin with increased markings.

A *stria* (stretch mark) is a streak-like linear atrophic pink, purple or white lesion of the skin caused by changes in the connective tissue.

Pigmentation, either more or less than surrounding skin, can develop after lesions heal.

Having identified the lesions as primary or secondary, adjectives can be used to describe them in terms of their other features.

• Colour (e.g. salmon-pink, lilac, violet).
• Sharpness of edge (e.g. well-defined, ill-defined).
• Surface contour (e.g. dome-shaped, umbilicated, spire-like; Fig. 3.2).
• Geometric shape (e.g. nummular, oval, irregular, like the coast of Maine).
• Texture (e.g. rough, silky, smooth, hard).
• Smell (e.g. foul-smelling).
• Temperature (e.g. hot, warm).

Dermatologists also use a few special adjectives which warrant definition.

• *Nummular* means round or coin-like.
• *Annular* means ring-like.
• *Circinate* means circular.
• *Arcuate* means curved.
• *Discoid* means disc-like.
• *Gyrate* means wave-like.
• *Retiform* and *reticulate* mean net-like.

To describe a skin lesion, use the term for the primary lesion as the noun, and the adjectives mentioned above to define it. For example, the lesions of psoriasis may appear as 'salmon-pink sharply demarcated nummular plaques covered by large silver polygonal scales'.

Try not to use the terms 'lesion' or 'area'. Why say 'papular lesion' when you can say papule? It is

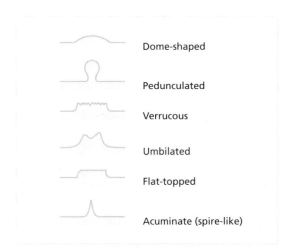

Dome-shaped

Pedunculated

Verrucous

Umbilated

Flat-topped

Acuminate (spire-like)

Fig. 3.2 Surface contours of papules.

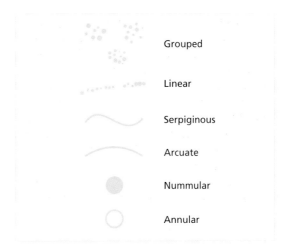

Grouped

Linear

Serpiginous

Arcuate

Nummular

Annular

Fig. 3.3 Configuration of lesions.

almost as bad as the ubiquitous term 'skin rash'. By the way, there are very few diseases that are truly 'maculopapular'. The term is best avoided except to describe some drug eruptions and viral exanthems. Even then, the terms 'scarlatiniform' (like scarlet fever —punctate, slightly elevated papules) or 'morbilliform' (like measles—a net-like blotchy slightly elevated pink exanthem) are more helpful.

Configuration

After unravelling the primary and secondary lesions, look for arrangements and configurations that can be, for example, discrete, confluent, grouped, annular, arcuate or dermatomal (Fig. 3.3). Note that while individual lesions may be annular, several individual lesions may arrange themselves into an annular configuration. Terms like annular, and other adjectives discussed under the morphology of individual lesions, can apply to their groupings too. The Köbner or isomorphic phenomenon is the induction of skin lesions by, and at the site of, trauma such as scratch marks or operative incisions.

Special tools and techniques

A *magnifying lens* is a helpful aid to diagnosis because subtle changes in the skin become more apparent when enlarged. One attached to spectacles will leave your hand free.

A *Wood's light*, emitting long wavelength ultraviolet radiation, will help with the examination of some skin conditions. Fluorescence is seen in some fungal infections (Chapter 14), erythrasma (p. 189) and pseudomonas infections. Some subtle disorders of pigmentation can be seen more clearly under Wood's light, e.g. the pale patches of tuberous sclerosis, low-grade vitiligo and pityriasis versicolor, and the darker *café-au-lait* patches of neurofibromatosis. The urine in hepatic cutaneous porphyria (p. 287) often fluoresces coral pink, even without solvent extraction of the porphyrins (see Fig. 19.10).

Diascopy is the name given to the technique in which a glass slide or clear plastic spoon is used to blanch vascular lesions and so to unmask their underlying colour.

Photography, conventional or digital, helps to record the baseline appearance of a lesion or rash, so that change can be assessed objectively at later visits. Small changes in pigmented lesions can be detected by analysing sequential digital images stored in computerized systems.

Dermatoscopy (epiluminescence microscopy, skin surface microscopy)

This non-invasive technique for diagnosing pigmented lesions *in vivo* has come of age in the last few years. It is particularly useful in the diagnosis of malignant melanomas. The lesion is covered with mineral oil, alcohol or water and then illuminated and observed at

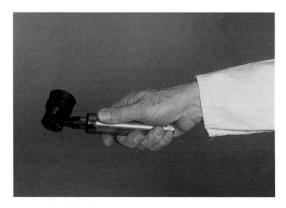

Fig. 3.4 A dermatoscope.

$10 \times$ magnification with a hand-held dermatoscope (Fig. 3.4). The fluid eliminates surface reflection and makes the horny layer translucent so that pigmented structures in the epidermis and superficial dermis and the superficial vascular plexus (p. 17) can be assessed. The dermatoscopic appearance of many pigmented lesions, including seborrhoeic warts, haemangiomas, basal cell carcinomas and most naevi and malignant melanomas is characteristic (Fig. 3.5). Images can be recorded by conventional or digital photography and sequential changes assessed. With formal training and practice, the use of dermatoscopy improves the accuracy with which pigmented lesions are diagnosed.

A dermatoscope can also be used to identify scabies mites in their burrows (p. 228).

> ### LEARNING POINTS
>
> 1 As Osler said: 'See and then reason, but see first'.
> 2 A correct diagnosis is the key to correct treatment.
> 3 The term 'skin rash' is as bad as 'gastric stomach'.
> 4 Avoid using too many long Latin descriptive names as a cloak for ignorance.
> 5 The history is especially important when the diagnosis is difficult.
> 6 Undress the patients and use a lens, even if it only gives you more time to think.
> 7 Remember the old adage that if you do not look in the mouth you will put your foot in it.

Assessment

Next try to put the disease into a general class; the titles of the chapters in this book are representative. Once classified, a differential diagnosis is usually forthcoming. Each diagnosis can then be considered on its merits, and laboratory tests may be used to confirm or refute diagnoses in the differential list. At this stage you must make a working diagnosis or formulate a plan to do so!

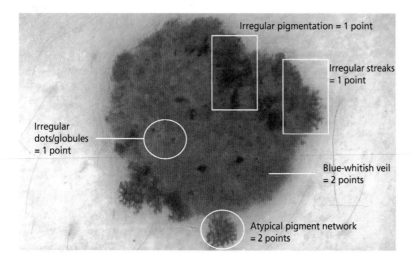

Fig. 3.5 Dermatoscopic appearance of a malignant melanoma.

Side-room and office tests

A number of tests can be performed in the practice office so that their results will be available immediately.

Potassium hydroxide preparations for fungal infections

If a fungal infection is suspected, scales or plucked hairs can be dissolved in an aqueous solution of 20% potassium hydroxide (KOH) containing 40% dimethyl sulphoxide (DMSO). The scale from the edge of a scaling lesion is vigorously scraped on to a glass slide with a No. 15 scalpel blade or the edge of a second glass slide. Other samples can include nail clippings, the roofs of blisters, hair pluckings, and the contents of pustules when a candidal infection is suspected. A drop or two of the KOH solution is run under the cover slip (Fig. 3.6). After 5–10 min the mount is examined under a microscope with the condenser lens lowered to increase contrast. Nail clippings take longer to clear—up to a couple of hours. With experience, fungal and candidal hyphae can be readily detected (Fig. 3.7). No heat is required if DMSO is included in the KOH solution.

Detection of a scabies mite

Burrows in an itchy patient are diagnostic of scabies. Retrieving a mite from the skin will confirm the diagnosis and convince a sceptical patient of the infestation. The burrow should be examined under a magnifying glass; the acarus is seen as a tiny black or grey dot at the most recent, least scaly end. It can

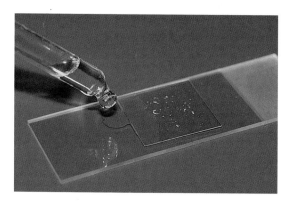

Fig. 3.6 Preparing a skin scraping for microscopy by adding potassium hydroxide (KOH) from a pipette.

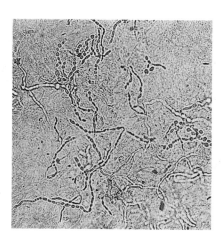

Fig. 3.7 Fungal hyphae in a KOH preparation. The polygonal shadows in the background are horny layer cells.

be removed by a sterile needle and placed on a slide within a marked circle. Alternatively, if mites are not seen, possible burrows can be vigorously scraped with a No. 15 scalpel blade, moistened with liquid paraffin or vegetable oil, and the scrapings transferred to a slide. Patients never argue the toss when confronted by a magnified mobile mite. Dermatoscopy (see above) can also be used to detect the scabies mite.

Cytology (Tzanck smear)

Cytology can aid diagnosis of viral infections such as herpes simplex and zoster, and of bullous diseases such as pemphigus. A blister roof is removed and the cells from the base of the blister are scraped off with a No. 10 or 15 surgical blade. These cells are smeared on to a microscope slide, air-dried and fixed with methanol. They are then stained with Giemsa, toluidine blue or Wright's stain. Acantholytic cells (Chapter 9) are seen in pemphigus and multinucleate giant cells are diagnostic of herpes simplex or varicella zoster infections (Chapter 14). Practice is needed to get good preparations. The technique remains popular in the USA but has fallen out of favour in the UK as histology, virological culture and electron microscopy have become more accessible.

Patch tests

Patch tests are invaluable in detecting the allergens responsible for allergic contact dermatitis (Chapter 7).

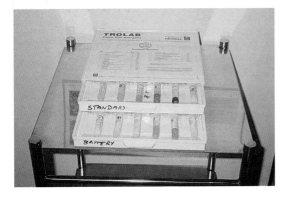

Fig. 3.8 Patch testing equipment. Syringes contain commercially prepared antigens, to be applied in aluminium cups.

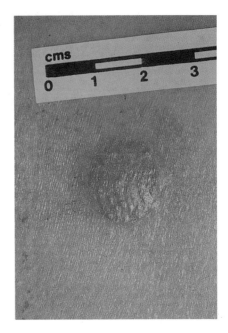

Fig. 3.9 A strong positive reaction to a rubber additive.

Either suspected individual antigens, or a battery of antigens which are common culprits, can be tested. Standard dilutions of the common antigens in appropriate bases are available commercially (Fig. 3.8). The test materials are applied to the back under aluminium discs or patches; the occlusion encourages penetration of the allergen. The patches are left in place for 48 h and then, after careful marking, are removed. The sites are inspected 10 min later, again at 96 h and sometimes even later if doubtful reactions require further assessment. The test detects type IV delayed hypersensitivity reactions (Chapter 2). The readings are scored according to the reaction seen.

NT Not tested.

0 No reaction.

± Doubtful reaction (minimal erythema).

+ Weak reaction (erythematous and maybe papular).

++ Strong reaction (erythematous and oedematous or vesicular; Fig. 3.9).

+++ Extreme reaction (erythematous and bullous).

IR Irritant reaction (variable, but often sharply circumscribed, with a glazed appearance and increased skin markings).

A positive patch test does not prove that the allergen in question has caused the current episode of contact dermatitis; the results must be interpreted in the light of the history and possible previous exposure to the allergen.

Patch testing requires attention to detail in applying the patches properly, and skill and experience in interpreting the results.

Prick testing

Prick testing is much less helpful in dermatology. It detects immediate (type I) hypersensitivity (Chapter 2) and patients should not have taken systemic antihistamines for at least 48 h before the test. Commercially prepared diluted antigens and a control are placed as single drops on marked areas of the forearm. The skin is gently pricked through the drops using separate sterile fine (e.g. Size 25 gauge, or smaller) needles. The prick should not cause bleeding. The drops are then removed with a tissue wipe. After 10 min the sites are inspected and the diameter of any wheal measured and recorded. A result is considered positive if the test antigen causes a wheal of 4 mm or greater (Fig. 3.10) and the control elicits negligible reaction. Like patch testing, prick testing should not be undertaken by those without formal training in the procedure. Although the risk of anaphylaxis is small, resuscitation facilities including adrenaline (epinephrine) and oxygen (p. 310) must be available. The relevance of positive results to the cause of the condition under investigation—usually urticaria or atopic dermatitis—is often debatable. Positive results should correlate with positive radioallergosorbent tests (RAST; p. 74) used to measure total and specific immunoglobulin E (IgE) levels to

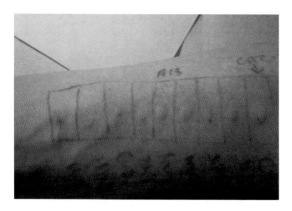

Fig. 3.10 Prick testing: many positive results in an atopic individual.

inhaled and ingested allergens. RAST tests, although more expensive, pose no risk of anaphylaxis and take up less of the patient's time in the clinic. They are now used more often than prick tests.

Skin biopsy

Biopsy (from the Greek *bios* meaning 'life' and *opsis* 'sight') of skin lesions is useful to establish or confirm a clinical diagnosis. A piece of tissue is removed surgically for histological examination and, sometimes, for other tests (e.g. culture for organisms). When used selectively, a skin biopsy can solve the most perplexing problem but, conversely, will be unhelpful in conditions without a specific histology (e.g. most drug eruptions, pityriasis rosea, reactive erythemas).

Skin biopsies may be *incisional*, when just part of a lesion is removed for laboratory examination or *excisional*, when the whole lesion is cut out. Excisional biopsy is preferable for most small lesions (up to 0.5 cm diameter) but incisional biopsy is chosen when the partial removal of a larger lesion is adequate for diagnosis, and complete removal might leave an unnecessary and unsightly scar. Ideally, an incisional biopsy should include a piece of the surrounding normal skin (Fig. 3.11) although this may not be possible if a small punch is used.

The main steps in skin biopsy are:
1 administration of local anaesthesia; and
2 removal of all (excision) or part (incision) of the lesion and repair of the defect made by a scalpel or punch.

Local anaesthetic

Lignocaine (lidocaine) 1–2% is used. Sometimes adrenaline 1 : 200 000 is added. This causes vasoconstriction, reduced clearance of the local anaesthetic and prolongation of the local anaesthetic effect. Plain lignocaine should be used on the fingers, toes and penis as the prolonged vasoconstriction produced by adrenaline can be dangerous here. Adrenaline is also best avoided in diabetics with small vessel disease, in those with a history of heart disease (including dysrhythmias), in patients taking non-selective α blockers and tricyclic antidepressants (because of potential interactions) and in uncontrolled hyperthyroidism. There are exceptions to these general rules and, undoubtedly, the total dose of local anaesthetic and/or adrenaline is important. Nevertheless, the rules should not be broken unless the surgeon is quite sure that the procedure that he or she is about to embark on is safe.

It is wise to avoid local anaesthesia during early pregnancy and to delay non-urgent procedures until after the first trimester.

As 'B' follows 'A' in the alphabet, get into the habit of checking the precise concentration of the lignocaine ± added adrenaline on the label *before* withdrawing it into the syringe and then, *before* injecting it, confirm that the patient has not had any previous allergic reactions to local anaesthetic.

Infiltration of the local anaesthetic into the skin around the area to be biopsied is the most widely used method. If the local anaesthetic is injected into the subcutaneous fat, it will be relatively pain-free, will produce a diffuse swelling of the skin and will take several minutes to induce anaesthesia. Intradermal injections are painful and produce a discrete wheal associated with rapid anaesthesia. The application of EMLA cream (eutectic mixture of local anaesthesia) to the operation site 2 h before giving a local anaesthetic to children helps to numb the initial prick.

Scalpel biopsy

This provides more tissue than a punch biopsy. It can be used routinely, but is especially useful for biopsying disorders of the subcutaneous fat, for obtaining specimens with both normal and abnormal skin for comparison (Fig. 3.11) and for removing small lesions *in toto* (excision biopsy, see p. 321). After selecting the lesion for biopsy, an elliptical piece of skin is excised.

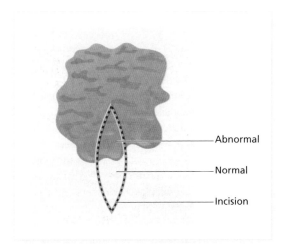

Fig. 3.11 Incision biopsy. This should include adjacent normal skin.

The specimen should include the subcutaneous fat. Removing the specimen with forceps may cause crush artefact, which can be avoided by lifting the specimen with either a Gillies hook or a syringe needle. The wound is then sutured; firm compression for 5 min stops oozing. Non-absorbable 3/0 sutures are used for biopsies on the legs and back, 5/0 for the face, and 4/0 for elsewhere. Stitches are usually removed from the face in 4 days, from the anterior trunk and arms in 7 days, and from the back and legs in 10 days. Some guidelines for skin biopsies are listed in Table 3.3.

Punch biopsy

The skin is sampled with a small (3–4 mm diameter) tissue punch. Lignocaine 1% is injected intradermally

Table 3.3 Guidelines for skin biopsies.

Sample a fresh lesion
Obtain your specimen from near the lesion's edge
Avoid sites where a scar would be conspicuous
Avoid the upper trunk or jaw line where keloids are most likely to form
Avoid the legs, where healing is slow
Avoid lesions over bony prominences, where infection is more likely
Use the scalpel technique for scalp disorders and diseases of the subcutaneous fat or vessels
Do not crush the tissue
Place in proper fixative
If two lesions are sampled, be sure they do not get mixed up or mislabelled. Label specimen containers before the biopsy is placed in them
Make sure that the patient's name, age and sex are clearly indicated on the pathology form
Provide the pathologist with a legible summary of the history, the site of the biopsy and a differential diagnosis
Discuss the results with the pathologist

first, and a cylinder of skin is incised with the punch by rotating it back and forth (Fig. 3.12). Skin is lifted up carefully with a needle or forceps and the base is cut off at the level of subcutaneous fat. The defect is cauterized or repaired with a single suture. The biopsy specimen must not be crushed with the forceps or critical histological patterns may be distorted.

The tissue can be sent to the pathologist with a summary of the history, a differential diagnosis and the patient's age. Close liaison with the pathologist is essential, because the diagnosis may only become apparent with knowledge of both the clinical and histological features.

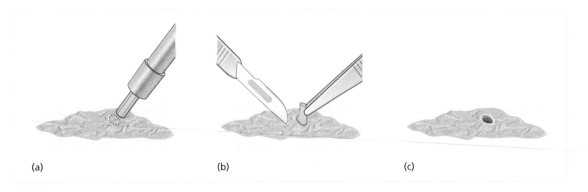

(a)   (b)   (c)

Fig. 3.12 Steps in taking a punch biopsy.

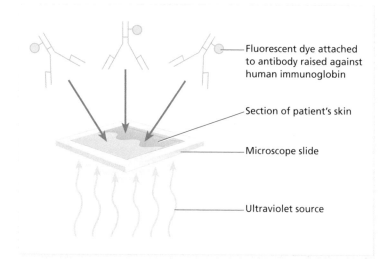

Fig. 3.13 Direct immunofluorescence detects antibodies in a patient's skin. Here immunoglobulin G (IgG) antibodies are detected by staining with a fluorescent dye attached to antihuman IgG.

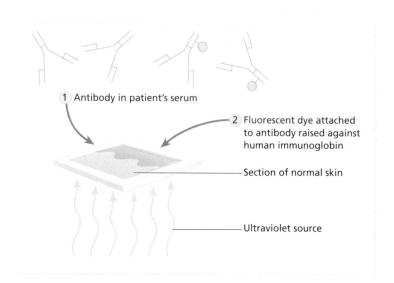

Fig. 3.14 Indirect immunofluorescence detects antibodies in a patient's serum. There are two steps. (1) Antibodies in this serum are made to bind to antigens in a section of normal skin. (2) Antibody raised against human immunoglobulin, conjugated with a fluorescent dye can then be used to stain these bound antibodies (as in the direct immunofluorescence test).

Laboratory tests

The laboratory is vital for the accurate diagnosis of many skin disorders. Tests include various assays of blood, serum and urine, bacterial, fungal and viral culture from skin and other specimens, immunofluorescent and immunohistological examinations (Figs 3.13 and 3.14), radiography, ultrasonography and other methods of image intensification. Specific details are discussed as each disease is presented.

Conclusions

Clinical dermatology is a visual specialty. You must see the disease, and understand what you are seeing. Look closely and thoroughly. Take time. Examine the whole body. Locate primary lesions and check configuration and distribution. Ask appropriate questions, especially if the diagnosis is difficult. Classify the disorder and list the differential diagnoses. Use the history, examination and laboratory tests to make a diagnosis

LEARNING POINTS

1 A biopsy is the refuge of a bankrupt mind when dealing with conditions that do not have a specific histology. Here, a return to the history and examination is more likely to reveal diagnostic clues than a pathologist.
2 If you do not remember the two essential checks before injecting local anaesthetic then read p. 37 again.

if this cannot be made by clinical features alone. Then treat. Refer the patient to a dermatologist if:

- you cannot make a diagnosis;
- the disorder does not respond to treatment;
- the disorder is unusual or severe; or
- you are just not sure.

Further reading

Cox, N.H. & Lawrence, C.M. (1998) *Diagnostic Problems in Dermatology*. Mosby Wolfe, Edinburgh.

Lawrence, C.M. & Cox, N.M. (2001) *Physical Signs in Dermatology*, 2nd edn. Mosby, Edinburgh.

Mutasim, D.F. and Adams, B.B. (2001) Immunofluorescence in dermatology. *Journal of the American Academy of Dermatology* **45**, 803–822.

Savin, J.A., Hunter, J.A.A. & Hepburn, N.C. (1997) *Skin Signs in Clinical Medicine: Diagnosis in Colour*. Mosby Wolfe, London.

Shelley, W.B. & Shelley, E.D. (1992) *Advanced Dermatologic Diagnosis*. W.B. Saunders, Philadelphia, PA.

Stolz, W. *et al.* (2002) *Color Atlas of Dermatoscopy*, 2nd edn. Blackwell Publishing, Oxford.

4 Disorders of keratinization

The complex but orderly processes of keratinization, and of cell cohesion and proliferation within the epidermis, have been described in Chapter 2. As they proceed, the living keratinocytes of the deeper epidermis change into the dead corneocytes of the horny layer, where they are stuck together by inter-cellular lipids. They are then shed in such a way that the surface of the normal skin does not seem scaly to the naked eye. Shedding balances production, so that the thickness of the horny layer does not alter. However, if keratinization or cell cohesion is abnormal, the horny layer may become thick or the skin surface may become dry and scaly. Such changes can be localized or generalized.

In this chapter we describe a variety of skin disorders that have as their basis a disorder of keratinization. During the last few years the molecular mechanisms underlying many of these have become clearer, including abnormal genetic coding for keratins, the enzymes involved in cell cohesion in the horny layer, and the molecules that are critical in the signalling pathway governing cell cohesion in the spinous layer.

The ichthyoses

The word ichthyosis comes from the Greek word for a fish. It is applied to disorders that share, as their main feature, a dry rough skin with marked scaling but no inflammation. Strictly speaking, the scales lack the regular overlapping pattern of fish scales, but the term is usefully descriptive and too well entrenched to be discarded. There are several types.

Ichthyosis vulgaris

Cause

Inherited as an autosomal dominant disorder, this condition is common and affects about 1 person in 300. The relevant gene may be concerned with the production of profilaggrin, a precursor of filaggrin, itself a component of keratohyalin granules.

Presentation

The dryness is usually mild and symptoms are few. The scales are small and branny, being most obvious on the limbs and least obvious in the major flexures. The skin creases of the palm may be accentuated. Keratosis pilaris (p. 44) is often present on the limbs.

Clinical course

The skin changes are not usually present at birth but develop over the first few years of life. Some patients improve in adult life, particularly during warm weather, but the condition seldom clears completely.

Complications

The already dry skin chaps in the winter and is easily irritated by degreasing agents. This should be taken into account in the choice of a career. Ichthyosis of this type is apt to appear in a stubborn combination with atopic eczema.

Differential diagnosis

It can usually be distinguished from less common types of ichthyosis on the basis of the pattern of inheritance and of the type and distribution of the scaling.

Investigations

None are usually needed.

Treatment

This is palliative. The dryness can be helped by the regular use of emollients, which are best applied after a shower or bath. Emulsifying ointment, soft white paraffin, E45 and unguentum merck are all quite suitable (Formulary 1, p. 328) and the selection depends on the patient's preference. Many find proprietary bath oils and creams containing urea or lactic acid helpful also (Formulary 1, p. 331).

X-linked recessive ichthyosis

Cause

This less common type of ichthyosis is inherited as an X-linked recessive trait and therefore, in its complete form, is seen only in males, although some female carriers show mild scaling. The condition affects about 1 in 6000 males in the UK and is associated with a deficiency of the enzyme steroid sulphatase, which hydrolyses cholesterol sulphate. The responsible gene has been localized to the terminal part of the X chromosome at Xp 22.3 (see Chapter 21).

Presentation and course

In contrast to the delayed onset of the dominantly inherited ichthyosis vulgaris, scaling appears early, often soon after birth, and always by the first birthday. The scales are larger and browner (Fig. 4.1), involve the neck, and to a lesser extent the popliteal and antecubital areas, as well as the skin generally. The palms and soles are normal. There is no association with atopy or keratosis pilaris. The condition persists throughout life.

Complications

Corneal opacities may appear in adult life. Kallmann's syndrome is caused by the deletion of a part of the X chromosome that includes the gene for X-linked recessive ichthyosis, which is therefore one of its features. Other features of this contiguous gene disorder are hypogonadism, anosmia and neurological defects.

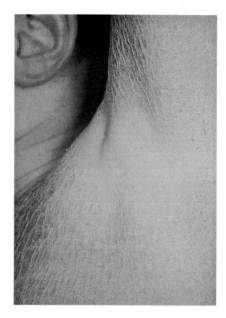

Fig. 4.1 Ichthyosis: large rather dark scales suggest the less common type inherited as a sex-linked recessive trait.

Differential diagnosis

This is as for ichthyosis vulgaris. It is helpful to remember that only males are affected. Bear Kallmann's syndrome in mind if there are other congenital abnormalities.

Investigations

None are usually needed. A few centres can measure steroid sulphatase in fibroblasts cultured from a skin biopsy.

Treatment

Oral aromatic retinoids are probably best avoided. Topical measures are as for ichthyosis vulgaris.

Collodion baby (Fig. 4.2)

This is a description and not a diagnosis. The bizarre skin charges are seen at birth. At first the stratum corneum is smooth and shiny, and the skin looks as though it has been covered with cellophane or collodion. Its tightness may cause ectropion and feeding difficulties. The shiny outer surface is shed within a few days leaving behind, most often, a non-bullous

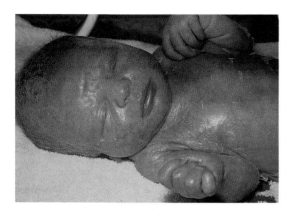

Fig. 4.2 A collodion baby who had an underlying non-bullous ichthyosiform erythroderma.

ichthyosiform erythroderma, and less often a lamellar ichthyosis. Problems with temperature regulation and high water loss through the skin in the early days of life are best dealt with by the use of a high humidity incubator. Regular applications of a greasy emollient also limit fluid loss and make the skin supple. The much rarer 'harlequin fetus' is covered with thick fissured hyperkeratosis. Ectropion is extreme and most affected infants die early.

Lamellar ichthyosis and non-bullous ichthyosiform erythroderma

Understandably, these rare conditions have often been confused in the past. Both may be inherited as an autosomal recessive trait, and in both the skin changes at birth are those of a collodion baby (see above). Later the two conditions can be distinguished by the finer scaling and more obvious redness of non-bullous ichthyosiform erythroderma. Both last for life and are sufficiently disfiguring for the long-term use of acitretin to be justifiable (Formulary 2, p. 349). Lamellar ichthyosis shows genetic heterogeneity: the most severe type is caused by mutations in the gene for keratinocyte transglutaminase, an enzyme that cross-links the cornified cell envelope, lying on chromosome 14q11.2.

Epidermolytic hyperkeratosis (bullous ichthyosiform erythroderma)

This rare condition is inherited as an autosomal dominant disorder. Shortly after birth the baby's skin becomes generally red and shows numerous blisters. The redness fades over a few months, and the tendency to blister also lessens, but during childhood a gross brownish warty hyperkeratosis appears, sometimes in a roughly linear form and usually worst in the flexures. The histology is distinctive: a thickened granular cell layer contains large granules, and clefts may be seen in the upper epidermis. The condition is caused by mutations in the genes (on chromosomes 12q13 and 17q21) controlling the production of keratins 1 and 10. A few patients with localized areas of hyperkeratosis with the same histological features have gonadal mosaicism, and so their children are at risk of developing the generalized form of the disorder. Treatment is symptomatic and antibiotics may be needed if the blisters become infected. Acitretin (Formulary 2, p. 349) has helped in severe cases.

Other ichthyosiform disorders

Sometimes ichthyotic skin changes are a minor part of a multisystem disease, but such associations are very rare. *Refsum's syndrome*, an autosomal recessive trait, is caused by deficiency of a single enzyme concerned in the breakdown of phytanic acid, which then accumulates in the tissues. The other features (retinal degeneration, peripheral neuropathy and ataxia) overshadow the minor dryness of the skin.

Rud's syndrome is an ichthyosiform erythroderma in association with mental retardation and epilepsy. In *Netherton's syndrome*, brittle hairs, with a so-called 'bamboo deformity', are present as well as a curious gyrate and erythematous hyperkeratotic eruption (ichthyosis linearis circumflexa). Other conditions are identified by confusing acronyms: IBIDS (also known as trichothiodystrophy) stands for Ichthyosis, Brittle hair, Impaired intelligence, Decreased fertility and Short stature; the KID syndrome consists of Keratitis, Ichthyosis and Deafness.

Acquired ichthyosis

It is unusual for ichthyosis to appear for the first time in adult life; but if it does, an underlying disease should be suspected. The most frequent is Hodgkin's disease. Other recorded causes include other lymphomas, leprosy, sarcoidosis, malabsorption and a poor diet. The skin may also appear dry in hypothyroidism.

Other disorders of keratinization

Keratosis pilaris

Cause

This common condition is inherited as an autosomal dominant trait, and is possibly caused by mutations in a gene lying on the short arm of chromosome 18. The abnormality lies in the keratinization of hair follicles, which become filled with horny plugs.

Presentation and course

The changes begin in childhood and tend to become less obvious in adult life. In the most common type, the greyish horny follicular plugs, sometimes with red areolae, are confined to the outer aspects of the thighs and upper arms, where the skin feels rough. Less often the plugs affect the sides of the face; perifollicular erythema and loss of eyebrow hairs may then occur. There is an association with ichthyosis vulgaris.

Complications

Involvement of the cheeks may lead to an ugly pitted scarring. Rarely, the follicles in the eyebrows may be damaged with subsequent loss of hair there.

Differential diagnosis

A rather similar pattern of widespread follicular keratosis (phrynoderma) can occur in severe vitamin deficiency. The lack is probably not just of vitamin A, as was once thought, but of several vitamins.

Investigations

None are needed.

Treatment

Treatment is not usually needed, although keratolytics such as salicylic acid or urea in a cream base may smooth the skin temporarily (Formulary 1, p. 331).

Keratosis follicularis (Darier's disease)

Cause

This rare condition is inherited as an autosomal dominant trait. Fertility tends to be low and many cases represent new mutations. The abnormal gene (on chromosome 12q23-q24.1) encodes for a molecule important in a signalling pathway that regulates cell–cell adhesion in the epidermis.

Presentation

The first signs usually appear in the mid-teens, sometimes after overexposure to sunlight. The characteristic lesions are small pink or brownish papules with a greasy scale (Fig. 4.3). These coalesce into warty plaques in a 'seborrhoeic' distribution (Fig. 4.4). Early lesions are often seen on the sternal and interscapular areas, and behind the ears. The severity of the condition varies greatly from person to person: sometimes the skin is widely affected. The abnormalities remain for life, often causing much embarrassment and discomfort.

Other changes include lesions looking like plane warts on the backs of the hands, punctate keratoses or

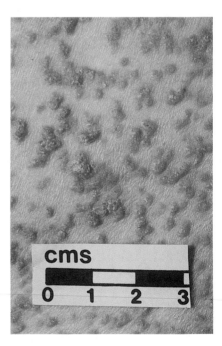

Fig. 4.3 The typical yellow-brown greasy papules of Darier's disease.

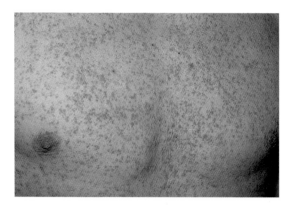

Fig. 4.4 Extensive Darier's disease, in this case made worse by sun exposure.

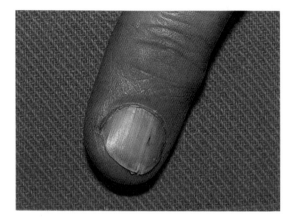

Fig. 4.5 The nail in Darier's disease. One or more longitudinal pale or pink stripes run over the lunule to the free margin where they end in a triangular nick.

pits on the palms and soles, cobblestone-like changes in the mouth, and a distinctive nail dystrophy in which white or pinkish lines or ridges run longitudinally to the free edge of the nail where they end in triangular nicks (Fig. 4.5).

Complications

Some patients are stunted. Personality disorders, including antisocial behaviour, are seen more often than would be expected by chance. An impairment of delayed hypersensitivity may be the basis for a tendency to develop widespread herpes simplex and bacterial infections. Bacterial overgrowth is responsible for the unpleasant smell of some severely affected patients.

Differential diagnosis

The distribution of the lesions may be similar to that of seborrhoeic eczema, but this lacks the warty papules of Darier's disease. The distribution differs from that of acanthosis nigricans (mainly flexural) and of keratosis pilaris (favours the outer upper arms and thighs). Other forms of folliculitis and Grover's disease (p. 111) can also cause confusion.

Investigations

The diagnosis should be confirmed by a skin biopsy, which will show characteristic clefts in the epidermis, and dyskeratotic cells.

Treatment

Severe and disabling disease can be dramatically alleviated by long-term acitretin (Formulary 2, p. 349). Milder cases need only topical keratolytics, such as salicylic acid, and the control of local infection (Formulary 1, p. 334).

Keratoderma of the palms and soles

Inherited types

Many genodermatoses share keratoderma of the palms and soles as their main feature; they are not described in detail here. The clinical patterns and modes of inheritance vary from family to family. Punctate, striate, diffuse and mutilating varieties have been documented, sometimes in association with metabolic disorders such as tyrosinaemia, or with changes elsewhere. The punctate type is caused by mutations in the keratin 16 gene on chromosome 17q12-q21; the epidermolytic type by mutations in the gene for keratin 9, found only on palms and soles.

The most common pattern is a diffuse one, known also as tylosis (Fig. 4.6), which is inherited as an autosomal dominant trait. In a few families these changes have been associated with carcinoma of the oesophagus, but in most families this is not the case.

Treatment tends to be unsatisfactory, but keratolytics such as salicylic acid and urea can be used in higher concentrations on the palms and soles than elsewhere (Formulary 1, p. 331).

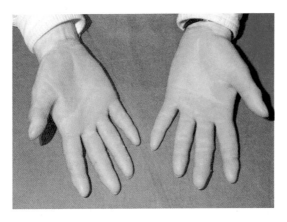

Fig. 4.6 Tylosis.

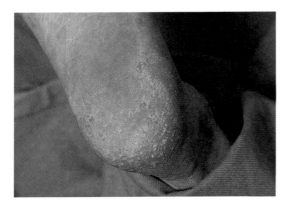

Fig. 4.7 Keratoderma climactericum—thickly keratotic skin, especially around the heels. Painful fissures are a problem.

Acquired types

It is not uncommon for normal people to have a few inconspicuous punctate keratoses on their palms, and it is no longer thought that these relate to internal malignancy, although palmar keratoses caused by arsenic may have this association. Black patients are prone to keratotic papules along their palmar creases.

Keratoderma of the palms and soles may be part of the picture of some generalized skin diseases such as pityriasis rubra pilaris (p. 67) and lichen planus (p. 64).

A distinctive pattern (keratoderma climactericum) is sometimes seen in middle-aged women at about the time of the menopause. It is most marked around the borders of the heels where painful fissures form and interfere with walking (Fig. 4.7). Regular paring and the use of keratolytic ointments are often more helpful than attempts at hormone replacement, and the condition tends to settle over a few years. Acitretin in low doses may be worth a trial.

Knuckle pads

Cause

Sometimes these are familial; usually they are not. Trauma seems not to be important.

Presentation

Fibromatous and hyperkeratotic areas appear on the backs of many finger joints, usually beginning in late childhood and persisting thereafter. There may be an association with Dupuytren's contracture.

Differential diagnosis

Occupational callosities, granuloma annulare and viral warts should be considered.

Investigations

A biopsy may be helpful in the few cases of genuine clinical difficulty.

Treatment

None, including surgery, is satisfactory.

Callosities and corns

Both are responses to pressure. A callosity is a more diffuse type of thickening of the keratin layer, which seems to be a protective response to widely applied repeated friction or pressure. Callosities are often occupational; e.g. they are seen on the hands of manual workers. Usually painless, they need no therapy.

Corns have a central core of hard keratin, which can hurt if forced inwards. They appear where there is high local pressure, often between bony prominences and shoes. Favourite areas include the backs of the toe joints, and the soles under prominent metatarsals. 'Soft corns' arise in the third or fourth toe clefts when the toes are squeezed together by tight shoes; such corns are often macerated.

The main differential is from hyperkeratotic warts, but these will show tiny bleeding points when pared down, whereas a corn has only its hard compacted avascular core surrounded by a more diffuse thickening of opalescent keratin.

The right treatment for corns is to eliminate the pressure that caused them, but patients may be slow to accept this. While regular paring reduces the symptoms temporarily, well-fitting shoes are essential. Corns under the metatarsals can be helped by soft spongy soles, but sometimes need orthopaedic alteration of weight bearing. Especial care is needed with corns on ischaemic or diabetic feet, which are at greater risk of infection and ulceration.

Further reading

Dunnill, M.G. (1998) The molecular basis of inherited disorders of keratinization. *Hospital Medicine* **59**, 17–22.

Hernandez-Martin, A., Gonzalez-Sarmiento, R. & De Unamuno, P. (1999) X-linked ichthyosis: an update. *British Journal of Dermatology* **141**, 617–627.

Ishida-Yamamoto, A., Tanaka, H., Nakane, H., Takahashi, H. & Iizuka, H. (1998) Inherited disorders of epidermal keratinization. *Journal of Dermatological Science* **18** (3), 139–154.

Ratnavel, R.C. & Griffiths, W.A.D. (1997) The inherited palmoplantar keratodermas. *British Journal of Dermatology* **137**, 485–490.

Sakuntabhai, A., Burge, S., Monk, S. & Hovnanian, A. (1999) Spectrum of novel ATP2A2 mutations in patients with Darier's disease. *Human Molecular Genetics* **8**, 1611–1619.

5   Psoriasis

One to three per cent of most populations have psoriasis, which is most prevalent in European and North American white people, uncommon in American black people and almost non-existent in American Indians. It is a chronic non-infectious inflammatory skin disorder, characterized by well-defined erythematous plaques bearing large adherent silvery scales. It can start at any age but is rare under 10 years, and appears most often between 15 and 40 years. Its course is unpredictable but is usually chronic with exacerbations and remissions.

Cause and pathogenesis

The precise cause of psoriasis is still unknown. However, there is often a genetic predisposition, and sometimes an obvious environmental trigger.

There are two key abnormalities in a psoriatic plaque: hyperproliferation of keratinocytes; and an inflammatory cell infiltrate in which neutrophils and TH-1 type T lymphocytes predominate. Each of these abnormalities can induce the other, leading to a vicious cycle of keratinocyte proliferation and inflammatory reaction; but it is still not clear which is the primary defect. Perhaps the genetic abnormality leads first to keratinocyte hyperproliferation that, in turn, produces a defective skin barrier (p. 11) allowing the penetration by, or unmasking of, hidden antigens to which an immune response is mounted. Alternatively, the psoriatic plaque might reflect a genetically determined reaction to different types of trauma (e.g. physical wounds, environmental irritants and drugs) in which the healing response is exaggerated and uncontrolled.

To prove the primary role of an immune reaction, putative antigens (e.g. bacteria, viruses or autoantigens) that initiate the immune response will have to be identified. This theory postulates that the increase in keratinocyte proliferation is caused by inflammatory cell mediators or signalling. Theories about the pathogenesis of psoriasis tend to tag along behind fashions in cell biology, and this idea is currently in vogue.

Genetics

A child with one affected parent has a 16% chance of developing the disease, and this rises to 50% if both parents are affected. Genomic imprinting (p. 301) may explain why psoriatic fathers are more likely to pass on the disease to their children than are psoriatic mothers. If non-psoriatic parents have a child with psoriasis, the risk for subsequent children is about 10%. In one study, the disorder was concordant in 70% of monozygotic twins but in only 20% of dizygotic ones. These figures are useful for counselling but psoriasis does not usually follow a simple Mendelian pattern of inheritance. The mode of inheritance has therefore to be categorized as genetically complex, implying a polygenic inheritance.

Psoriasis is also genetically heterogeneous. Early onset psoriasis shows an obvious hereditary element and linkage analysis (p. 300) revealed the first psoriasis susceptibility locus (S1), on 6p—close to the major histocompatibility complex Class I (MHC-I) region, but probably not HLA-C itself. The risk of those with the HLA-CW6 genotype developing psoriasis is 20 times that of those without it; 10% of CW6+ individuals will develop psoriasis. Other MHC-I associated diseases include Behçet's disease, ulcerative colitis and anterior uveitis. Interestingly, T-cell mediation is also seen in these diseases. The hereditary element and the HLA associations are much weaker in late-onset psoriasis.

In 1994, a second psoriasis susceptibility locus (S2) was discovered on 17q, incidentally next to a Crohn's disease susceptibility gene. Since then three more susceptibility loci have been confirmed (on 4q, 1q and 3q) and a few more await verification. It is unlikely to be coincidental that two of these loci (6p.21 and 1q.21–23) include genes that encode enzymes involved in cornification (p. 10).

This large number of genetic linkages suggests that 'psoriasis' may in fact be a phenotypic expression of several different genetic aberrations, all characterized by well-defined erythematous and scaly plaques, which are clinically indistinguishable. This idea fits the view that psoriasis is a multifactorial disease with a complex genetic trait, and that an individual's predisposition to it is determined by a large number of genes, each of which has only a low penetrance. Clinical expression of the disease is brought about by subsequent environmental stimuli.

Epidermal cell kinetics

The increased epidermal proliferation of psoriasis is caused by an excessive number of germinative cells entering the cell cycle rather than by a decrease in cell cycle time. The growth fraction (p. 8) approaches 100%, compared with 30% in normal skin. The epidermal turnover time (p. 8) is greatly shortened, to less than 10 days as compared with 60 days in normal skin. This epidermal hyperproliferation accounts for many of the metabolic abnormalities associated with psoriasis. It is not confined to obvious plaques: similar but less marked changes occur in the apparently normal skin of psoriatics as well.

The exact mechanism underlying this increased epidermal proliferation is uncertain. Cyclic guanosine monophosphate (cGMP), arachidonic acid metabolites, polyamines, calmodulin and plasminogen activator are all increased in psoriatic plaques but theories based on their prime involvement have neither stood the test of time nor provided useful targets for therapeutic intervention. Perhaps the underlying abnormality is a genetic defect in the control of keratinocyte growth. γ-Interferon (IFN-γ) inhibits growth and promotes the differentiation of normal keratinocytes by the phosphorylation and activation of the transcription factor STAT-1α but IFN-γ fails to activate STAT-1α in psoriatic keratinocytes. These proliferate out

of control, rather like a car going too fast because the accelerator is stuck, which cannot be stopped by putting a foot on the brake. Similarly, subnormal activation of another transcription factor, NFκB, may also be important for the formation of psoriatic plaques, as the absence of NFκB activity in gene knock-out mice has been shown to lead to epidermal hyperproliferation.

Others think that psoriasis is caused by a genetic defect of retinoid signalling and that is why it improves with retinoid treatment. In this context, there are two families of retinoid receptors in the epidermis: retinoic acid receptors (RARs) and retinoid X receptors (RXRs). Receptor-specific retinoids are now available that bind to RARs, reduce keratinocyte proliferation, normalize differentiation and reduce infiltration by inflammatory cells.

Altered epidermal maturation

During normal keratinization the profile of keratin types in an epidermal cell changes as it moves from the basal layer (K5 and K14) towards the surface (K1 and K10; p. 11). K6 and K16 are produced in psoriasis but their presence is secondary and non-specific, merely a result of increased epidermal proliferation.

Inflammation

Psoriasis differs from the ichthyoses (p. 41) in its accumulation of inflammatory cells, and this could be an immunological response to as yet unknown antigens. Certain interleukins and growth factors are elevated, and adhesion molecules are expressed or up-regulated in the lesions. Immune events may well have a primary role in the pathogenesis of the disease of psoriasis and a hypothetical model might run as follows.

1 Keratinocytes are stimulated by various insults (e.g. trauma, infections, drugs, ultraviolet radiation) to release IL-1, IL-8 and IL-18.

2 IL-1 up-regulates the expression of intercellular adhesion molecule-1 (ICAM-1) and E selectin on vascular endothelium in the dermal papillae. CLA positive memory T lymphocytes accumulate in these papillary vessels because their lymphocyte function-associated antigen (LFA-1) sticks to adhesion molecules that are expressed on the vascular endothelium (p. 27).

3 IL-8 from keratinocytes attracts T lymphocytes and neutrophils to migrate from papillary vessels into the epidermis where the T cells are held by adhesion of their LFA-1 with ICAM-1 on keratinocytes.

4 T cells accumulating in the epidermis are activated as a result of their interactions with Langerhans cells (possibly presenting unmasked retroviral or mycobacterial antigens or antigens shared by streptococci and keratinocytes; p. 20) and keratinocytes (p. 19). Activated T cells release IL-2, IFN-γ and tumour necrosis factor-α (TNF-α).

5 IL-2 ensures proliferation of the local T cells.

6 IFN-γ and TNF-α induce keratinocytes to express HLA-DR, to up-regulate their ICAM-1 expression and to produce further IL-6, IL-8 and TGF-α.

7 TGF-α acts as an autocrine mediator and attaches to epidermal growth factor (EGF) receptors inducing keratinocyte proliferation. IL-6 and transforming growth factor-α (TNF-α) also have keratinocyte mitogenic properties.

Bacterial exotoxins produced by *Staphylococcus aureus* and certain streptococci can act as superantigens (p. 21) and promote marked T-cell proliferation. This appears to be a key mechanism in the pathogenesis of guttate psoriasis.

Cyclosporin (p. 61) inhibits T-helper cell function and improves psoriasis. This fits in with the idea that psoriasis is a T-cell-driven disease. However, psoriasis is made worse by HIV infection; this paradox is hard to explain as the T-helper lymphocyte is a major target for the HIV retrovirus.

Neutrophils have also attracted attention, and some believe that psoriasis is a neutrophil-driven disease. Circulating neutrophils are activated, particularly in acute flares. They accumulate in the skin after sticking to endothelial cells (ICAM-1–MAC-1 family interaction). They then migrate through the layers of the epidermis up to the horny layer forming (Munro's) microabscesses, under the influence of chemotactic factors produced by activated keratinocytes, including IL-8, Gro-α and leukotriene-B4. Scales of psoriasis also contain chemotactic factors and these provoke visible collections of subcorneal neutrophils as seen in pustular psoriasis (p. 53).

The dermis

The dermis is abnormal in psoriasis. If psoriatic skin is grafted on to athymic mice, both epidermis and dermis must be present for the graft to sustain its psoriasis. The dermal capillary loops in psoriatic plaques are abnormally dilated and tortuous, and these changes come before epidermal hyperplasia in the development of a new plaque. Fibroblasts from psoriatics replicate more rapidly *in vitro* and produce more glycosaminoglycans than do those from non-psoriatics.

Precipitating factors

These include the following.

1 Trauma—if the psoriasis is active, lesions can appear in skin damaged by scratches or surgical wounds (the Köbner phenomenon; Fig. 5.1).

2 Infection—tonsillitis caused by β-haemolytic streptococci often triggers guttate psoriasis. AIDS often worsens it, or precipitates explosive forms.

3 Hormonal—psoriasis frequently improves in pregnancy only to relapse postpartum. Hypocalcaemia secondary to hypoparathyroidism is a rare precipitating cause.

4 Sunlight—improves most psoriatics but 10% become worse.

5 Drugs—antimalarials, β blockers, IFN-α and lithium may worsen psoriasis. Psoriasis may 'rebound' after withdrawal of treatment with systemic steroids or potent topical steroids. The case against non-steroidal anti-inflammatory drugs (NSAIDS) remains unproven.

6 Cigarette smoking and alcohol—the effects of confounding variables have been difficult to unravel in most epidemiological studies but there is growing

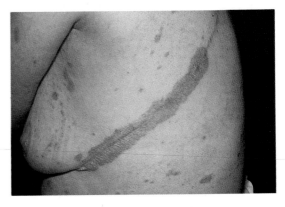

Fig. 5.1 The Köbner phenomenon seen after a recent thoracotomy operation.

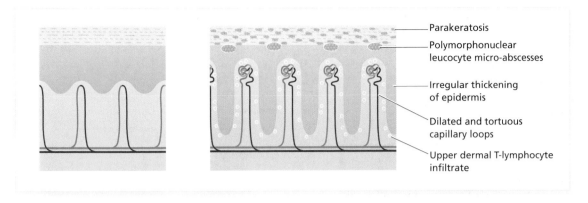

Parakeratosis

Polymorphonuclear
leucocyte micro-abscesses

Irregular thickening
of epidermis

Dilated and tortuous
capillary loops

Upper dermal T-lymphocyte
infiltrate

Fig. 5.2 Histology of psoriasis (right) compared with normal skin (left).

evidence that both have an independent effect in pre-cipitating or maintaining psoriasis.

7 Emotion—emotional upsets seem to cause some exacerbations.

Histology (Fig. 5.2)

The main changes are the following.

1 Parakeratosis (nuclei retained in the horny layer).

2 Irregular thickening of the epidermis, but thinning over dermal papillae is apparent clinically when bleeding is caused by scratching and the removal of scales (Auspitz's sign).

3 Polymorphonuclear leucocyte microabscesses (described originally by Munro).

4 Dilated and tortuous capillary loops in the dermal papillae.

5 T-lymphocyte infiltrate in upper dermis.

Presentation

Common patterns

Plaque pattern

This is the most common type. Lesions are well demarcated and range from a few millimetres to several centimetres in diameter (Fig. 5.3). The lesions are pink or red with large dry silvery-white polygonal scales (like candle grease). The elbows, knees, lower back and scalp are sites of predilection (Fig. 5.4).

Guttate pattern

This is usually seen in children and adolescents and may be the first sign of the disease, often triggered by streptococcal tonsillitis. Numerous small round red macules come up suddenly on the trunk and soon become scaly (Fig. 5.5). The rash often clears in a few months but plaque psoriasis may develop later.

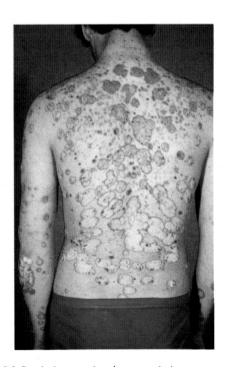

Fig. 5.3 Psoriasis: extensive plaque psoriasis.

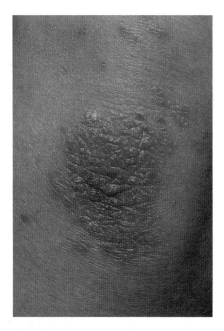

Fig. 5.4 Psoriasis favours the extensor aspects of the knees and elbows.

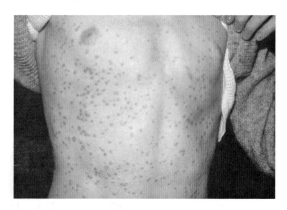

Fig. 5.5 Guttate psoriasis.

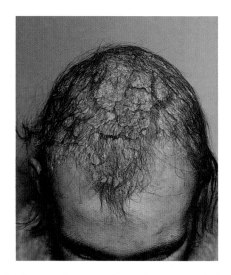

Fig. 5.6 Untreated severe and extensive scalp psoriasis.

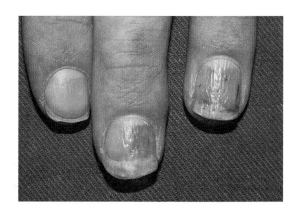

Fig. 5.7 Thimble-like pitting of nails with onycholysis.

Scalp

The scalp is often involved. Areas of scaling are interspersed with normal skin; their lumpiness is more easily felt than seen (Fig. 5.6). Frequently, the psoriasis overflows just beyond the scalp margin. Significant hair loss is rare.

Nails

Involvement of the nails is common, with 'thimble pitting' (Fig. 5.7), onycholysis (separation of the nail from the nail bed; Fig. 5.8) and sometimes subungual hyperkeratosis.

Flexures

Psoriasis of the submammary, axillary and anogenital folds is not scaly although the glistening sharply demarcated red plaques (Fig. 5.9), often with fissuring in the depth of the fold, are still readily recognizable. Flexural psoriasis is most common in women and in the elderly, and is more common among HIV-infected individuals than uninfected ones.

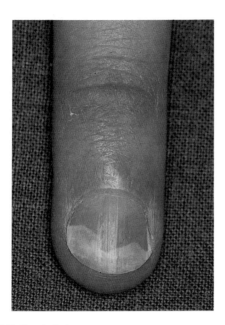

Fig. 5.8 Onycholysis.

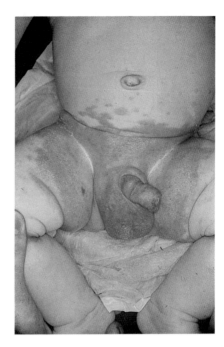

Fig. 5.10 An irritant napkin rash now turning into napkin psoriasis.

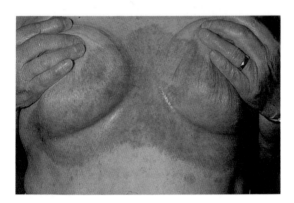

Fig. 5.9 Sharply defined glistening erythematous patches of flexural psoriasis.

Palms and soles

Palmar psoriasis may be hard to recognize as its lesions are often poorly demarcated and barely erythematous. The fingers may develop painful fissures.

Less common patterns

Napkin psoriasis

A psoriasiform spread outside the napkin (nappy/diaper) area may give the first clue to a psoriatic tend-

ency in an infant (Fig. 5.10). Usually it clears quickly but there is an increased risk of ordinary psoriasis developing in later life.

Localized pustular psoriasis (palmo-plantar pustulosis)

This is a recalcitrant, often painful condition which some regard as a separate entity. It affects the palms and soles, which become studded with numerous sterile pustules, 3–10 mm in diameter, lying on an erythematous base. The pustules change to brown macules or scales (Figs 5.11 and 5.12). Generalized pustular psoriasis is a rare but serious condition, with fever and recurrent episodes of pustulation within areas of erythema.

Erythrodermic psoriasis

This is also rare and can be sparked off by the irritant effect of tar or dithranol, by a drug eruption or by the withdrawal of potent topical or systemic steroids. The skin becomes universally and uniformly red with variable scaling (Fig. 5.13). Malaise is accompanied by shivering and the skin feels hot and uncomfortable.

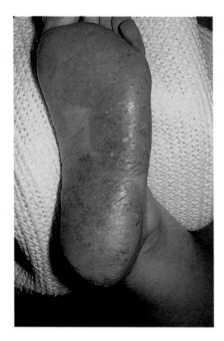

Fig. 5.11 Pustular psoriasis of the sole.

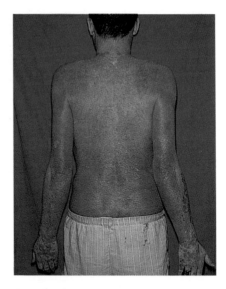

Fig. 5.13 Erythrodermic psoriasis.

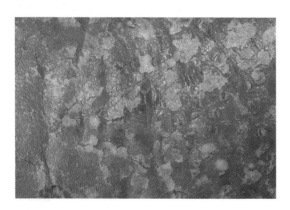

Fig. 5.12 A closer view of pustules on the sole.

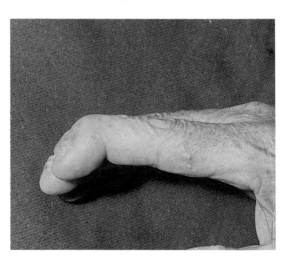

Fig. 5.14 Fixed flexion deformity of distal interphalangeal joints following arthropathy.

Complications

Psoriatic arthropathy

Arthritis occurs in about 5% of psoriatics. Several patterns are recognized. Distal arthritis involves the terminal interphalangeal joints of the toes and fingers, especially those with marked nail changes (Fig. 5.14). Other patterns include involvement of a single large joint; one which mimics rheumatoid arthritis and may become mutilating (Fig. 5.15); and one where the brunt is borne by the sacro-iliac joints and spine. Tests for rheumatoid factor are negative and nodules are absent. In patients with spondylitis and sacroiliitis there is a strong correlation with the presence of HLA-B27.

Differential diagnosis

Discoid eczema (p. 89)

Lesions are less well defined and may be exudative or crusted, lack 'candle grease' scaling, and may be extremely itchy. Lesions do not favour scalp, extensor

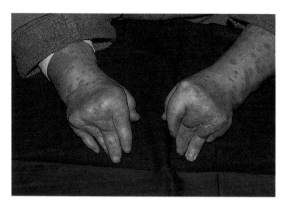

Fig. 5.15 Rheumatoid-like changes associated with severe psoriasis of hands.

aspects of elbows and knees but rather the trunk and proximal parts of the extremities.

Seborrhoeic eczema (p. 87)

Scalp involvement is more diffuse and less lumpy. Intervening areas of normal scalp skin are unusual.

Flexural plaques are less well defined and more exudative. There may be signs of seborrhoeic eczema elsewhere, such as in the eyebrows, nasolabial folds or on the chest.

Pityriasis rosea (p. 63)

This may be confused with guttate psoriasis but the lesions, which are oval rather than round, tend to run along rib lines. Scaling is of collarette type and a herald plaque may precede the rash. Lesions are usually confined to the upper trunk.

Secondary syphilis (p. 194)

There is usually a history of a primary chancre. The scaly lesions are brownish and characteristically the palms and soles are involved. Oral changes, patchy alopecia, condylomata lata and lymphadenopathy complete the picture.

Cutaneous T-cell lymphoma (p. 280)

The lesions, which tend to persist, are not in typical locations and are often annular, arcuate, reniform or show bizarre outlines. Atrophy or poikiloderma may be present and individual lesions may vary in their thickness.

Tinea unguium (p. 215)

This is often confused with nail psoriasis but is more asymmetrical and there may be obvious tinea of neighbouring skin. Uninvolved nails are common. Pitting is not seen and nails tend to be crumbly and discoloured at their free edge.

Investigations

1 Biopsy is seldom necessary.
2 Throat swabbing for β-haemolytic streptococci is needed in guttate psoriasis.
3 Skin scrapings and nail clippings may be required to exclude tinea.
4 Radiology and tests for rheumatoid factor are helpful in assessing arthritis.

Treatment

The need for this depends both on the patient's own perception of his or her disability, and on the doctor's objective assessment of how severe the skin disease is. The two do not always tally.

General measures

Explanations and reassurances must be geared to the patient's or the parent's intelligence. Information leaflets help to reinforce verbal advice. The doctor as well as the patient should keep the disease in perspective, and treatment must never be allowed to be more troublesome than the disease itself. The disease is not contagious. At present there is no cure for psoriasis; all treatments are suppressive and aimed at either inducing a remission or making the condition more tolerable. However, spontaneous remissions will occur in 50% of patients. Treatment for patients with chronic stable plaque psoriasis is relatively simple and may be safely administered by the family practitioner. However, systemic treatment for severe psoriasis should be monitored by a dermatologist. No treatment, at present, alters the overall course of the disease.

Physical and mental rest help to back up the specific management of acute episodes. Concomitant anxiety and depression should be treated on their own merits (see Table 5.1 for appropriate treatments).

Table 5.1 Treatment options in psoriasis.

Type of psoriasis	Treatment of choice	Alternative treatments
Stable plaque	Vitamin D analogue Local retinoid Local steroid Dithranol	Coal tar
Extensive stable plaque (> 30% surface area) recalcitrant to local therapy	UVB PUVA PUVA + acitretin	Methotrexate Cyclosporin A Acitretin Sulfasalazine Mycophenolate mofetil
Widespread small plaque	UVB	Vitamin D analogue Coal tar
Guttate	Systemic antibiotic Emollients while erupting; then UVB	Weak tar preparation Mild local steroid
Facial	Tacrolimus Mild to moderately potent local steroid	
Flexural	Tacrolimus Vitamin D analogue (caution: may irritate) Mild to moderately potent local steroid + anticandidal/fungal	
Pustular psoriasis of hands and feet	Moderately potent or potent local steroid Local retinoid	Acitretin Topical PUVA
Acute erythrodermic, unstable or generalized pustular	Inpatient treatment with ichthammol paste Local steroid may be used initially with or without wet compresses	Acitretin Methotrexate Cyclosporin A

Main types of treatment

These can be divided into four main categories: local, ultraviolet radiation, systemic and combined. Broad recommendations are listed in Table 5.1, but most physicians will have their own favourites. In many ways it is better to become familiar with a few remedies than dabble with many. The management of patients with psoriasis is an art as well as a science and few other skin conditions benefit so much from patience and experience—of both patients and doctors.

Local treatments

Vitamin D analogues

Ultraviolet radiation helps many patients with psoriasis (see below), perhaps by increasing the production of cholecalciferol in the skin (p. 12). Calcipotriol and tacacitol are analogues of chlolecalciferol, which do not cause hypercalcaemia and calciuria when used topically in the recommended dose. Both can be used for mild to moderate psoriasis affecting less than 40% of the skin. They work by influencing vitamin D receptors in keratinocytes, reducing epidermal proliferation and restoring a normal horny layer. They also inhibit the synthesis of polyamines (p. 49).

Calcipotriol (calcipotriene, USA)

Patients like calcipotriol because it is odourless, colourless and does not stain. It seldom clears plaques of psoriasis completely, but does reduce their scaling and thickness. Local and usually transient irritation may occur with the recommended twice-daily application. One way of lessening this is to combine the use of calcipotriol with that of a moderately potent steroid, the calcipotriol being applied in the evening and the steroid in the morning (see Topical corticosteroids below). Calcipotriol should not be used on the face. Up to 100 g/week calcipotriol may be used but the manufacturer's recommendations should be consulted when it is used in children over 6 years old.

Our current practice, which may be unnecessary, is still to check the blood calcium and phosphate levels every 6 months, especially if the psoriasis is widespread or the patient has had calcified renal stones in the past.

Tacalcitol

Tacalcitol ointment (not available in the USA) is applied sparingly once daily at bedtime, the maximum amount being 10 g/day. As with calcipotriol, irritation —often transient—may occur. The drug should not be used for longer than a year at a time and is not yet recommended for children.

Local retinoids

Tazarotene is a topically active retinoid. It has a selective affinity for RARs and, when bound to these, improves psoriasis by reducing keratinocyte proliferation, normalizing the disturbed differentiation and lessening the infiltrate of dermal inflammatory cells. It is recommended for chronic stable plaque psoriasis on the trunk and limbs covering up to 20% of the body. It is applied sparingly once a day, in the evening, and can be used for courses of up to 12 weeks. It seldom clears psoriasis but reduces the induration, scaling and redness of plaques. It is available as either a 0.05% or 0.1% gel. Like the vitamin D analogues, its main side-effect is irritation. If this occurs, the strength should be reduced to 0.05%; if irritation persists, applications should be cut to alternate days and a combination treatment with a local steroid considered.

In the USA, tazarotene is licensed for children aged 12 years and over; in Europe it is currently licensed only for adults over 18 years old. The drug should not be used in pregnancy or during lactation. Females of childbearing age should use adequate contraception during therapy.

Topical corticosteroids

Practice varies from centre to centre and from country to country. Many dermatologists, particularly in the

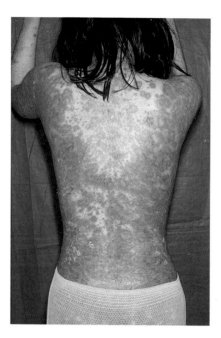

Fig. 5.16 Unstable psoriasis following long-term use of a potent topical steroid.

USA, find topical corticosteroids most helpful and use them as the mainstay of their long-term management of stable plaque psoriasis. Patients like them because they are clean and reduce scaling and redness.

In our view such usage is safe, but only under proper supervision by doctors well aware of problems such as dermal atrophy, tachyphylaxis, early relapses, the occasional precipitation of unstable psoriasis (Fig. 5.16) and, rarely, in extensive cases, of adrenal suppression caused by systemic absorption. A commitment by the prescriber to keep the patient under regular clinical review is especially important if more than 50 g/week of a moderately potent topical corticosteroid preparation is being used. Combined tar–steroid preparations may also be helpful (Formulary 1, p. 333).

The regular use of topical corticosteroids is less controversial under the following circumstances.
1 In 'limited choice' areas such as the face, ears, genitals and flexures where tar and dithranol are seldom tolerated (mildly potent steroid preparations should be used if possible).
2 For patients who cannot use vitamin D analogues, tar or dithranol because of allergic or irritant reactions (moderately potent preparations, except for 'no choice' areas where mildly potent ones should be used if possible).

3 For unresponsive psoriasis on the scalp, palms and soles (moderately potent, potent and very potent—but only in the short term—preparations).
4 For patients with minor localized psoriasis (moderately potent or potent preparations).

A combination ointment of calcipotriol and betamethasone diproprionate (a potent corticosteroid) has recently been marketed in the UK. The maximum dose should not exceed 15g/day or 100g/week and the ointment should not be applied for longer than 4 weeks.

Dithranol (anthralin)

Dithranol is rarely used in the USA nowadays but remains popular in the UK. Like coal tar it inhibits DNA synthesis, but some of its benefits may be brought about by the formation of free radicals of oxygen.

Dithranol is more tricky to use than coal tar. It has to be applied carefully, to the plaques only; and, if left on for more than 30 min, must be covered with gauze dressings. It is irritant, so treatment should start with a weak (0.1%) preparation, thereafter the strength can be stepped up at weekly intervals. Dithranol stronger than 1% is seldom necessary. Irritation of the surrounding skin can be lessened by the application of a protective bland paste, e.g. zinc paste.

Dithranol stains normal skin, but the purple-brown discoloration peels off after a few days. It also stains bathtubs, clothes—and anything else it touches. One popular regimen is to apply dithranol daily for 5 days in the week; after 1 month many patients will be clear.

Short contact therapy, in which dithranol is applied for no longer than 30 min, is also effective. Initially a test patch of psoriasis is treated with a 0.1% dithranol cream, left on for 20 min and then washed off. If there is no undue reaction, the application can be extended the next day and, if tolerated, can be left on for 30 min. After the cream is washed off, a bland application such as soft white paraffin or emulsifying ointment is applied. Depending on response, the strength of the dithranol can be increased from 0.1 to 2% over 2–3 weeks. Suitable preparations are listed in Formulary 1 (p. 337).

Dithranol is too irritant to apply to the face, the inner thighs, genital region or skin folds. Special care must be taken to avoid contact with the eyes. Recent research has shown that applying triethanolamine after the dithranol has been removed reduces inflammation and staining without diminishing the therapeutic effect.

Coal tar preparations

Crude coal tar and its distillation products have been used to treat psoriasis for many years. Their precise mode of action is uncertain but tar does inhibit DNA synthesis.

Many preparations are available but it is wise to become familiar with a few. The less refined tars are smelly, messy and stain clothes, but are more effective than the cleaner refined preparations. Tar emulsions can also be added to the bath. Suitable preparations are listed in Formulary 1 (p. 337). Surprisingly, no increase in skin cancer has been found in patients treated for long periods with tar preparations; it has even been suggested that psoriatics are less likely than normal to develop skin cancer.

Ultraviolet radiation

Most patients improve with natural sunlight and should be encouraged to sunbathe. During the winter, courses of artificial ultraviolet radiation (UVB), as an outpatient or at home, may help (Fig. 5.17). Both broadband UVB and narrow band UVB (311 nm) can be used. Treatments should be given by an expert, twice to three times weekly for 8 weeks. Goggles should be worn. The initial dose is calculated either by establishing the skin type (p. 233) or by determining

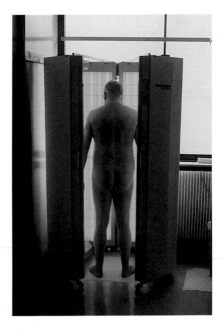

Fig. 5.17 Ultraviolet radiation therapy.

the minimal dose of UVB that causes erythema in a test patch 24 h after radiation. The initial small dose is increased incrementally after each exposure providing it is well tolerated. The number of treatments and doses employed should be recorded. The main risk of UVB therapies in the short term is acute phototoxicity (sunburn-like reaction) and, in the long term, the induction of skin cancer.

Special situations

Scalp psoriasis

This is often recalcitrant. Oily preparations containing 3% salicylic acid are useful (Formulary 1, p. 338). They should be rubbed into the scalp three times a week and washed out with a tar shampoo 4–6 h later. If progress is slow, they can be left on for one or two nights before shampooing. Salicylic acid and tar combinations are also effective.

Guttate psoriasis

A course of penicillin V or erythromycin is indicated for any associated streptococcal throat infection. Bland local treatment is often enough as the natural trend is towards remission. Suitable preparations include emulsifying ointment and zinc and ichthammol cream. Tar–steroid preparations are reasonable alternatives. A course of ultraviolet therapy (UVB) may be helpful after the eruptive phase is over.

Eruptive/unstable psoriasis

Bland treatment is needed and rest is important. Tar, dithranol and ultraviolet therapy are best avoided. Suitable preparations include emulsifying ointment and zinc and ichthammol cream.

Systemic treatment

A systemic approach should be considered if extensive psoriasis (more than 20% of the body surface) fails to improve with prolonged courses of tar or dithranol. As the potential side-effects are great, local measures should be given a good trial first. The most commonly used systemic treatments are photochemotherapy with psoralen and ultraviolet A (PUVA) treatment, retinoids, methotrexate, hydroxyurea (hydroxycarbamide), sulfasalazine, mycophenolate mofetil and cyclosporin.

Photochemotherapy (PUVA)

In this ingenious therapy, a drug is photo-activated in the skin by ultraviolet radiation. An oral dose of 8-methoxypsoralen (8-MOP) or 5-methoxypsoralen (5-MOP) is followed by exposure to long-wave ultraviolet radiation (UVA: 320–400 nm). The psoralen reaches the skin and, in the presence of UVA, forms photo-adducts with DNA pyrimidine bases and cross-links between complementary DNA strands; this inhibits DNA synthesis and epidermal cell division.

The 8-MOP (crystalline formulation 0.6–0.8 mg/kg body weight or liquid formulation 0.3–0.4 mg/kg) or 5-MOP (1.2–1.6 mg/kg) is taken 1–2 h before exposure to a bank of UVA tubes mounted in a cabinet similar to that seen in Fig. 5.17. Psoralens may also be administered in bath water for those unable to tolerate the oral regimen. The initial exposure is calculated either by determining the patient's minimal phototoxic dose (the least dose of UVA that after ingestion of 8-MOP produces a barely perceptible erythema 72 h after testing) or by assessing skin colour and ability to tan. The usual starting dose is from 0.5 J/cm^2 (skin type I: always burns and never tans) to 2.0 J/cm^2 (skin type IV: never burns and always tans). Treatment is given two or three times a week with increasing doses of UVA, depending on erythema production and the therapeutic response. Protective goggles are worn during radiation and UVA opaque plastic glasses must be used after taking the tablets and for 24 h after each treatment (see below). All phototherapy equipment should be serviced and calibrated regularly by trained personnel. An accurate record of each patient's cumulative dosage and number of treatments should be kept.

Clearance takes 5–10 weeks. Thereafter it is often possible to keep the skin clear by PUVA once a fortnight or every 3 weeks. However, as the side-effects of PUVA relate to its cumulative dose (see below), maintenance therapy should not be used unless alternative treatments prove to be unsatisfactory. As far as possible, PUVA therapy is avoided in younger patients.

Side effects Painful erythema is the most common side-effect but the risk of this can be minimized by careful dosimetry. One-quarter of patients itch during and immediately after radiation; fewer feel nauseated after taking 8-MOP. 5-MOP, not yet available in the USA, is worth trying if these effects become intolerable. Long-term side-effects include premature ageing of the skin (with mottled pigmentation, scattered lentigines, wrinkles and atrophy), cutaneous malignancies (usually after a cumulative dose greater than 1000 J or after more than 250 treatments) and, theoretically at least, cataract formation. The use of UVA blocking glasses (see above) for 24 h after each treatment should protect against the latter. The long-term side-effects relate to the total amount of UVA received over the years; this must be recorded and kept as low as possible, without denying treatment when it is clearly needed.

Retinoids

Acitretin (10–25 mg daily; Formulary 2, p. 349) is an analogue of vitamin A, and is one of the few drugs helpful in pustular psoriasis. It is also used to thin down thick hyperkeratotic plaques. Minor side-effects are frequent and dose-related. They include dry lips, mouth, vagina and eyes, peeling of the skin, pruritus, thinning of the hair, and unpleasant paronychia. All settle on stopping or reducing the dosage of the drug, but the use of emollients and artificial tears is often recommended.

Acitretin can be used on its own for long periods, but regular blood tests are needed to exclude abnormal liver function and the elevation of serum lipids (mainly triglycerides but also cholesterol). Yearly X-rays should detect bone spurs and ossification of ligaments, especially the paraspinal ones (disseminated interstitial skeletal hyperostosis (DISH) syndrome). Children, and those with persistently abnormal liver function tests or hyperlipidaemia, should not be treated.

The most important side-effect is teratogenicity and acitretin should not normally be prescribed to women of childbearing age. If, for unavoidable clinical reasons, it is still the drug of choice, effective oral contraceptive measures must be taken and, in view of the long half-life of its metabolite, these should continue for 2 years after treatment has ceased. Blood donation should be avoided for a similar period.

Retinoids and PUVA act synergistically and are often used together in the so-called Re-PUVA regimen. This clears plaque psoriasis quicker than PUVA alone, and needs a smaller cumulative dose of UVA. The standard precautions for both PUVA and retinoid treatment should, of course, still be observed.

Methotrexate

This folic acid antagonist (Formulary 2, p. 348) inhibits DNA synthesis during the S phase of mitosis. After an initial trial dose of 2.5 mg, in an adult of average weight, the drug is given orally once a week and the dose increased gradually to a maintenance one of 7.5–15 mg/week. This often controls even aggressive psoriasis. The drug is eliminated largely by the kidneys and so the dose must be reduced if renal function is poor. Aspirin and sulphonamides displace the drug from binding with plasma albumin, and frusemide (furosemide) decreases its renal clearance: note must therefore be taken of concurrent drug therapy (Formulary 2, p. 348) and the dose reduced accordingly. Minor and temporary side-effects, such as nausea and malaise, are common in the 48 h after administration. The most serious drawback to this treatment is hepatic fibrosis, the risk of which is greatly increased in those who drink an excessive amount of alcohol. Unfortunately, routine liver function tests and scans cannot predict this reliably, and a liver biopsy to exclude active liver disease is advised for those with risk factors. Exceptions are made for patients over 70 years old and when only short-term treatment with methotrexate is anticipated. Liver biopsy before treatment, or early in the course of therapy, should be repeated after every cumulative dose of 1.5–2 g, especially in less than perfectly healthy drinking adults. Blood checks to exclude marrow suppression, and to monitor renal and liver function, should also be performed—weekly at the start of treatment, with the interval being slowly increased to monthly or every other month depending on when stable maintenance therapy is established.

The drug is teratogenic and should not be given to females in their reproductive years. Oligospermia has been noted in men and fertility may be lowered; however, a child fathered by a man on methotrexate can be expected to be normal. Folic acid, 5 mg daily, taken on days when the patient does not have methotrexate, can lessen nausea and reduce marrow suppression. Methotrexate should not be taken at the same time as systemic steroids or cyclosporin.

Cyclosporin

Cyclosporin inhibits cell-mediated immune reactions. It blocks resting lymphocytes in the G_0 or early G_1 phase of the cell cycle and inhibits lymphokine release, especially that of IL-2.

Cyclosporin is effective in severe psoriasis, but patients needing it should be under the care of specialists. The initial daily dose is 3–4 mg/kg/day and not more

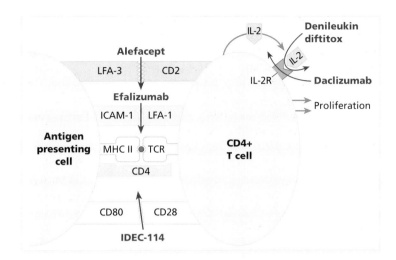

Fig. 5.18 Therapeutic targets to reduce T-helper cell proliferation in psoriasis. Proprietary names of experimental drugs given beside arrows.

than 5 mg/kg/day. With improvement the dose can often be reduced but the side-effects of long-term treatment include hypertension, kidney damage and persistent viral warts with a risk of skin cancer. Blood pressure and renal function should be assessed carefully before starting treatment. The serum creatinine should be measured two or three times before starting therapy to be sure of the baseline and then every other week for the first 3 months of therapy. Thereafter, if the results are stable, the frequency of testing will depend on the dosage (monthly for > 2.5 mg/kg/day or every other month for < 2.5 mg/kg/day). The dosage should be reduced if the serum creatinine concentration rises to 30% above the baseline level on two occasions within 2 weeks. If these changes do not reverse themselves when the dosage has been reduced for 1 month, then the drug should be stopped.

Hypertension is a common side-effect of cyclosporin: nearly 50% of patients develop a systolic blood pressure over 160 mmHg and/or a diastolic blood pressure over 95 mmHg. Usually these rises are mild or moderate, and respond to concomitant treatment with a calcium channel blocker, such as nifedipine. If this cannot be tolerated, an angiotensin-converting enzyme inhibitor should be used under specialist supervision. Diuretics, which may themselves worsen renal function, and β blockers, which may themselves worsen psoriasis, should probably be avoided. Cyclosporin interacts with a number of drugs (Formulary 2, p. 347) and these should be avoided.

It is also advisable to watch levels of cholesterol, triglycerides, potassium and magnesium, and advise patients that they will become hirsute and that they

may develop gingival hyperplasia. Treatment with cyclosporin should not continue for longer than 1 year without careful assessment and close monitoring.

Other systemic drugs

Antimetabolites such as mycophenolate mofetil, 6-tioguanine, azathioprine and hydroxyurea help psoriasis, but less than methotrexate; they tend to damage the marrow rather than the liver. Regular blood monitoring is again essential. Sulfasalazine occasionally helps psoriasis.

Combination therapy

If psoriasis is resistant to one treatment, a combination of treatments used together may be the answer. Combination treatments can even prevent side-effects by allowing less of each drug to be used. Common combinations include topical vitamin D analogues with either local steroids or UVB, dithranol following a tar bath and UVB (Ingram regimen) and coal tar following a tar bath and UVB (Goeckerman regimen).

Rotational therapy may also minimize the toxicity of some treatments—an example would be PUVA, methotrexate, acitretin and cyclosporin, each used separately for 1–2 years before moving on to the next treatment.

Future treatments

The development of retinoids and vitamin D analogues over the last decade has heralded a resurgence of interest in new treatments for psoriasis. The idea

LEARNING POINTS

1 Discuss a treatment plan with the patient. Consider disability, cost, time, mess and risk of systemic therapy to general health.
2 The treatment must not be worse than the disease.
3 Do not aggravate eruptive psoriasis.
4 Never use systemic steroids.
5 Avoid the long-term use of potent or very potent topical corticosteroids.
6 Never promise a permanent cure, but be encouraging.
7 Great advances have been made over the last 20 years in the treatment of severe psoriasis, but patients taking modern systemic agents require careful monitoring.

of using a weekly injection to control psoriasis is no longer a pipe-dream. The immunologically based pathogenesis of psoriasis presents many targets for therapeutic exploitation; most involve inhibiting the proliferation of T-helper lymphocytes (Fig. 5.18), others block key cytokines such as TNF-α (e.g. with infliximab or etanercept), or inhibit the adhesion of inflammatory cells to the endothelium of dermal vessels (e.g. with antibodies against E selectin). Pati-

ents are already participating in trials of humanized monoclonal antibodies. Even vaccination with pathogenic T cells or T-cell receptor peptides is no longer science fiction.

Further reading

Griffiths, C. & Barker, J. (1999) *Key Advances in the Effective Management of Psoriasis*. Royal Society of Medicine Press, London.

Halpern, S.M. *et al.* (2000) Guidelines for topical PUVA: a report of a workshop of the British Photodermatology Group. *British Journal of Dermatology* **142**, 22–31.

van der Kerkhof, P.C.M. (1999) *Textbook of Psoriasis*. Blackwell Science, Oxford.

Kirby, B. and Griffiths, C.E.M. (2002) Novel immune-based therapies for psoriasis. *British Journal of Dermatology* **146**, 546–551.

Kragballe, K. (2000) *Vitamin D in Dermatology*. Marcel Dekker, Basel.

Lebwohl, M. & Ali, S. (2001) Treatment of psoriasis. I. Topical therapy and phototherapy. *Journal of the American Academy of Dermatology*, **45**, 487–498.

Lebwohl, M. & Ali, S. (2001) Treatment of psoriasis. II. Systemic therapies. *Journal of the American Academy of Dermatology*, **45**, 649–661.

Roenick, H.H. & Maibach, H.I. (1998) *Psoriasis*. Marcel Dekker, New York.

Other papulosquamous disorders

Psoriasis is not the only skin disease that is sharply marginated and scaly. Table 6.1 lists some of the most common ones. Eczema can also be raised and scaly, but is usually poorly marginated and fissures, crusts or lichenifies (Chapter 7). Psoriasis is discussed in Chapter 5.

Pityriasis rosea

Cause

The cause of pityriasis rosea is not known. An infectious agent has always seemed likely but has not yet been proven: human herpesvirus 7 is the latest suspect. The disorder seems not to be contagious.

Presentation

Pityriasis rosea is common, particularly during the winter. It mainly affects children and young adults,

Table 6.1 Some important papulosquamous diseases.

Psoriasis
Pityriasis rosea
Lichen planus
Pityriasis rubra pilaris
Parapsoriasis
Mycosis fungoides
Pityriasis lichenoides
Discoid lupus erythematosus
Tinea
Nummular eczema
Seborrhoeic dermatitis
Secondary syphilis
Drug eruptions

and second attacks are rare. Most patients develop one plaque (the 'herald' or 'mother' plaque) before the others (Fig. 6.1). It is larger (2–5 cm in diameter) than later lesions, and is rounder, redder and more scaly. After several days many smaller plaques appear, mainly on the trunk, but some also on the neck and extremities. About half of the patients complain of itching. An individual plaque is oval, salmon pink and shows a delicate scaling, adherent peripherally as a collarette. The configuration of such plaques is often characteristic. Their longitudinal axes run down and out from the spine (Fig. 6.2), along the lines of the ribs. Purpuric lesions are rare.

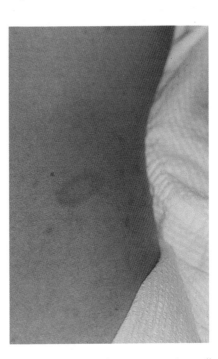

Fig. 6.1 The herald plaque of pityriasis rosea is usually on the trunk and is larger than the other lesions. Its annular configuration is shown well here.

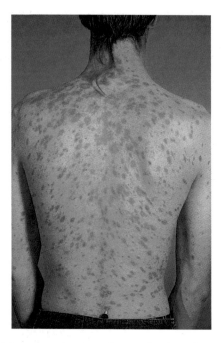

Fig. 6.2 An extensive pityriasis rosea showing a 'fir tree' distribution on the back.

Course

The herald plaque precedes the generalized eruption by several days. Subsequent lesions enlarge over the first week or two. A minority of patients have systemic symptoms such as aching and tiredness. The eruption lasts between 2 and 10 weeks and then resolves spontaneously, sometimes leaving hyperpigmented patches that fade more slowly.

Differential diagnosis

Although herald plaques are often mistaken for ringworm, the two disorders most likely to be misdiagnosed early in the general eruption are guttate psoriasis and secondary syphilis. Tinea corporis and pityriasis versicolor can be distinguished by the microscopical examination of scales (p. 35), and secondary syphilis by its other features (mouth lesions, palmar lesions, condyloma lata, lymphadenopathy, alopecia) and by serology. Gold and captopril are the drugs most likely to cause a pityriasis rosea-like drug reaction, but barbiturates, penicillamine, some antibiotics and other drugs can also do so.

Investigations

Because secondary syphilis can mimic pityriasis rosea so closely, testing for syphilis is usually wise.

Treatment

No treatment is curative, and active treatment is seldom needed. A moderately potent topical steroid or calamine lotion will help the itching. One per cent salicylic acid in soft white paraffin or emulsifying ointment reduces scaling. Sunlight or artificial UVB often relieves pruritus and may hasten resolution.

Lichen planus

Cause

The precise cause of lichen planus is unknown, but the disease seems to be mediated immunologically. Lymphocytes abut the epidermal basal cells and damage them. Chronic graft-vs.-host disease can cause an eruption rather like lichen planus in which histoincompatibility causes lymphocytes to attack the epidermis. Lichen planus is also associated with autoimmune disorders, such as alopecia areata, vitiligo and ulcerative colitis, more commonly than would be expected by chance. Drugs too can cause lichen planus (see below). Some patients with lichen planus also have a hepatitis B or C infection—but lichen planus itself is not infectious.

Presentation

Typical lesions are violaceous or lilac-coloured, intensely itchy, flat-topped papules that usually arise on the extremities, particularly on the volar aspects

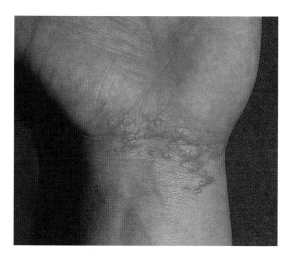

Fig. 6.3 Shiny flat-topped papules of lichen planus. Note the Wickham's striae.

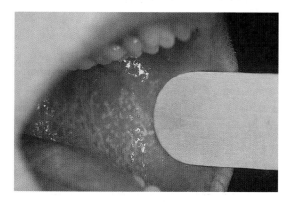

Fig. 6.4 Lichen planus: classic white lacy network lying on the buccal mucosa.

Table 6.2 Variants of lichen planus.

Annular
Atrophic
Bullous
Follicular
Hypertrophic (Fig. 6.5)
Ulcerative

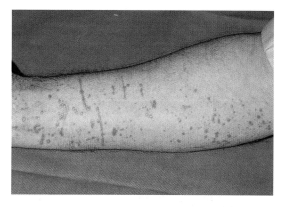

Fig. 6.5 Lichen planus: striking Köbner effect on the forearm.

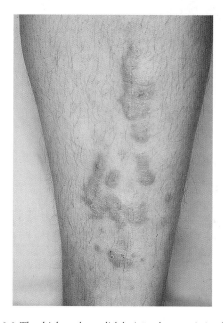

Fig. 6.6 The thickened purplish lesions characteristic of hypertrophic lichen planus on the shins.

of the wrists and legs (Fig. 6.3). A close look is needed to see a white streaky pattern on the surface of these papules (Wickham's striae). White asymptomatic lacy lines, dots, and occasionally small white plaques, are also found in the mouth, particularly inside the cheeks, in about 50% of patients (Fig. 6.4), and oral lesions may be the sole manifestation of the disease. The genital skin may be similarly affected (see Fig. 13.37). Variants of the classical pattern are rare and often difficult to diagnose (Table 6.2). Curiously, although the skin plaques are usually itchy, patients rub rather than scratch, so that excoriations are uncommon. As in psoriasis, the Köbner phenomenon may occur (Fig. 6.5). The nails are usually normal, but in about 10% of patients show changes ranging from fine longitudinal grooves to destruction of the entire nail fold and bed (see Fig. 13.26). Scalp lesions can cause a patchy scarring alopecia.

Course

Individual lesions may last for many months and the eruption as a whole tends to last about 1 year. However, the hypertrophic variant of the disease, with thick warty lesions usually around the ankles (Fig. 6.6), often lasts for many years. As lesions resolve, they become darker, flatter and leave discrete brown or grey macules. About one in six patients will have a recurrence.

Complications

Nail and hair loss can be permanent. The ulcerative form of lichen planus in the mouth may lead to squamous cell carcinoma. Ulceration, usually over bony prominences, may be disabling, especially if it is on the soles. Any association with liver disease is probably caused by the coexisting hepatitis infections mentioned above.

Differential diagnosis

Lichen planus should be differentiated from the other papulosquamous diseases listed in Table 6.1. Lichenoid drug reactions can mimic lichen planus closely. Gold and other heavy metals have often been implicated. Other drug causes include antimalarials, β blockers, non-steroidal anti-inflammatory drugs, para-aminobenzoic acid, thiazide diuretics and peni-

cillamine. Contact with chemicals used to develop colour film can also produce similar lesions. It may be hard to tell lichen planus from generalized discoid lupus erythematosus if only a few large lesions are present, or if the eruption is on the palms, soles or scalp. Wickham's striae or oral lesions favour the diagnosis of lichen planus. Oral candidiasis (p. 000) can also cause confusion.

Investigations

The diagnosis is usually obvious clinically. The histology is characteristic (Fig. 6.7), so a biopsy will confirm the diagnosis if necessary.

Treatment

Treatment can be difficult. If drugs are suspected as the cause, they should be stopped and unrelated ones substituted. Potent topical steroids will sometimes relieve symptoms and flatten the plaques. Systemic steroid courses work too, but are recommended only in special situations (e.g. unusually extensive involvement, nail destruction or painful and erosive oral lichen planus). Treatment with photochemotherapy with psoralen and ultraviolet A (PUVA; p. 59) or with narrow-band UVB (p. 58) may reduce pruritus and help to clear up the skin lesions. Acitretin (Formulary 2, p. 349) has also helped some patients with stubborn lichen planus. Antihistamines may blunt the itch. Mucous membrane lesions are usually asymptomatic and do not require treatment; if they do, then applications of a corticosteroid or tacrolimus in a gel base may be helpful.

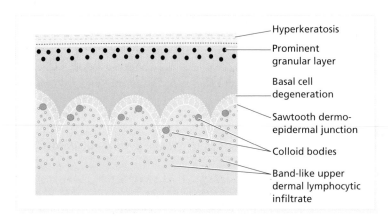

Fig. 6.7 Histology of lichen planus.

Pityriasis rubra pilaris

Cause

Several types have been described, but their causes are unknown. A defect in vitamin A metabolism was once suggested but has been disproved. The familial type has an autosomal dominant inheritance.

Presentation

The familial type develops gradually in childhood and persists throughout life. The more common acquired type begins in adult life with redness and scaling of the face and scalp. Later, red or pink areas grow quickly and merge, so that patients with pityriasis rubra pilaris are often erythrodermic. Small islands of skin may be 'spared' from this general erythema, but even here the follicles may be red and plugged with keratin (Fig. 6.8). Similarly, the generalized plaques, although otherwise rather like psoriasis, may also show follicular plugging.

Course

The palms and soles become thick, smooth and yellow. They often fissure rather than bend. The acquired form of pityriasis rubra pilaris generally lasts for 6–18 months, but may recur. Even when the plaques have gone, the skin may retain a rough scaly texture with persistent small scattered follicular plugs.

Complications

There are usually no complications. However, widespread erythroderma causes the patients to tolerate cold poorly.

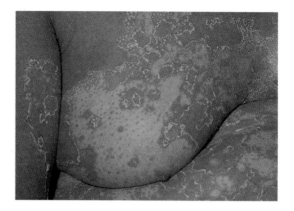

Fig. 6.8 Pityriasis rubra pilaris. Note the red plugged follicles, seen even in the 'spared' areas.

Differential diagnosis

Psoriasis is the disorder closest in appearance to pityriasis rubra pilaris, but lacks its slightly orange tinge. The thickening of the palms and soles, the follicular erythema in islands of uninvolved skin, and follicular plugging within the plaques, especially over the knuckles, are other features that help to separate them.

Investigations

A biopsy may help to distinguish psoriasis from pityriasis rubra pilaris; but, even so, the two disorders share many histological features.

Treatment

The disorder responds slowly to systemic retinoids such as acitretin (in adults, 25–50 mg/day for 6–8 months; p. 349). Oral methotrexate in low doses, once a week may also help (p. 348). Topical steroids and keratolytics (e.g. 2% salicylic acid in soft white paraffin) reduce inflammation and scaling, but usually do not suppress the disorder completely. Systemic steroids are not indicated.

Parapsoriasis and premycotic eruption

Parapsoriasis is a contentious term, which many would like to drop. We still find it useful clinically for lesions that look a little like psoriasis but which scale subtly

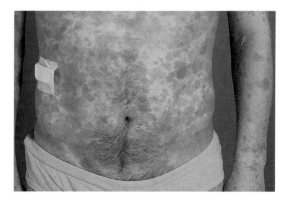

Fig. 6.9 A bizarre eruption: its persistence and variable colour suggested a prelymphomatous eruption. Biopsy confirmed this.

rather than grossly, and which persist despite anti-psoriasis treatment. It is worth trying to distinguish a benign type of parapsoriasis from a premycotic type, which is a forerunner of mycosis fungoides, a cutaneous T-cell lymphoma (Fig. 6.9)—although they can look alike early in their development. However, even the term 'premycotic' is disputed, as some think that these lesions are mycosis fungoides right from the start, preferring the term 'patch stage cutaneous T-cell lymphoma' (p. 280).

Cause

The cause is otherwise unknown.

Presentation

Pink scaly well-marginated plaques appear, typically on the buttocks, breasts, abdomen or flexural skin. The distinguishing features of the small-plaque (benign) and large-plaque (premycotic/prelymphomatous) types are given in Table 6.3. Perhaps the most important

point to look for is the presence of poikiloderma (atrophy, telangiectasia and reticulate pigmentation) in the latter type. Both conditions are stubborn in their response to topical treatment, although often responding temporarily to PUVA. Itching is variable.

Complications

Patients with suspected premycotic/prelymphomatous eruptions should be followed up carefully, even though the development of cutaneous T-cell lymphoma may not occur for years. If poikiloderma or induration develops, the diagnosis of a cutaneous T-cell lymphoma becomes likely.

Differential diagnosis

This includes psoriasis, tinea and nummular (discoid) eczema. In contrast to psoriasis and pityriasis rosea, the lesions of parapsoriasis, characteristically, are asymmetrical. Topical steroids can cause atrophy and confusion.

Investigations

Several biopsies should be taken if a premycotic eruption is suspected, if possible from thick or atrophic untreated areas. These may suggest an early cutaneous T-cell lymphoma, with bizarre mononuclear cells both in the dermis and in microscopic abscesses within the epidermis. Electron microscopy may show abnormal lymphocytes with convoluted nuclei in the dermis or epidermis, although the finding of these cells, especially in the dermis, is non-specific. DNA probes can determine monoclonality of the T cells within the lymphoid infiltrate of mycosis fungoides based on rearrangements of the T-cell receptor genes (p. 19). The use of these probes and of immunophenotyping

Parapsoriasis (benign type)	Premycotic/prelymphomatous eruptions
Smaller plaques	Larger
Yellowish	Not yellow—pink, or slightly violet, or brown
Sometimes finger-shaped lesions running around the trunk	Asymmetrical with bizarre outline
No atrophy	Atrophy ± poikiloderma
Responds to UVB	Responds better to PUVA
Remains benign although rarely clears	May progress to a cutaneous T-cell lymphoma

Table 6.3 Distinguishing features of parapsoriasis and premycotic/prelymphomatous eruptions.

helps to differentiate benign parapsoriasis from pre-mycotic/prelymphomatous eruptions.

Treatment

Treatment is controversial. Less aggressive treatments are used for the benign type of parapsoriasis. Usually, moderately potent steroids or ultraviolet radiation bring some resolution, but lesions tend to recur when these are stopped. For premycotic/prelymphomatous eruptions, treatment with PUVA (p. 59) or with topical nitrogen mustard paints, is advocated by some, although it is not clear that this slows down or prevents the development of a subsequent cutaneous T-cell lymphoma.

Pityriasis lichenoides

Pityriasis lichenoides is uncommon. It occurs in two forms. The numerous small circular scaly macules and papules of the chronic type are easy to confuse with guttate psoriasis (p. 51). However, their scaling is distinctive in that single silver-grey scales surmount the lesions (mica scales). The acute type is characterized by papules that become necrotic and leave scars like those of chickenpox. More often than not there are a few lesions of the chronic type in the acute variant and vice versa. UVB radiation can reduce the number of lesions and spontaneous resolution occurs eventually.

Other papulosquamous diseases

Discoid lupus erythematosus is typically papulosquamous; it is discussed with subacute cutaneous lupus erythematosus in Chapter 10. Fungus infections are nummular and scaly and can appear papulosquamous or eczematous; they are dealt with in Chapter 14. Seborrhoeic and nummular discoid eczema are discussed in Chapter 7. Secondary syphilis is discussed in Chapter 14.

Erythroderma/exfoliative dermatitis

Sometimes the whole skin becomes red and scaly (see Fig. 5.13). The disorders that can cause this are listed in Table 6.4. The best clue to the underlying cause is a history of a previous skin disease. Sometimes

Table 6.4 Some causes of erythroderma/exfoliative dermatitis.

Psoriasis
Pityriasis rubra pilaris
Ichthyosiform erythroderma
Pemphigus erythematosus
Contact, atopic, or seborrhoeic eczema
Reiter's syndrome
Lymphoma (including the Sézary syndrome)
Drug eruptions
Crusted (Norwegian) scabies

LEARNING POINTS

The dangers of erythroderma are the following.
1 Poor temperature regulation.
2 High-output cardiac failure.
3 Protein deficiency.

the histology is helpful but often it is non-specific. 'Erythroderma' is the term used when the skin is red with little or no scaling, while the term 'exfoliative dermatitis' is preferred if scaling predominates.

Most patients have lymphadenopathy, and many have hepatomegaly as well. If the condition becomes chronic, tightness of the facial skin leads to ectropion, scalp and body hair may be lost, and the nails become thickened and may be shed too. Temperature regulation is impaired and heat loss through the skin usually makes the patient feel cold and shiver. Oedema, high output cardiac failure, tachycardia, anaemia, failure to sweat and dehydration can occur. Treatment is that of the underlying condition.

Further reading

Bhattacharya, M., Kaur, I. & Kumar, B. (2000) Lichen planus: a clinical and epidemiological study. *Journal of Dermatology* 27, 576–582.

Clayton, B.D., Jorrizzo, J.L. & Hitchcock, M.G. (1997) Adult pityriasis rubra pilaris: a 10-year case series. *Journal of the American Academy of Dermatology* 36, 959–964.

Savin, J.A. (1991) Oral lichen planus. *British Medical Journal* 302, 544–545.

7 Eczema and dermatitis

The disorders grouped under this heading are the most common skin conditions seen by family doctors, and make up some 20% of all new patients referred to our clinics.

Terminology

The word 'eczema' comes from the Greek for 'boiling' —a reference to the tiny vesicles (bubbles) that are often seen in the early acute stages of the disorder, but less often in its later chronic stages. 'Dermatitis' means inflammation of the skin and is therefore, strictly speaking, a broader term than eczema—which is just one of several possible types of skin inflammation.

In the past too much time has been devoted to trying to distinguish between these two terms. To us, they mean the same thing. This approach is now used by most dermatologists, although many stick to the term eczema when talking to patients for whom 'dermatitis' may carry industrial and compensation overtones, which can stir up unnecessary legal battles. In this book contact eczema is the same as contact dermatitis; seborrhoeic eczema the same as seborrhoeic dermatitis, etc.

Classification of eczema

This is a messy legacy from a time when little was known about the subject. As a result, some terms are based on the appearance of lesions, e.g. discoid eczema and hyperkeratotic eczema, while others reflect outmoded or unproven theories of causation, e.g. infective eczema and seborrhoeic eczema. Classification by site, e.g. flexural eczema and hand eczema, is equally unhelpful.

Eczema is a reaction pattern. Many different stimuli can make the skin react in the same way, and several

of these may be in action at the same time (Fig. 7.1). This can make it hard to be sure which type of eczema is present; and even experienced dermatologists admit that they can only classify some two-thirds of the cases they see. To complicate matters further, the physical signs that make up eczema, although limited, can be jumbled together in an infinite number of ways, so that no two cases look alike.

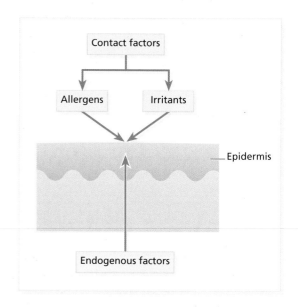

Fig. 7.1 The causes of eczema.

Table 7.1 Eczema—a working classification.

Mainly caused by exogenous (contact) factors	Irritant
	Allergic
	Photodermatitis (Chapter 16)
Other types of eczema	Atopic
	Seborrhoeic
	Discoid (nummular)
	Pompholyx
	Gravitational (venous, stasis)
	Asteatotic
	Neurodermatitis
	Juvenile plantar dermatosis
	Napkin (diaper) dermatitis

> **LEARNING POINT**
>
> Time spent thinking about contact factors may well help even those patients with the most blatantly 'constitutional' types of eczema.

One time-honoured subdivision of eczema is into exogenous (or contact) and endogenous (or constitutional) types. However, it is now clear that this is too simple. Different types of eczema often overlap, e.g. when a contact eczema is superimposed on a gravitational one. Even atopic eczema, the type most widely accepted as endogenous, is greatly influenced by external 'flare factors'—and itself predisposes to the development of irritant contact dermatitis, e.g. caused by soap. Nevertheless, it is still true that any rational approach to any patient with eczema must include a search for remediable environmental factors.

A working classification of eczema is given in Table 7.1.

Pathogenesis

The pathways leading to an eczematous reaction are likely to be common to all subtypes and to involve similar inflammatory mediators (prostaglandins, leukotrienes and cytokines; p. 21). Helper T cells, sometimes activated by superantigens from *Staphylococcus aureus*, predominate in the inflammatory infiltrate. One current view is that epidermal cytokines

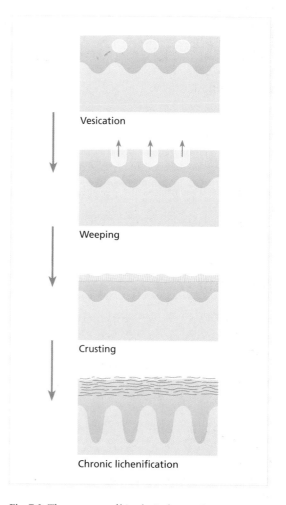

Fig. 7.2 The sequence of histological events in eczema.

help to produce spongiosis (p. 22); and that their secretion by keratinocytes can be elicited by T lymphocytes, irritants, bacterial products and other stimuli (see Fig. 2.11).

Histology (Fig. 7.2)

The clinical appearance of the different stages of eczema mirrors their histology. In the acute stage, oedema in the epidermis (spongiosis) progresses to the formation of intraepidermal vesicles, which may coalesce into larger blisters or rupture. The chronic stages of eczema show less spongiosis and vesication but more thickening of the prickle cell layer (acanthosis) and horny layers (hyperkeratosis and parakeratosis).

These changes are accompanied by a variable degree of vasodilatation and infiltration with lymphocytes.

Clinical appearance

The different types of eczema have their own distinguishing marks, and these will be dealt with later; most share certain general features, which it is convenient to consider here. The absence of a sharp margin is a particularly important feature that separates eczema from most papulosquamous eruptions.

Acute eczema

Acute eczema (Figs 7.3 and 7.4) is recognized by its:
• weeping and crusting;
• blistering—usually with vesicles but, in fierce cases, with large blisters;
• redness, papules and swelling—usually with an ill-defined border; and
• scaling.

Chronic eczema

Chronic eczema may show all of the above changes but in general is:
• less vesicular and exudative;
• more scaly, pigmented and thickened;
• more likely to show lichenification (Fig. 7.5)—a dry leathery thickened state, with increased skin markings, secondary to repeated scratching or rubbing; and
• more likely to fissure.

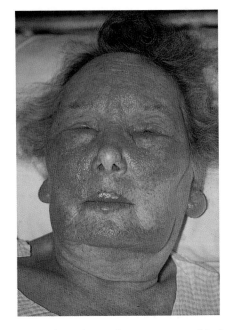

Fig. 7.4 Vesicular and crusted contact eczema of the face (cosmetic allergy).

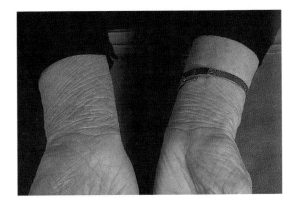

Fig. 7.5 Lichenification of the wrists—note also the increased skin markings on the palms ('atopic palms').

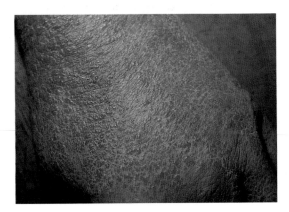

Fig. 7.3 Acute vesicular contact eczema of the hand.

LEARNING POINTS

1 Eczema is like jazz; it is hard to define—but it should be easy to recognize if you bear in mind the physical signs listed above.
2 If it does not itch, it is probably not eczema.

Complications

Heavy bacterial colonization is common in all types of eczema but overt infection is most troublesome in the seborrhoeic, nummular and atopic types. Local superimposed allergic reactions to medicaments can provoke dissemination, especially in gravitational eczema.

All severe forms of eczema have a huge effect on the quality of life. An itchy sleepless child can wreck family life. Eczema can interfere with work, sporting activities and sex lives. Jobs can be lost through it.

Differential diagnosis

This falls into two halves. First, eczema has to be separated from other skin conditions that look like it. Table 7.2 plots a way through this maze. Always

Table 7.2 Is the rash eczematous?

Atypical physical signs? Could be eczema but consider other erythemato-squamous eruptions			
↓			
Sharply marginated, strong colour, very scaly? Points of elbows and knees involved?	Yes →	Likely to be psoriasis (Chapter 5)	→ Can be confused with seborrhoeic eczema and neurodermatitis on the scalp, with seborrhoeic eczema in the flexures, and discoid eczema on the limbs. Look for confirmatory nail and joint changes. Ask about family history
↓No			
Itchy social contacts? Face spared? Burrows found? Genitals and nipples affected?	Yes →	This is scabies (p. 227)	→ Ensure all contacts are treated adequately—whether itchy or not
↓No			
Mouth lesions? Violaceous tinge? Shiny flat topped papules?	Yes →	Could be lichen planus (p. 64)	→ Also consider lichenoid drug eruptions
↓No			
Annular lesions with active scaly edges?	Yes →	Probably a fungal infection (Chapter 14)	→ More likely if the rash affects the groin, or is asymmetrical, perhaps affecting the palm of one hand only; and not doing well with topical steroids. Look at scales, cleared with potassium hydroxide, under a microscope or send scrapings to mycology laboratory. Check for contact with animals and for thickened toe nails
↓No			
Localized to palms and soles? Obvious pustules?	Yes →	Probably palmoplantar pustulosis (p. 53)	→ Expect poor response to most topical treatments
↓No			
Unusually swollen; on the face?	Yes →	Consider angioedema (p. 97) or erysipelas (p. 192)	→ Needs rapid treatment with antihistamines or antibiotics
↓No			
Consider dermatitis herpetiformis, not the various pityriases (rosea, versicolor, and rubra pilaris) and drug eruptions (Chapter 22)			

remember that eczemas are scaly, with poorly defined margins.

Occasionally a biopsy is helpful in confirming a diagnosis of eczema, but it will not determine the cause or type. Once the diagnosis of eczema becomes solid, look for clinical pointers towards an external cause. This determines both the need for investigations and the best line of treatment. Sometimes an eruption will follow one of the well-known patterns of eczema, such as the way atopic eczema picks out the skin behind the knees, and a diagnosis can then be made readily enough. Often, however, this is not the case, and the history then becomes especially important.

A contact element is likely if:
• there is obvious contact with known irritants or allergens;
• the eruption clears when the patient goes on holiday, or at the weekends;
• the eczema is asymmetrical, or has a linear or rectilinear configuration; or
• the rash picks out the eyelids, external ear canals, hands and feet, the skin around stasis ulcers, or the peri-anal skin.

Investigations

Each pattern of eczema needs a different line of inquiry.

Exogenous eczema

Here the main decision is whether or not to undertake patch testing (p. 35) to confirm allergic contact dermatitis and to identify the allergens responsible for it. In patch testing, standardized non-irritating concentrations of common allergens are applied to the normal skin of the back. If the patient is allergic to the allergen, eczema will develop at the site of contact after 48–96 h. Patch testing with irritants is of no value in any type of eczema, but testing with suitably diluted allergens is essential in suspected allergic contact eczema. The technique is not easy. Its problems include separating irritant from allergic patch test reactions, and picking the right allergens to test. If legal issues depend on the results, testing should be carried out by a dermatologist who will have the standard equipment and a suitable selection of properly standardized allergens (see Fig. 3.7). Patch testing can be used to confirm a suspected allergy or, by the use of a battery of common sensitizers, to discover unsuspected allergies, which then have to be assessed in the light of the history and the clinical picture. A visit to the home or workplace may help with this.

Photopatch testing is more specialized and facilities are only available in a few centres. A chemical is applied to the skin for 24 h and then the site is irradiated with a suberythema dose of ultraviolet irradiation; the patches are inspected for an eczematous reaction 48 h later.

Other types of eczema

The only indication for patch testing here is when an added contact allergic element is suspected. This is most common in gravitational eczema; neomycin, framycetin, lanolin or preservative allergy can perpetuate the condition and even trigger dissemination. Ironically rubber gloves, so often used to protect eczematous hands, can themselves sensitize.

The role of prick testing in atopic eczema is discussed on p. 36.

Patients with atopic dermatitis often have multiple type I reactions to foods, danders, pollens, dusts and moulds. Some find the measurement of serum total immunoglobulin E (IgE), and of IgE antibodies specific to certain antigens, not only useful in diagnosing the atopic state, but also helpful when advising on the role of dietary and environmental allergens in causing or perpetuating atopic dermatitis, particularly in children. Total and specific IgE antibodies are measured by a radioallergosorbent test (RAST). Prick and RAST testing give similar results but many now prefer the more expensive RAST test as it carries no risk of anaphylaxis, is easier to perform and is less time consuming.

If the eczema is worsening despite treatment, or if there is much crusting, heavy bacterial colonization may be present. Opinions vary about the value of cultures for bacteria and candida, but antibiotic treatment may be helpful. Scrapings for microscopical examination (p. 35) and culture for fungus will rule out tinea if there is clinical doubt—as in some cases of discoid eczema.

Finally, malabsorption should be considered in otherwise unexplained widespread pigmented atypical patterns of endogenous eczema.

Treatment

Acute weeping eczema

This does best with rest and liquid applications. Non-steroidal preparations are helpful and the techniques used will vary with the facilities available and the site of the lesions. In general practice a simple and convenient way of dealing with weeping eczema of the hands or feet is to use thrice daily 10-min soaks in a cool 0.65% aluminium acetate solution (Formulary 1, p. 329)—saline or even tap water will do almost as well—each soaking being followed by a smear of a corticosteroid cream or lotion and the application of a non-stick dressing or cotton gloves. One reason for dropping the dilute potassium permanganate solution that was once so popular is because it stains the skin and nails brown.

Wider areas on the trunk respond well to corticosteroid creams and lotions. However, traditional remedies such as exposure and frequent applications of calamine lotion, and the use of half-strength magenta paint for the flexures are also effective.

An experienced doctor or nurse can teach patients how to use wet dressings, and supervise this. The aluminium acetate solution, saline or water, can be applied on cotton gauze, under a polythene covering, and changed twice daily. Details of wet wrap techniques are given below. Rest at home will help too.

Wet wrap dressings

This is a labour-intensive, but highly effective technique, of value in the treatment of troublesome atopic eczema in children. After a bath, a corticosteroid is applied to the skin and then covered with two layers of tubular dressing—the inner layer already soaked in warm water, the outer layer being applied dry. Cotton pyjamas or a T-shirt can be used to cover these, and the dressings can then be left in place for several hours. The corticosteroid may be one that is rapidly metabolized after systemic absorption such as a beclomethasone (beclometasone) diproprionate ointment diluted to 0.025% (available only in the UK). Alternatives include 1 or 2.5% hydrocortisone cream for children and 0.025 or 0.1 % triamcinolone cream for adults. The bandages can be washed and reused. The evaporation of fluid from the bandages cools the skin and provides rapid relief of itching. With improvement, the frequency of the dressings can be cut down and a moisturiser can be substituted for the corticosteroid. Parents can be taught the technique by a trained nurse, who must follow up treatment closely. Parents easily learn how to modify the technique to suit the needs of their own child. Side-effects seem to be minimal.

Subacute eczema

Steroid lotions or creams are the mainstay of treatment; their strength is determined by the severity of the attack. Vioform, bacitracin, fusidic acid, mupirocin or neomycin (see Formulary 1, p. 334) can be incorporated into the application if an infective element is present, but watch out for sensitization to neomycin, especially when treating gravitational eczema.

Chronic eczema

This responds best to steroids in an ointment base, but is also often helped by non-steroid applications such as ichthammol and zinc cream or paste.

The strength of the steroid is important (Fig. 7.6). Nothing stronger than 0.5 or 1% hydrocortisone ointment should be used on the face or in infancy. Even in adults one should be reluctant to prescribe more than 200 g/week of a mildly potent steroid, 50 g/week of a moderately potent or 30 g/week of a potent one for long periods. Very potent topical steroids should not be used long-term.

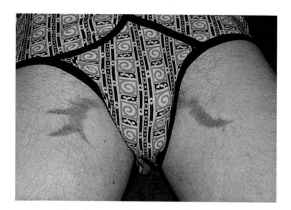

Fig. 7.6 Stretch marks following the use of too potent topical steroids to the groin.

Bacterial superinfection may need systemic antibiotics but can often be controlled by the incorporation of antibiotics, e.g. fusidic acid, mupirocin, neomycin or chlortetracycline, or antiseptics, e.g. Vioform, into the steroid formulation. Many proprietary mixtures of this type are available in the UK. Chronic localized hyperkeratotic eczema of the palms or soles can be helped by salicylic acid (1–6% in emulsifying ointment) or stabilized urea preparations (Formulary 1, p. 328).

Systemic treatment

Short courses of systemic steroids may occasionally be justified in extremely acute and severe eczema, particularly when the cause is known and already eliminated (e.g. allergic contact dermatitis from a plant such as poison ivy). However, prolonged systemic steroid treatment should be avoided in chronic cases, particularly in atopic eczema. Hydroxyzine, doxepin, trimeprazine and other antihistamines (Formulary 2, p. 344) may help at night. Systemic antibiotics may be needed in widespread bacterial superinfection. However, *Staphylococcus aureus* routinely colonizes all weeping eczemas, and most dry ones as well. Simply isolating it does not automatically prompt a prescription for an antibiotic, although if the density of organisms is high, usually manifest as extensive crusting, then systemic antibiotics can help.

Common patterns of eczema

Irritant contact dermatitis

This accounts for more than 80% of all cases of contact dermatitis, and for the vast majority of industrial cases. However, it can also occur in children, e.g. as a reaction to a bubble bath, play dough or lip-licking (Fig. 7.7).

Cause

Strong irritants elicit an acute reaction after brief contact and the diagnosis is then usually obvious. Prolonged exposure, sometimes over years, is needed for weak irritants to cause dermatitis, usually of the hands and forearms (Fig. 7.8). Detergents, alkalis, solvents, cutting oils and abrasive dusts are common

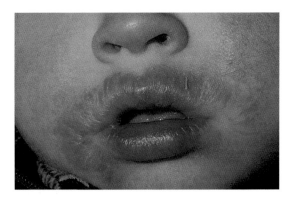

Fig. 7.7 Licking the lips as a nervous habit has caused this characteristic pattern of dry fissured irritant eczema.

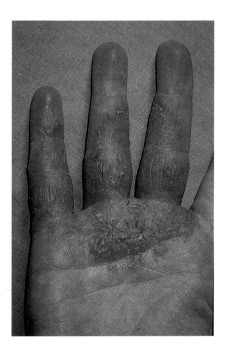

Fig. 7.8 Typical chronic hand eczema—irritants have played a part here.

culprits. There is a wide range of susceptibility: those with very dry or fair skins are especially vulnerable. Past or present atopic dermatitis doubles the risk of irritant hand eczema developing.

Course

The need to continue at work, or with housework, often stops the skin regaining its normal barrier function. Even under ideal circumstances this may take several months. All too often therefore irritant eczema, probably reversible in the early stages, becomes chronic.

Complications

The condition may lead to loss of work.

Differential diagnosis

It is often hard to differentiate irritant from allergic contact dermatitis, and from atopic eczema of the hands—the more so as atopic patients are especially prone to develop irritant eczema.

Investigations

Patch testing with irritants is not helpful and may be misleading; but patch testing to a battery of common allergens (p. 35) is worthwhile if an allergic element is suspected. Even if the results are negative, patch testing is not a waste of time, and provides a valuable opportunity to educate patients about their condition.

Treatment

Management is based upon avoidance of the irritants responsible for the condition, but often this is not possible and the best that can be achieved is reduced exposure by the use of protective gloves and clothing. The factory doctor or nurse can often advise here. Washing facilities at work should be good. Barrier creams seldom help established cases, and dirty hands should not be cleaned with harsh solvents.

Prevention is better than cure because, once started, irritant eczema can persist long after contact with offending substances has ceased, despite the vigorous use of emollients and topical corticosteroids. Vulnerable people should be advised to avoid jobs that carry an especially heavy exposure to skin irritants (see Table 7.4). If the right person can be placed in the right job, fewer trainee hairdressers and mechanics will find out the hard way that their skins are easily

Table 7.3 The allergens in our battery and what they mean.

Allergen	Common sources	Comments
Metals		
The classic metal allergy for men is still to chrome, present in cement. In the past, more women than men have been allergic to nickel but the current fashion for men to have their ears and other parts of their body pierced is changing this		
Chrome	Cement; chromium plating processes; antirust paints; tattoos (green) and some leathers. Sensitization follows contact with chrome salts rather than chromium metal	A common problem for building site workers. In Scandinavia putting iron sulphate into cement has been shown to reduce its allergenicity by making the chrome salts insoluble
Nickel	Nickel-plated objects, especially cheap jewellery. Remember jean studs	The best way of becoming sensitive is to pierce your ears. Nickel is being taken out of some good costume jewellery. Stainless steel is relatively safe
Cobalt	A contaminant of nickel and occurs with it	Eruption similar to that of nickel allergy. The main allergen for those with metal on metal arthroplasties
Cosmetics		
Despite attempts to design 'hypoallergenic' cosmetics, allergic reactions are still seen. The most common culprits are fragrances, followed by preservatives, dyes and lanolin		
Fragrance mix	An infinite variety of cosmetics, sprays and toiletries	Any perfume will contain many ingredients. This convenient mix picks up some 80% of perfume allergies. Some perfume allergic subjects also react to balsam of Peru, tars or colophony

Continued p. 78

Table 7.3 (*cont'd*)

Allergen	Common sources	Comments
Balsam of Peru	Used in some scented cosmetics. Also in some spices and suppositories, e.g. Anusol	May indicate allergy to perfumes also. Can cross-react with colophony, orange peel, cinnamon and benzyl benzoate
Paraphenylene diamine (PPD)	Dark dyes for hair and clothing	Few heed the manufacturer's warning to patch test themselves before dyeing their hair. May cross-react with other chemicals containing the 'para' group, e.g. some local anaesthetics, sulphonamides or para-aminobenzoic acid (in some sunscreens)
Wool alcohols	Anything with lanolin in it	Common cause of reactions to cosmetics and topical medicaments. The newer purified lanolins cause fewer problems
Cetosteryl alcohol	Emollient, and base for many cosmetics	Taking over now as a vehicle from lanolin

Preservatives and biocides
No one likes rancid cosmetics, or smelly cutting oils. Biocides are hidden in many materials to stop this sort of thing happening

Allergen	Common sources	Comments
Formaldehyde	Used as a preservative in some shampoos and cosmetics. Also in pathology laboratories and white shoes	Many pathologists are allergic to it. Quaternium 15 (see below) releases formaldehyde as do some formaldehyde resins
Parabens-mix	Preservatives in a wide variety of creams and lotions, both medical and cosmetic	Common cause of allergy in those who react to a number of seemingly unrelated creams
Chlorocresol	Common preservative	Cross reacts with chloroxylenol—a popular antiseptic
Kathon	Preservative in many cosmetics, shampoos, soaps and sunscreens	Also found in some odd places such as moist toilet papers, and washing-up liquids
Quaternium 15	Preservative in many topical medicaments and cosmetics	Releases formaldehyde and may cross-react with it
Imidazolidinyl urea	Common ingredient of moisturizers and cosmetics	Cosmetic allergy
Other biocides	In glues, paints, cutting oils, etc.	Responsible for some cases of occupational dermatitis

Medicaments
These may share allergens, such as preservatives and lanolin, with cosmetics (see above). In addition the active ingredients can sensitize, especially when applied long-term to venous ulcers, pruritus ani, eczema or otitis externa

Allergen	Common sources	Comments
Neomycin	Popular topical antibiotic. Safe in short bursts, e.g. for impetigo and cuts	Common sensitizer in those with leg ulcers. Simply swapping to another antibiotic may not always help as neomycin cross-reacts with framycetin and gentamycin
Quinoline mix	Used as an antiseptic in creams, often in combination with a corticosteroid	Its aliases include Vioform and chinoform
Ethylenediamine dihydrochloride	Stabilizer in some topical steroid mixtures (e.g. Mycolog and the alleged active ingredient in fat removal creams). A component in aminophylline. A hardener for epoxy resin	Cross-reacts with some antihistamines, e.g. hydroxyzine

Continued

Table 7.3 (*cont'd*)

Allergen	Common sources	Comments
Benzocaine	A local anaesthetic which lurks in some topical applications, e.g. for piles and sunburn	Dermatologists seldom recommend using these preparations—they have seen too many reactions
Tixocortol pivalate	Topical steroid	A marker for allergy to various topical steroids. Hydrocortisone allergy exists. Think of this when steroid applications seem to be making things worse
Budesonide	Topical steroid	Testing with both tixocortol pivalate and budesonide will detect 95% of topical steroid allergies

Rubber
Rubber itself is often not the problem: but it has to be converted from soft latex (p. 96) to usable rubber by adding vulcanizers to make it harder, accelerators to speed up vulcanization, and antioxidants to stop it perishing in the air. These additives are allergens

Mercapto-mix	Chemicals used to harden rubber	Diagnosis is often obvious: sometimes less so. Remember shoe soles, rubber bands and golf club grips
Thiuram-mix	Another set of rubber accelerators	Common culprit in rubber glove allergy
Black rubber mix	All black heavy-duty rubber, e.g. tyres, rubber boots, squash balls	These are paraphenylene diamine derivatives, cross-reacting with PPD dyes (see above)
Carba mix	Mainly in rubber gloves	Patch testing with rubber chemicals occasionally sensitizes patients to them

Plants
In the USA, the Rhus family (poison ivy and poison oak) are important allergens: in Europe, *Primula obconica* holds pride of place. Both cause severe reactions with streaky erythema and blistering. The Rhus antigen is such a potent sensitizer that patch testing with it is unwise. Other reaction patterns include a lichenified dermatitis of exposed areas from chrysanthemums, and a fingertip dermatitis from tulip bulbs

Primin	Allergen in *Primula obconica*	More reliable than patch testing to *Primula* leaves
Sesquiterpene lactone mix	Compositae plant allergy	Picks up chrysanth allergy. Flying pollen affects exposed parts and reactions can look like light sensitivity

Resins
Common sensitizers such as epoxy resins can cause trouble both at home, as adhesives, and in industry

Epoxy resin	Common in 'two-component' adhesive mixtures (e.g. Araldite). Also used in electrical and plastics industries	'Cured' resin does not sensitize. A few become allergic to the added hardener rather than to the resin itself
Paratertiary butylphenol formaldehyde resin	Used as an adhesive, e.g. in shoes, wrist watch straps, prostheses, hobbies	Cross-reacts with formaldehyde. Depigmentation has been recorded
Colophony	Naturally occurring and found in pine sawdust. Used as an adhesive in sticking plasters, bandages. Also found in various varnishes, paper and rosin	The usual cause of sticking plaster allergy; also of dermatitis of the hands of violinists who handle rosin

irritated. Moderately potent topical corticosteroids and emollients are valuable, but are secondary to the avoidance of irritants and protective measures.

Allergic contact dermatitis

Cause

The mechanism is that of delayed (type IV) hypersensitivity, which is dealt with in detail on p. 26. It has the following features.
- Previous contact is needed to induce allergy.
- It is specific to one chemical and its close relatives.
- After allergy has been established, all areas of skin will react to the allergen.
- Sensitization persists indefinitely.
- Desensitization is seldom possible.

Allergens

In an ideal world, allergens would be replaced by less harmful substances, and some attempts are already being made to achieve this. A whole new industry has arisen around the need for predictive patch testing before new substances or cosmetics are let out into the community. Similarly, chrome allergy is less of a problem now in enlightened countries that insist on adding ferrous sulphate to cement to reduce its water-soluble chromate content. However, contact allergens will never be abolished completely and family doctors still need to know about the most common ones and where to find them (Table 7.3). It is not possible to guess which substances are likely to sensitize just by looking at their formulae. In fact, most allergens are relatively simple chemicals that have to bind to protein to become 'complete' antigens. Their ability to sensitize varies—from substances that can do so after a single exposure (e.g. poison ivy), to those that need prolonged exposure (e.g. chrome—bricklayers take an average of 10 years to become allergic to it).

Presentation and clinical course

The original site of the eruption gives a clue to the likely allergen but secondary spread may later obscure this. Easily recognizable patterns exist. Nickel allergy, for example, gives rise to eczema under jewellery, bra

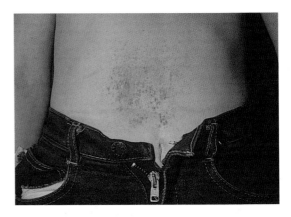

Fig. 7.9 Contact eczema caused by allergy to nickel in a jean stud.

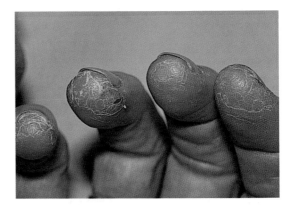

Fig. 7.10 Dry fissured eczema of the fingertips caused by handling garlic.

clips and jean studs (Fig. 7.9). The lax skin of the eyelids and genitalia is especially likely to become oedematous. Possible allergens are numerous and to spot the less common ones in the environment needs specialist knowledge. Table 7.3 lists some common allergens and their distribution.

Allergic contact dermatitis should be suspected if:
1 certain areas are involved, e.g. the eyelids, external auditory meati, hands (Fig. 7.10) or feet, and around gravitational ulcers;
2 there is known contact with the allergens mentioned in Table 7.3; or
3 the individual's work carries a high risk, e.g. hairdressing, working in a flower shop, or dentistry.

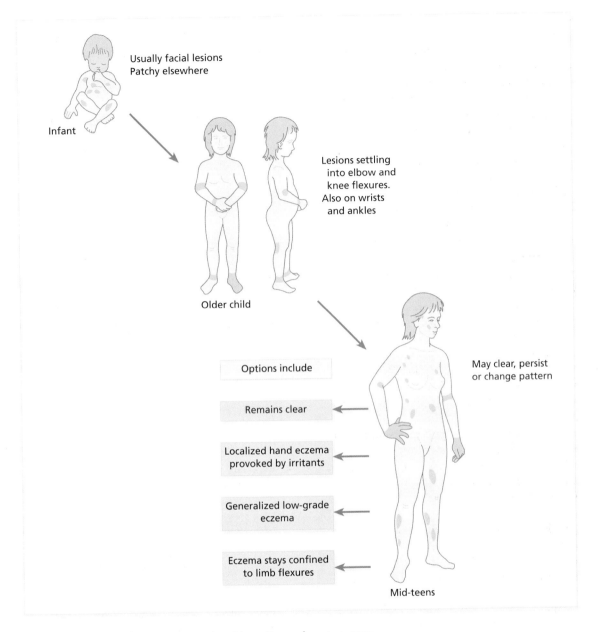

Fig. 7.12 The pattern of atopic eczema varies with age. It may clear at any stage.

ical picture. Affected children may sleep poorly, be hyperactive and sometimes manipulative, using the state of their eczema to get what they want from their parents. Luckily, the condition remits spontaneously before the age of 10 years in at least two-thirds of affected children, although it may come back at times of stress. Eczema and asthma may seesaw, so that while one improves the other may get worse.

Diagnostic criteria

Useful diagnostic criteria have been developed in the UK recently (Table 7.5).

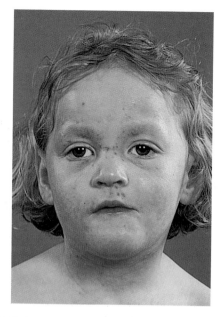

Fig. 7.13 Atopic eczema in a child: worse around the eyes due to rubbing. (Courtesy of Dr Olivia Schofield, The Royal Infirmary of Edinburgh, Edinburgh, UK.)

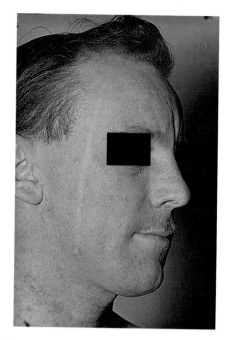

Fig. 7.15 Trivial scratching has led to striking white dermographism.

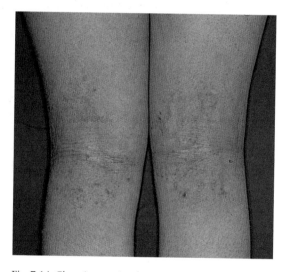

Fig. 7.14 Chronic excoriated atopic eczema behind the knees.

Table 7.5 Diagnostic criteria for atopic eczema.

Must have:
A chronically itchy skin (or report of scratching or rubbing in a child)

Plus three or more of the following:
History of itchiness in skin creases such as folds of the elbows, behind the knees, fronts of ankles or around the neck (or the cheeks in children under 4 years)
History of asthma or hay fever (or history of atopic disease in a first-degree relative in children under 4 years)
General dry skin in the past year
Visible flexural eczema (or eczema affecting the cheeks or forehead and outer limbs in children under 4 years)
Onset in the first 2 years of life (not always diagnostic in children under 4 years)

Complications

Overt bacterial infection is troublesome in many patients with atopic eczema (Fig. 7.16). They are also especially prone to viral infections, most dangerously with widespread herpes simplex (eczema herpeticum; Fig. 7.17), but also with molluscum contagiosum and warts. Growth hormone levels rise during deep sleep (stages 3 and 4), but these stages may not be reached during the disturbed sleep of children with severe atopic eczema and as a consequence they may grow poorly. The absorption of topical steroids can contribute to this too.

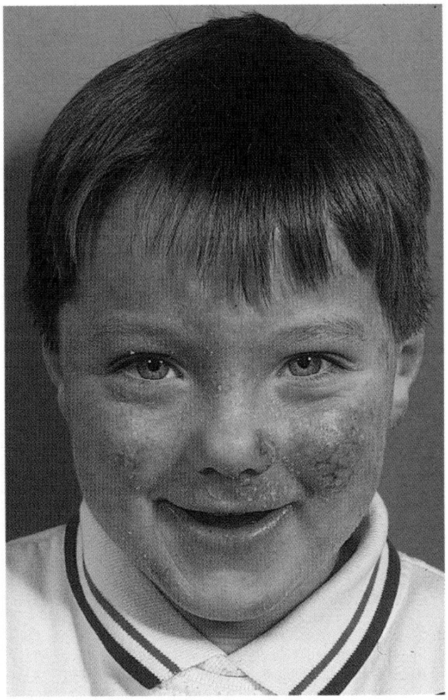

Fig. 7.16 Facial eczema in a young boy worsening recently. Crusting on the cheeks and upper lip points to possible bacterial superinfection. (Courtesy of Dr Olivia Schofield, The Royal Infirmary of Edinburgh, Edinburgh, UK.)

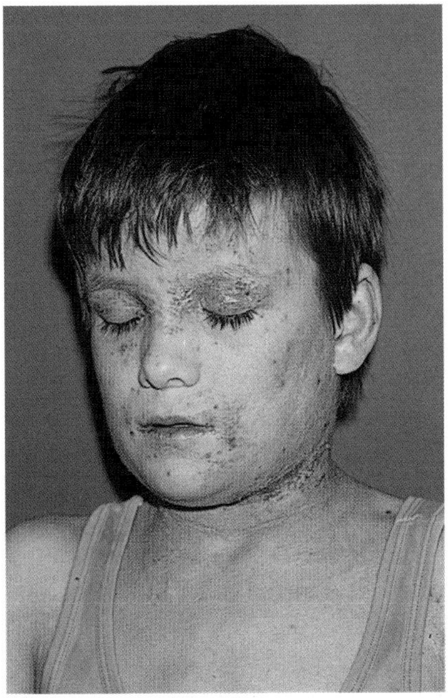

Fig. 7.17 Infected facial eczema—herpes simplex was isolated.

Investigations

Prick testing (see Fig. 3.10) demonstrates immediate-type hypersensitivity and is helpful in the investigation of asthma and hay fever. However, the value of prick testing in atopic eczema remains controversial. Often the finding of multiple positive reactions, and a high IgE level, does little more than support a doubtful clinical diagnosis without leading to fruitful lines of treatment.

Treatment

Management here is complex and should include the following.

• Explanation, reassurance and encouragement. Many patients and parents benefit from an introduction to the National Eczema Society in the UK or the National Eczema Association for Science and Education or the Inflammatory Skin Institute in the USA.

• The avoidance of exacerbating factors such as irritants (e.g. woollen clothing next to the skin) and later of careers such as hairdressing and engineering, which would inevitably lead to much exposure to irritants. Also avoid extremes of temperature, and contact with soaps and detergents.

• The judicious use of topical steroids and other applications as for other types of chronic eczema (p. 75 and Table 7.6). A technique useful for extensive and troublesome eczema, particularly in children, is that of 'wet wrap' dressings—see above (p. 75). A nurse who is expert in applying such dressings is an asset to any practice (Fig. 7.18).

Tacrolimus (Formulary 1, p. 334) is a macrolide immunosuppressant produced by a streptomycete. It is used systemically in kidney, liver and heart transplantation. Trials of tacrolimus in ointment form have shown that it can be a quick and highly successful topical treatment for moderate to severe atopic eczema. The preparation seems to be safe in use, with a

Table 7.6 Principles of treatment with topical corticosteroids.

Use the weakest steroid that controls the eczema effectively
Review their use regularly: check for local and systemic side-effects
In primary care, avoid using potent and very potent steroids for children with atopic eczema
Be wary of repeat prescriptions

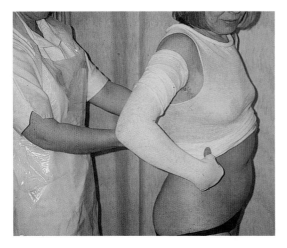

Fig. 7.18 Protective tubular gauze dressings being applied over a topical steroid ointment.

transient burning sensation being the most common side-effect; however, it decreases with usage. Some use topical steroids briefly, to improve the eczema, before starting tacrolimus ointment, hoping in this way to decrease the incidence and severity of this burning sensation. Systemic absorption is low, and skin atrophy is not a problem. Local infection might be troublesome and the development of skin cancer, especially on exposed treated areas, is a concern when the drug is used for prolonged periods. Perhaps more information and experience are required before tacrolimus can be hailed as a revolutionary new treatment for the treatment of inflammatory skin disorders—but the results so far look highly impressive. Topical tacrolimus is now available as Protopic ointment (Formulary 1, p. 334).

Pimecrolimus (Formulary 1, p. 334) is another topical immunosuppressant and a derivative of askamycin. Clinical trials in atopic eczema have been encouraging and it can be used in patients older than 3 months. Its action is very similar to that of tacrolimus and time will tell if either preparation is superior.
• The regular use of bland emollients, either directly to the skin or in the form of oils to be used in the bath. Some of these can also be used as soap substitutes. A list of suitable preparations is given in Formulary 1 (p. 328). Some rules governing the use of emollients are given in Table 7.7.
• Those with an associated ichthyosis should generally use ointments rather than creams.
• The scratch–itch cycle can often be interrupted by occlusive bandaging, e.g. with a 1% ichthammol paste bandage. Nails should be kept short.

Table 7.7 Winning ways with emollients.

Make sure they are applied when the skin is moist
Prescribe plenty (at least 500 g/week for the whole skin of an adult and 250 g/week for the whole skin of a child) and ensure they are used at least 3–4 times a day
For maximal effect, combine the use of creams, ointments, bath oils and emollient soap substitutes

• Sedative antihistamines, e.g. trimeprazine or hydroxyzine (Formulary 2, p. 345) are of value if sleep is interrupted, but histamine release is not the main cause of the itching, so the newer non-sedative antihistamines help less than might be expected.
• Acute flares are often induced by the surface proliferation of staphylococci, even without frank sepsis. A month's course of a systemic antibiotic, e.g. erythromycin, may then be helpful.
• Allergen avoidance: prick tests confirm that most sufferers from atopic eczema have immediate hypersensitivity responses to allergens in the faeces of house dust mites. Sometimes, but not always, measures to reduce contact with these allergens help eczema. These measures should include encasing the mattress in a dustproof bag, washing the duvets and pillows every 3 months at a temperature greater than 55°C, and thorough and regular vacuuming in the bedroom, where carpets should preferably be avoided.
• Do not keep pets to which there is obvious allergy.
• The role of diet in atopic eczema is even more debatable, and treatments based on changing the diet of sufferers are often disappointing. Similarly, it is not certain that the avoidance of dietary allergens (e.g. cow's milk and eggs) by a pregnant or lactating woman lessens the risk of her baby developing eczema. It may still be wise to breastfeed children at special risk for 6 months.
• Routine inoculations are permissible during quiet phases of the eczema. However, children who are allergic to eggs should not be inoculated against measles, influenza and yellow fever.
• Those with active herpes simplex infections should be avoided to cut the risk of developing eczema herpeticum.
• In stubborn cases UVB, UVA-1 (340–400 nm) or even PUVA therapy may be useful.
• Cyclosporin: severe and unresponsive cases may be helped by short courses under specialist supervision (Formulary 2, p. 347).

• Chinese herbal remedies: properly conducted trials have given promising results but difficulties remain. The active ingredients within these complex mixtures of herbs have still not been identified. We have some hope for the future but currently do not prescribe these treatments for our patients.

Seborrhoeic eczema

Presentation and course

The term covers at least three common patterns of eczema, mainly affecting hairy areas, and often showing characteristic greasy yellowish scales. These patterns may merge together (Fig. 7.19).

1 A red scaly or exudative eruption of the scalp, ears (Fig. 7.20), face (Fig. 7.21) and eyebrows. May be associated with chronic blepharitis and otitis externa.

2 Dry scaly 'petaloid' lesions of the presternal (Fig. 7.22) and interscapular areas. There may also be extensive follicular papules or pustules on the trunk (seborrhoeic folliculitis or pityrosporum folliculitis).

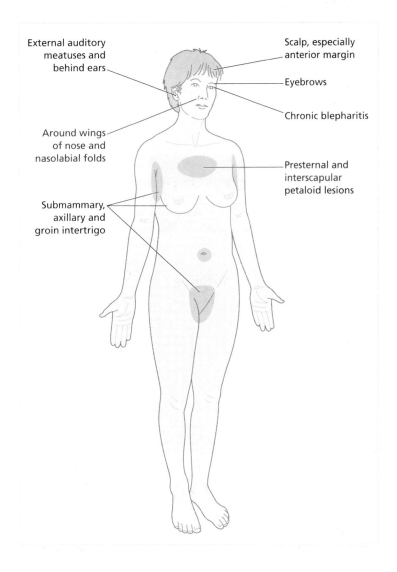

Fig. 7.19 Areas most often affected by seborrhoeic eczema.

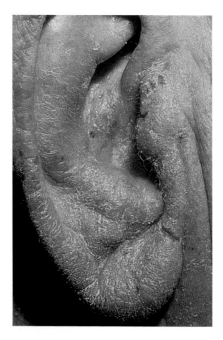

Fig. 7.20 Dry scaly seborrhoeic eczema of the ear.

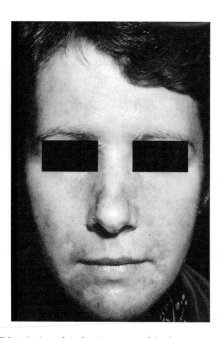

Fig. 7.21 Active seborrhoeic eczema of the face.

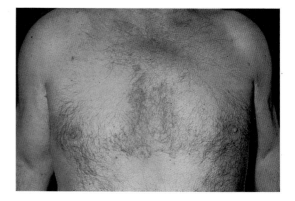

Fig. 7.22 Typical presternal patch of seborrhoeic eczema.

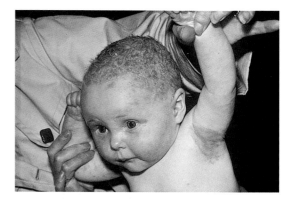

Fig. 7.23 Infantile seborrhoeic eczema.

3 Intertriginous lesions of the armpits, umbilicus or groins, or under spectacles or hearing aids.

Cause

This condition is not obviously related to seborrhoea. It may run in some families, often affecting those with a tendency to dandruff. The success of treatments directed against yeasts has suggested that overgrowth of the pityrosporum yeast skin commensals plays an important part in the development of seborrhoeic eczema. This fits well with the fact that seborrhoeic eczema is often an early sign of AIDS, and that it responds to antiyeast agents such as topical ketoconazole shampoo or cream.

Seborrhoeic eczema may affect infants (Fig. 7.23) but is most common in adult males. In infants it clears quickly but in adults its course is unpredictable and may be chronic or recurrent. Some particularly severe cases have occurred in patients with AIDS (p. 211 and Fig. 14.35).

Complications

May be associated with furunculosis. In the intertriginous type, superadded *Candida* infection is common.

Investigations

None are usually needed, but bear possible HIV infection and Parkinson's disease in mind.

Treatment

Therapy is suppressive rather than curative and patients should be told this. Topical imidazoles (Formulary 1, p. 335) are perhaps the first line of treatment. Two per cent sulphur and 2% salicylic acid in aqueous cream is often helpful and avoids the problem of topical steroids. It may be used on the scalp overnight and removed by a medicated shampoo, which may contain ketoconazole, tar, salicylic acid, sulphur, zinc or selenium sulphide (Formulary 1, p. 329). A topical lithium preparation (Formulary 1, p. 339) may help the facial rash. For intertriginous lesions a weak steroid–antiseptic or steroid–antifungal combination (Formulary 1, p. 332) is often effective. For severe and unresponsive cases a short course of oral itraconazole may be helpful.

Discoid (nummular) eczema

Cause

No cause has been established but chronic stress is often present. A reaction to bacterial antigens has been suspected as the lesions often yield staphylococci on culture, and as steroid–antiseptic or steroid–antibiotic mixtures do better than either separately.

Presentation and course

This common pattern of endogenous eczema classically affects the limbs of middle-aged males. The lesions are multiple, coin-shaped, vesicular or crusted, highly itchy plaques (Fig. 7.24), usually less than 5 cm across. The condition tends to persist for many months, and recurrences often appear at the site of previous plaques.

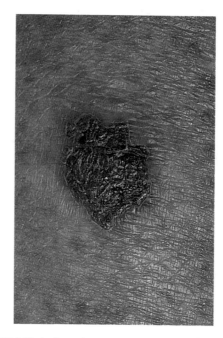

Fig. 7.24 Vesicular and weeping patch of discoid eczema.

Investigations

None are usually needed.

Treatment

With topical steroid–antiseptic or steroid–antibiotic combinations (see above).

Pompholyx

Cause

The cause is usually unknown, but pompholyx is sometimes provoked by heat or emotional upsets. In subjects allergic to nickel, small amounts of nickel in food may trigger pompholyx. The vesicles are not plugged sweat ducts, and the term 'dyshidrotic eczema' should now be dropped.

Presentation and course

In this tiresome and sometimes very unpleasant form of eczema, recurrent bouts of vesicles or larger blisters appear on the palms, fingers (Fig. 7.25) and/or the soles of adults. Bouts lasting a few weeks recur at

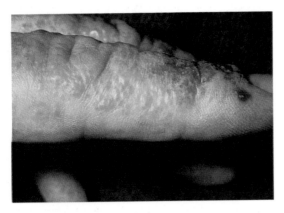

Fig. 7.25 Pompholyx vesicles along the side of a finger.

irregular intervals. Secondary infection and lymphangitis are a recurrent problem for some patients.

Investigations

None are usually needed: sometimes a pompholyx-like eruption of the hands can follow acute tinea pedis (an ide reaction). If this is suspected, scrapings or blister roofs, not from the hand lesions but from those on the feet, should be sent for mycological examination. Swabs from infected vesicles should be cultured for bacterial pathogens.

Treatment

As for acute eczema of the hands and feet (p. 75). Appropriate antibiotics should be given for bacterial infections. Aluminium acetate or potassium permanganate soaks, followed by applications of a very potent corticosteroid cream, are often helpful.

Gravitational (stasis) eczema

Cause

Often, but not always, accompanied by obvious venous insufficiency.

Presentation and course

A chronic patchy eczematous condition of the lower legs, sometimes accompanied by varicose veins, oedema and haemosiderin deposition (Fig. 7.26). When

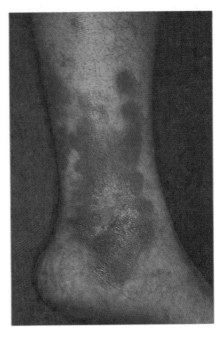

Fig. 7.26 Chronic gravitational eczema, perhaps with a superimposed contact dermatitis from a local medication.

severe it may spread to the other leg or even become generalized.

Complications

Patients often become sensitized to local antibiotic applications or to the preservatives in medicated bandages. Excoriations may lead to ulcer formation.

Treatment

This should include the elimination of oedema by elevation, pressure bandages or diuretics. A moderately potent topical steroid may be helpful, but stronger ones are best avoided. Bland applications, e.g. Lassar's paste or zinc cream BNF, or medicated bandages (Formulary 1, p. 338) are useful but stasis eczema is liable to persist, despite surgery to the underlying veins.

Asteatotic eczema

Cause

Many who develop asteatotic eczema in old age will always have had a dry skin and a tendency to chap.

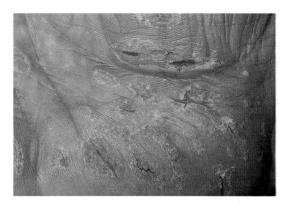

Fig. 7.28 It is often hard to tell palmar lichen simplex from hyperkeratotic fissured eczema, as shown here.

Localized neurodermatitis (lichen simplex)

Cause

The skin is damaged as a result of repeated rubbing or scratching, as a habit or in response to stress, but there is no underlying skin disorder.

Presentation and course

Usually occurs as a single fixed itchy lichenified plaque (Fig. 7.28). Favourite areas are the nape of the neck in women, the legs in men, and the anogenital area in both sexes. Lesions may resolve with treatment but tend to recur either in the same place or elsewhere.

Investigations

None are usually needed.

Treatment

Potent topical steroids or occlusive bandaging, where feasible, help to break the scratch–itch cycle. Tranquillizers are often disappointing.

Juvenile plantar dermatosis (Fig. 7.29)

Cause

This condition is thought to be related to the impermeability of modern socks and shoe linings with

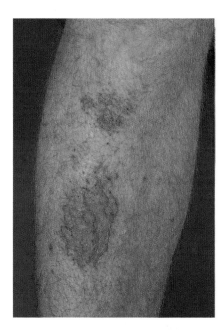

Fig. 7.27 Asteatotic eczema with network of fine fissures in the stratum corneum.

Other contributory factors include the removal of surface lipids by over-washing, the low humidity of winter and central heating, the use of diuretics, and hypothyroidism.

Presentation and course

Often unrecognized, this common and itchy pattern of eczema occurs usually on the legs of elderly patients. Against a background of dry skin, a network of fine red superficial fissures creates a 'crazy paving' appearance (Fig. 7.27).

Investigations

None are usually needed. Very extensive cases may be part of malabsorption syndromes, zinc deficiency or internal malignancy.

Treatment

Can be cleared by the use of a mild or moderately potent topical steroid in a greasy base, and aqueous cream as a soap substitute for the area. Baths should be restricted until clearance. Thereafter, daily use of unmedicated emollients (Formulary 1, p. 328) usually prevents recurrence.

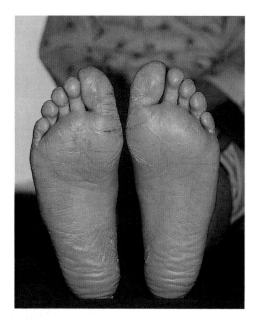

Fig. 7.29 The shiny skin and fissures of juvenile plantar dermatosis.

subsequent sweat gland blockage, and so has been called the 'toxic sock syndrome'! Some feel the condition is a manifestation of atopy.

Presentation and course

The skin of the weight-bearing areas of the feet, particularly the forefeet and undersides of the toes, becomes dry and shiny with deep painful fissures that make walking difficult. The toe webs are spared. Onset can be at any time after shoes are first worn, and even if untreated the condition clears in the early teens.

Investigations

Much time has been wasted in patch testing and scraping for fungus.

Treatment

The child should use a commercially available cork insole in all shoes, and stick to cotton or wool socks. An emollient such as emulsifying ointment or 1% ichthammol paste, or an emollient containing lactic acid, is as good as a topical steroid.

Napkin (diaper) dermatitis

Cause

The most common type of napkin eruption is irritant in origin, and is aggravated by the use of waterproof plastic pants. The mixture of faecal enzymes and ammonia produced by urea-splitting bacteria, if allowed to remain in prolonged contact with the skin, leads to a severe reaction. The overgrowth of yeasts is another aggravating factor. The introduction of modern disposable napkins has, over the last few years, helped to reduce the number of cases sent to our clinics.

Presentation

The moist, often glazed and sore erythema affects the napkin area generally (Fig. 7.30), with the exception of the skin folds, which tend to be spared.

Complications

Superinfection with *Candida albicans* is common, and this may lead to small erythematous papules or vesicopustules appearing around the periphery of the main eruption.

Differential diagnosis

The sparing of the folds helps to separate this condition from infantile seborrhoeic eczema and candidiasis.

Treatment

It is never easy to keep this area clean and dry, but this is the basis of all treatment. Theoretically, the child should be allowed to be free of napkins as much as possible but this may lead to a messy nightmare. On both sides of the Atlantic disposable nappies (diapers) have largely replaced washable ones. The superabsorbent type is best and should be changed regularly, especially in the middle of the night. When towelling napkins are used they should be washed thoroughly and changed frequently. The area should be cleaned at each nappy change with aqueous cream and water. Protective ointments, e.g. zinc and castor oil ointment, or silicone protective ointments, are often useful

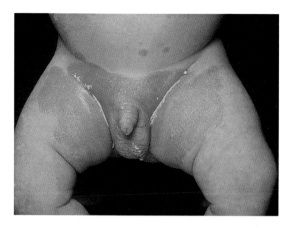

Fig. 7.30 Irritant napkin erythema with a hint of sparing of the skin folds.

(Formulary 1, p. 331), as are topical imidazole preparations that stop yeast growth. Potent steroids should be avoided but combinations of hydrocortisone with antifungals or antiseptics (Formulary 1, p. 332) are often useful.

Further reading

Bieber, T. and Leung, D.Y.M. (2002) *Atopic Dermatitis.* Marcel Dekker, New York.

Bourke, J., Coulson, I. and English, J. (2001) Guidelines for care of contact dermititis. *British Journal of Dermatology* **145**, 877–885.

Bridgett, C., Norén, P. & Staughton, R. (1996) *Atopic Skin Disease: a Manual for Practitioners.* Wrightson Biomedical, Petersfield.

Hanifin, J. and Saurat, J.-H. (2001) Understanding atopic dermatitis pathophysiology and etiology. *Journal of the American Academy of Dermatology,* Suppl. 45/1.

Hanifin, J.M. (2001) 1996 Tacrolimus ointment: advancing the treatment of atopic dermatitis. *Journal of the American Academy of Dermatology,* Suppl. 44/1.

Kanerva, L., Elsner, P., Wahlberg, J.E. & Maibach, H.I. (2000) *Handbook of Occupational Dermatology.* Springer, Berlin.

Rycroft, R.J.G., Menne, T., Frosch, P. & Lepoittevin, J.-P. (2001) *Textbook of Contact Dermatitis,* 3rd edn. Springer, Berlin.

8 Reactive erythemas and vasculitis

Blood vessels can be affected by a variety of insults, both exogenous and endogenous. When this occurs, the epidermis remains unaffected, but the skin becomes red or pink and often oedematous. This is a reactive erythema. If the blood vessels are damaged more severely, as in vasculitis, purpura or larger areas of haemorrhage mask the erythematous colour.

Urticaria (hives, 'nettle-rash')

Urticaria is a common reaction pattern in which pink, itchy or 'burning' swellings (wheals) can occur anywhere on the body. Individual wheals do not last longer than 24 h, but new ones may continue to appear for days, months or even years. Traditionally, urticaria is divided into acute and chronic forms, based on the duration of the disease rather than of individual wheals. Urticaria that persists for more than 6 weeks is classified as chronic. Most patients with chronic urticaria, other than those with an obvious physical cause, have what is often known as 'ordinary urticaria'.

Cause

The signs and symptoms of urticaria are caused by mast cell degranulation, with release of histamine (Fig. 8.1). The mechanisms underlying this may be

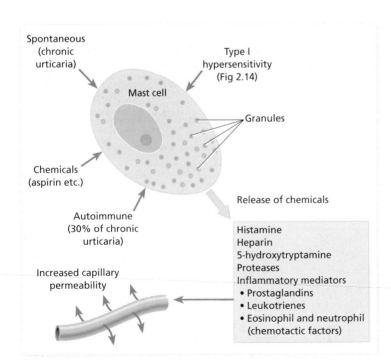

Fig. 8.1 Ways in which a mast cell can be degranulated and the ensuing reaction.

Table 8.1 The main types of urticaria.

Physical
   cold
   solar
   heat
   cholinergic
   dermographism (immediate pressure urticaria)
   delayed pressure
Hypersensitivity
Autoimmune
Pharmacological
Contact

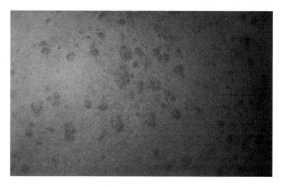

Fig. 8.2 Typical small transient wheals of cholinergic urticaria—in this case triggered by exercise.

different but the end result, increased capillary permeability leading to transient leakage of fluid into the surrounding tissue and development of a wheal, is the same (Fig. 8.1). For example, up to half of those patients with chronic urticaria have circulating antibodies directed against the high affinity immunoglobulin E (IgE) receptor on mast cells whereas the reaction in others in this group may be caused by immediate IgE-mediated hypersensitivity (see Fig. 2.14), direct degranulation by a chemical or trauma, or even spontaneous degranulation.

Classification

The various types of urticaria are listed in Table 8.1. They can often be identified by a careful history; laboratory tests are less useful. The duration of the wheals is an important pointer. Contact and physical urticarias, with the exception of delayed pressure urticaria, start shortly after the stimulus and go within an hour. Individual wheals of other forms resolve within 24 h.

Physical urticarias

Cold urticaria

Patients develop wheals in areas exposed to cold, e.g. on the face when cycling or freezing in a cold wind.

A useful test in the clinic is to reproduce the reaction by holding an ice cube, in a thin plastic bag to avoid wetting, against forearm skin. A few cases are associated with the presence of cryoglobulins, cold agglutinins or cryofibrinogens.

Solar urticaria

Wheals occur within minutes of sun exposure. Some patients with solar urticaria have erythropoietic protoporphyria (p. 287); most have an IgE-mediated urticarial reaction to sunlight.

Heat urticaria

In this condition wheals arise in areas after contact with hot objects or solutions.

Cholinergic urticaria

Anxiety, heat, sexual excitement or strenuous exercise elicits this characteristic response. The vessels overreact to acetylcholine liberated from sympathetic nerves in the skin. Transient 2–5 mm follicular macules or papules (Fig. 8.2) resemble a blush or viral exanthem. Some patients get blotchy patches on their necks.

Dermographism (Fig. 8.3)

This is the most common type of physical urticaria, the skin mast cells releasing extra histamine after rubbing or scratching. The linear wheals are therefore an exaggerated triple response of Lewis. They can readily be reproduced by rubbing the skin of the back lightly at different pressures, or by scratching the back with a fingernail or blunt object.

Delayed pressure urticaria

Sustained pressure causes oedema of the underlying skin and subcutaneous tissue 3–6 h later. The swelling

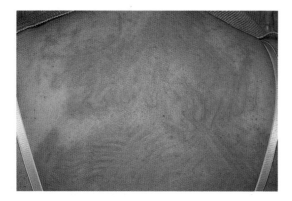

Fig. 8.3 Dermographism: a frenzy of scratching by an already dermographic individual led to this dramatic appearance.

may last up to 48 h and kinins or prostaglandins rather than histamine probably mediate it. It occurs particularly on the feet after walking, on the hands after clapping and on the buttocks after sitting. It can be disabling for manual labourers.

Other types of urticaria

Hypersensitivity urticaria

This common form of urticaria is caused by hypersensitivity, often an IgE-mediated (type I) allergic reaction (Chapter 2). Allergens may be encountered in ten different ways (the 10 'I's listed in Table 8.2).

Autoimmune urticaria

Some patients with chronic urticaria have an autoimmune disease with IgG antibodies to IgE or to

Table 8.2 The 10 'I's of antigen encounter in hypersensitive urticaria.

Ingestion
Inhalation
Instillation
Injection
Insertion
Insect bites
Infestations
Infection
Infusion
Inunction (contact)

FcIgE receptors on mast cells. Here the autoantibody acts as antigen to trigger mast cell degranulation.

Pharmacological urticaria

This occurs when drugs cause mast cells to release histamine in a non-allergic manner (e.g. aspirin, non-steroidal anti-inflammatory drugs (NSAIDs), angiotensin-converting enzyme (ACE) inhibitors and morphine).

Contact urticaria

This may be IgE-mediated or caused by a pharmacological effect. Wheals occur most often around the mouth. Foods and food additives are the most common culprits but drugs, animal saliva, caterpillars and plants may cause the reaction. Recently, latex allergy has become a significant public health concern.

Latex allergy

Possible reactions to the natural rubber latex of the *Hevea brasiliensis* tree include irritant dermatitis, contact allergic dermatitis (Chapter 7) and type I allergy (Chapter 2). Reactions associated with the latter include hypersensitivity urticaria (both by contact and by inhalation), hay fever, asthma, anaphylaxis and, rarely, death.

Medical latex gloves became universally popular after precautions were introduced to protect against HIV and hepatitis B infections. The demand for the gloves increased and this led to alterations in their manufacture and to a flood of high allergen gloves on the market. Cornstarch powder in these gloves bound to the latex proteins so that the allergen became airborne when the gloves were put on. Individuals at increased risk of latex allergy include health care workers, those undergoing multiple surgical procedures (e.g. spina bifida patients) and workers in mechanical, catering and electronic trades. Around 1–6% of the general population is believed to be sensitized to latex.

Latex reactions should be treated on their own merits (see below for urticaria, p. 312 and Fig. 22.5 for anaphylaxis and Chapter 7 for dermatitis). Prevention of latex allergy is equally important. Non-latex (e.g. vinyl) gloves should be worn by those not handling infectious material (e.g. caterers) and, if latex gloves are chosen for those handling infectious material, then powder-free low allergen ones should be used.

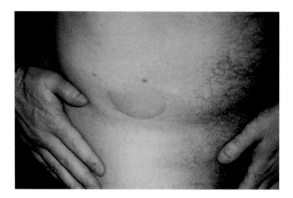

Fig. 8.4 A classic wheal.

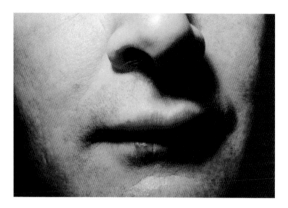

Fig. 8.6 Angioedema of the upper lip.

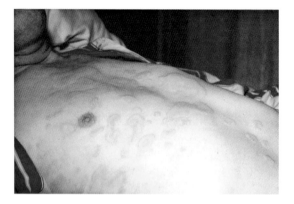

Fig. 8.5 Severe and acute urticaria caused by penicillin allergy.

Presentation

Most types of urticaria share the sudden appearance of pink itchy wheals, which can come up anywhere on the skin surface (Figs 8.4 and 8.5). Each lasts for less than a day, and most disappear within a few hours. Lesions may enlarge rapidly and some resolve centrally to take up an annular shape. In an acute anaphylactic reaction, wheals may cover most of the skin surface. In contrast, in chronic urticaria only a few wheals may develop each day.

Angioedema is a variant of urticaria that primarily affects the subcutaneous tissues, so that the swelling is less demarcated and less red than an urticarial wheal. Angioedema most commonly occurs at junctions between skin and mucous membranes (e.g. peri-orbital, peri-oral and genital; Fig. 8.6). It may be associated with swelling of the tongue and laryngeal mucosa. It sometimes accompanies chronic urticaria and its causes may be the same.

Course

The course of an urticarial reaction depends on its cause. If the urticaria is allergic, it will continue until the allergen is removed, tolerated or metabolized. Most such patients clear up within a day or two, even if the allergen is not identified. Urticaria may recur if the allergen is met again. At the other end of the scale, only half of patients attending hospital clinics with chronic urticaria and angioedema will be clear 5 years later. Those with urticarial lesions alone do better, half being clear after 6 months.

Complications

Urticaria is normally uncomplicated, although its itch may be enough to interfere with sleep or daily activities and to lead to depression. In acute anaphylactic reactions, oedema of the larynx may lead to asphyxiation, and oedema of the tracheo-bronchial tree may lead to asthma.

Differential diagnosis

There are two aspects to the differential diagnosis of urticaria. The first is to tell urticaria from other eruptions that are not urticaria at all. The second is to define the type of urticaria, according to Table 8.1. Insect bites or stings (Fig. 8.7) and infestations commonly elicit urticarial responses, but these may have a central punctum and individual lesions may last longer than 24 h. Erythema multiforme can mimic an annular urticaria. A form of vasculitis (urticarial vasculitis, p. 103) may resemble urticaria, but individual lesions last for longer than 24 h and may leave

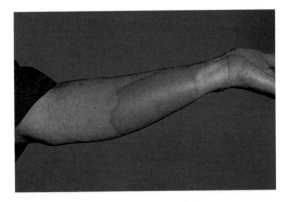

Fig. 8.7 A massive urticarial reaction to a wasp sting.

Table 8.3 Some endogenous causes of urticaria.

Infection
    Viral (e.g. hepatitis, infectious mononucleosis, HIV infection during seroconversion)
    Bacterial
    Mycoplasma
Intestinal parasites
Connective tissue disorders
Hypereosinophilic syndrome (unexplained eosinophilia with multiple internal organ involvement, especially cardiac)
Hyperthyroidism
Cancer
Lymphomas

Table 8.4 Some exogenous causes of urticaria.

Drugs, both topical and systemic
Foods and food additives
Bites
Inhalants
Pollens
Insect venoms
Animal dander

bruising in their wake. Some bullous diseases, such as dermatitis herpetiformis, bullous pemphigoid and pemphigoid gestationis, begin as urticarial papules or plaques, but later bullae make the diagnosis obvious. On the face, erysipelas can be distinguished from angioedema by its sharp margin, redder colour and accompanying pyrexia. Hereditary angioedema must be distinguished from the angioedema accompanying urticaria as their treatments are completely different.

Hereditary angioedema

Recurrent attacks of abdominal pain and vomiting, or massive oedema of soft tissues, which may involve the larynx, characterize this autosomal dominant condition. Urticaria does not accompany the tissue swellings. Tooth extraction, cheek biting and other forms of trauma may precipitate an attack. A deficiency of an inhibitor to C1 esterase allows complement consumption to go unchecked so that vasoactive mediators are generated. To confirm the diagnosis, serum C1 esterase inhibitor level and C4 level should both be checked as the level of C1 esterase inhibitor is not always depressed (there is a type where the inhibitor is present but does not work).

Investigations

The investigations will depend upon the presentation and type of urticaria. Many of the physical urticarias can be reproduced by appropriate physical tests. It is important to remember that antihistamines should be stopped for at least 3 days before these are undertaken.

Almost invariably, more is learned from the history than from the laboratory. The history should include details of the events surrounding the onset of the eruption. A review of systems may uncover evidence of an underlying disease. Careful attention should be paid to drugs, remembering that self-prescribed ones can also cause urticaria. Over-the-counter medications (such as aspirin and herbal remedies) and medications given by other routes (Table 8.2) can produce wheals.

If a patient has acute urticaria and its cause is not obvious, investigations are often deferred until it has persisted for a few weeks; then a physical examination (if not already carried out) and screening tests such as a complete blood count, erythrocyte sedimentation rate (ESR), routine biochemical screen, chest X-ray and urine analysis are worthwhile. If the urticaria continues for 2–3 months, the patient should probably be referred to a dermatologist for further evaluation. In general, the focus of such investigations will be on internal disorders associated with urticaria (Table 8.3) and on external allergens (Table 8.4). Even after extensive evaluation and environmental change, the cause cannot always be found.

In some patients with acute or contact urticaria, allergy testing in the form of radioallergosorbant tests (RAST) or prick tests (Chapter 3), using only allergens suggested by the history, can sometimes be of help. Many patients with chronic urticaria are sure that their problems could be solved by intensive allergy tests, and ask repeatedly for them, but this is seldom worthwhile.

Treatment

The ideal is to find a cause and then to eliminate it. In addition, aspirin—in any form—should be banned. The treatment for each type of urticaria is outlined in Table 8.5. In general, antihistamines are the mainstays of symptomatic treatment. Cetirizine 10 mg/day and loratadine 10 mg/day, both with half-lives of around 12 h, are useful. If necessary, these can be supplemented

Table 8.5 Some types of urticaria and their management.

Type	Treatment
Cold urticaria	Avoid cold
	Protective clothing
	Antihistamines
Solar urticaria	Avoid sun exposure
	Protective clothing
	Sunscreens and sun blocks
	Beta-carotene
	Antihistamines
Cholinergic urticaria	Avoid heat
	Minimize anxiety
	Avoid excessive exercise
	Anticholinergics
	Antihistamines
	Tranquillizers
Dermographism	Avoid trauma
	Antihistamines
Hereditary angioedema	Avoid trauma
	Attenuated androgenic steroids as prophylaxis
	Tracheotomy may be necessary
Hypersensitivity urticarias	Remove cause
	Antihistamines (H1 + H2)
	Sympathomimetics
	Systemic steroids (rarely justified)
	Avoid aspirin-containing drugs

with shorter acting antihistamines, e.g. hydroxyzine 10–25 mg up to every 6 h (Formulary 2, p. 345) and acrivastine, 8 mg three times daily. Alternatively they can be combined with a longer acting antihistamine (such as chlorpheniramine maleate 12 mg sustained-release tablets every 12 h) so that peaks and troughs are blunted, and histamine activity is blocked throughout the night. If the eruption is not controlled, the dose of hydroxyzine can often be increased and still tolerated. H2-blocking antihistamines (e.g. cimetidine) may add a slight benefit if used in conjunction with an H1 histamine antagonist. Chlorpheniramine or diphenhydramine are often used during pregnancy because of their long record of safety, but cetirizine, loratidine and mizolastine should be avoided. Sympathomimetic agents can help urticaria, although the effects of adrenaline (epinephrine) are short lived. Pseudoephedrine (30 or 60 mg every 4 h) or terbutaline (2.5 mg every 8 h) can sometimes be useful adjuncts.

A tapering course of systemic corticosteroids may be used, but only when the cause is known and there are no contraindications, and certainly not as a panacea to control chronic urticaria or urticaria of unknown cause. For the treatment of anaphylaxis see p. 312.

Erythema multiforme

Cause

In erythema multiforme, the victim has usually reacted to an infection, often herpes simplex, or to a drug,

Table 8.6 Some causes of erythema multiforme.

Viral infections, especially:
    herpes simplex
    hepatitis A, B and C
    mycoplasma
    orf
Bacterial infections
Fungal infections
    coccidioidomycosis
Parasitic infestations
Drugs
Pregnancy
Malignancy, or its treatment with radiotherapy
Idiopathic

but other factors have occasionally been implicated
(Table 8.6).

Presentation

The symptoms of an upper respiratory tract infection
may precede the eruption. Typically, annular non-
scaling plaques appear on the palms, soles, forearms
and legs. They may be slightly more purple than the
wheals of ordinary urticaria. Individual lesions enlarge
but clear centrally. A new lesion may begin at the same
site as the original one, so that the two concentric
plaques look like a target (Fig. 8.8). Some lesions
blister. The Stevens–Johnson syndrome is a severe variant of erythema multiforme associated with fever and
mucous membrane lesions. The oral mucosa, lips and
bulbar conjunctivae are most commonly affected, but
the nares, penis, vagina, pharynx, larynx and tracheo-
bronchial tree may also be involved (Fig. 8.9).

Course

Crops of new lesions appear for 1 or 2 weeks, or
until the responsible drug or other factor has been
eliminated. Individual lesions last several days, and
this differentiates them from the more fleeting lesions
of an annular urticaria. The site of resolved lesions
is marked transiently by hyperpigmentation, particularly in pigmented individuals. A recurrent variant of
erythema multiforme exists, characterized by repeated
attacks; this merges with a rare form in which lesions
continue to develop over a prolonged period, even
for years.

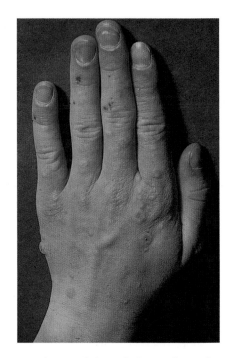

Fig. 8.8 Erythema multiforme: bullous and target lesions
occurring in a favourite site.

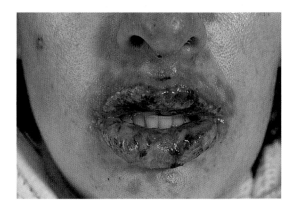

Fig. 8.9 Stevens–Johnson type of erythema multiforme. The
eyelids were also severely involved.

Complications

There are usually no complications. However, severe
lesions in the tracheo-bronchial tree of patients with
Stevens–Johnson syndrome can lead to asphyxia, and
ulcers of the bulbar conjunctiva to blindness. Corneal
ulcers, anterior uveitis and panophthalmitis may also

occur. Genital ulcers can cause urinary retention, and phimosis or vaginal stricture after they heal.

Differential diagnosis

Erythema multiforme can mimic the annular variant of urticaria as described above. However, target lesions are pathognomonic of erythema multiforme. Its acral distribution, the way individual lesions last for more than 24 h, their purple colour and the involvement of mucous membranes all help to identify erythema multiforme. Other bullous disorders may enter the differential diagnosis (Chapter 9).

Investigations

The histology of erythema multiforme is distinctive. Its main features are epidermal necrosis and dermal changes, consisting of endothelial swelling, a mixed lymphohistiocytic perivascular infiltrate and papillary dermal oedema. The abnormalities may be predominantly epidermal or dermal, or a combination of both; they probably depend on the age of the lesion biopsied.

Most investigations are directed towards identifying a cause. A careful history helps rule out a drug reaction. Tzanck smears (p. 35) or culture of suspicious prodromal vesicles may identify a precipitating herpes simplex infection, which usually is almost healed by the time the erythema multiforme erupts. A chest X-ray and serological tests should identify mycoplasmal pneumonia. A search for other infectious agents, neoplasia, endocrine causes or collagen disease is sometimes necessary, especially when the course is prolonged or recurrent. About 50% of cases have no demonstrable provoking factor.

Treatment

The best treatment for erythema multiforme is to identify and remove its cause. In mild cases, only symptomatic treatment is needed and this includes the use of antihistamines.

The Stevens–Johnson syndrome, on the other hand, may demand immediate consultation between dermatologists and specialists in other fields such as ophthalmology, urology and infectious diseases, depending on the particular case. Intravenous infusions of human gammaglobulin seem to be worthwhile. The use of

systemic steroids to abort Stevens–Johnson syndrome is debatable, but many believe that a short course (e.g. prednisolone 80 mg/day in divided doses in an adult) helps. However, the dose should be tapered rapidly or stopped because prolonged treatment in the Stevens–Johnson syndrome has been linked, controversially, with a high complication rate. Good nursing care with attention to the mouth and eyes is essential. The prevention of secondary infection, maintenance of a patent airway, good nutrition, and proper fluid and electrolyte balance are important.

Herpes simplex infections should be suspected in recurrent or continuous erythema multiforme of otherwise unknown cause. Treatment with oral acyclovir 200 mg three to five times daily or valciclovir 500 mg twice daily (Formulary 2, p. 344) may prevent attacks, both of herpes simplex and of the recurrent erythema multiforme which follows it.

Erythema nodosum

Erythema nodosum is an inflammation of the subcutaneous fat (a panniculitis). It is an immunological reaction, elicited by various bacterial, viral and fungal infections, malignant disorders, drugs and by a variety of other causes (Table 8.7).

Presentation

The characteristic lesion is a tender red nodule developing alone or in groups on the legs and forearms or, rarely, on other areas such as the thighs, face, breasts or other areas where there is fat (Fig. 8.10). Some patients also have painful joints and fever.

Table 8.7 Some causes of erythema nodosum.

Infections
  Bacteria (e.g. streptococci, tuberculosis, brucellosis,
  leprosy, yersinia)
  Viruses
  Mycoplasma
  Rickettsia
  Chlamydia
  Fungi (especially coccidioidomycosis)
Drugs (e.g. sulphonamides, oral contraceptive agents)
Systemic disease (e.g. sarcoidosis, ulcerative colitis, Crohn's
  disease, Behçet's disease)

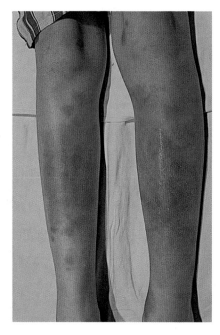

Fig. 8.10 Erythema nodosum: large painful dusky plaques on the shins. Always investigate this important reaction pattern (see text).

Course

Lesions usually resolve in 6–8 weeks. In the interim, lesions may enlarge and new ones may occur at other sites. Like other reactive erythemas, erythema nodosum may persist if its cause is not removed.

Complications

The nodules may be so tender that walking is difficult. Erythema nodosum leprosum occurs when lepromatous leprosy patients establish cell-mediated immunity to *Mycobacterium leprae*. These patients have severe malaise, arthralgia and fever.

Differential diagnosis

The differential diagnosis of a single tender red nodule is extensive and includes trauma, infection (early cellulitis or abscess) and phlebitis.

When lesions are multiple or bilateral, infection becomes less likely unless the lesions are developing in a sporotrichoid manner (p. 200). Other causes of a nodular panniculitis, which may appear like erythema nodosum, include panniculitis from pancreatitis, cold, trauma, injection of drugs or other foreign substances, withdrawal from systemic steroids, lupus erythematosus, superficial migratory thrombophlebitis, polyarteritis nodosa and a deficiency of α_1-antitrypsin. Some people use the term nodular vasculitis to describe a condition like erythema nodosum that lasts for more than 6 months.

Investigations

Erythema nodosum demands a careful history, physical examination, a chest X-ray, throat culture for streptococcus, a Mantoux test and an antistreptolysin-O (ASO) titre. If the results are normal, and there are no symptoms or physical findings to suggest other causes, extensive investigations can be deferred because the disease will usually resolve.

Treatment

The ideal treatment for erythema nodosum is to identify and eliminate its cause if possible. For example, if culture or an ASO test confirms a streptococcal infection, a suitable antibiotic should be recommended. Bed rest is also an important part of treatment. NSAIDs such as aspirin, indomethacin or ibuprofen may be helpful. Systemic steroids are usually not needed. For reasons that are not clear, potassium iodide in a dosage of 400–900 mg/day can help, but should not be used for longer than 6 months.

Vasculitis

Whereas the reactive erythemas are associated with some inflammation around superficial or deep blood

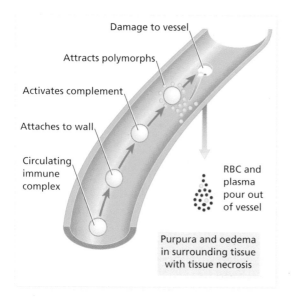

Fig. 8.11 Pathogenesis of vasculitis.

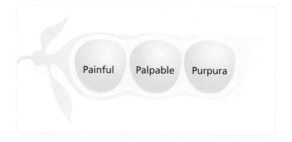

Fig. 8.12 The three 'P's of small vessel vasculitis.

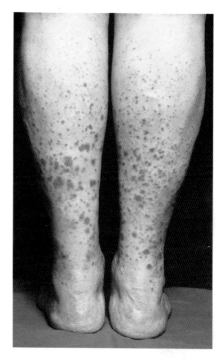

Fig. 8.13 The palpable purpuric lesions of small vessel vasculitis.

vessels, the term vasculitis is reserved for those showing inflammation within the vessel wall, with endothelial cell swelling, necrosis or fibrinoid change. The clinical manifestations depend upon the size of the blood vessel affected.

Leucocytoclastic (small vessel) vasculitis (Syn: allergic or hypersensitivity vasculitis, anaphylactoid purpura)

Cause

Immune complexes may lodge in the walls of blood vessels, activate complement and attract polymorphonuclear leucocytes (Fig. 8.11). Enzymes released from these can degrade the vessel wall. Antigens in these immune complexes include drugs, auto-antigens, and infectious agents such as bacteria.

Presentation

The most common presentation of vasculitis is painful palpable purpura (Fig. 8.12). Crops of lesions arise in dependent areas (the forearms and legs in ambulatory patients, or on the buttocks and flanks in bedridden ones; Fig. 8.13). Some have a small, livid or black centre, caused by necrosis of the tissue overlying the affected blood vessel.

Henoch–Schönlein purpura is a small vessel vasculitis associated with palpable purpura, arthritis and abdominal pain, often preceded by an upper respiratory tract infection. Children are most commonly, but not exclusively, affected.

Urticarial vasculitis is a small vessel vasculitis characterized by urticaria-like lesions which last for longer than 24 h, leaving bruising and then pigmentation (haemosiderin) at the site of previous lesions (Fig. 8.14). There may be foci of purpura in the wheals and other

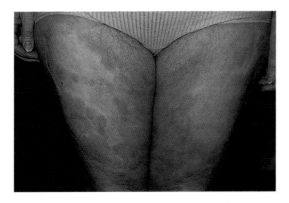

Fig. 8.14 Urticarial vasculitis: a combination of urticaria and bruising.

skin signs include angioedema. General features include malaise and arthralgia.

Course

The course of the vasculitis varies with its cause, its extent, the size of blood vessel affected, and the involvement of other organs.

Complications

Vasculitis may simply be cutaneous; alternatively, it may be systemic and then other organs will be damaged, including the kidney, central nervous system, gastrointestinal tract and lungs.

Differential diagnosis

Small vessel vasculitis has to be separated from other causes of purpura (p. 145) such as abnormalities of the clotting system and sepsis (with or without vasculitis). Vasculitic purpuras are raised (palpable). Occasionally, the vasculitis may look like urticaria if its purpuric element is not marked. Blanching such an urticarial papule with a glass slide may reveal subtle purpura.

Investigations

Investigations should be directed toward identifying the cause and detecting internal involvement. Questioning may indicate infections; myalgias, abdominal pain, claudication, mental confusion and mononeuritis may indicate systemic involvement. A physical exam-

ination, chest X-ray, ESR and biochemical tests monitoring the function of various organs are indicated. However, the most important test is urine analysis, checking for proteinuria and haematuria, because vasculitis can affect the kidney subtly and so lead to renal insufficiency.

Skin biopsy will confirm the diagnosis of small vessel vasculitis. The finding of circulating immune complexes, or a lowered level of total complement (CH50) or C4, will implicate immune complexes as its cause. Tests for hepatitis virus, cryoglobulins, rheumatoid factor and antinuclear antibodies may also be needed.

Direct immunofluorescence can be used to identify immune complexes in blood vessel walls, but is seldom performed because of false-positive and false-negative results, as inflammation may destroy the complexes in a true vasculitis and induce non-specific deposition in other diseases. Henoch–Schönlein vasculitis is confirmed if IgA deposits are found in the blood vessels of a patient with the clinical triad of palpable purpura, arthritis and abdominal pain.

Treatment

The treatment of choice is to identify the cause and eliminate it. In addition, antihistamines and bed rest sometimes help. Colchicine 0.6 mg twice daily or dapsone 100 mg daily may be worth a trial, but require monitoring for side-effects (Formulary 2, p. 352). Patients whose vasculitis is damaging the kidneys or other internal organs may require systemic corticosteroids or immunosuppressive agents such as cyclophosphamide.

Polyarteritis nodosa

Cause

This necrotizing vasculitis of large arteries causes skin nodules, infarctive ulcers and peripheral gangrene.

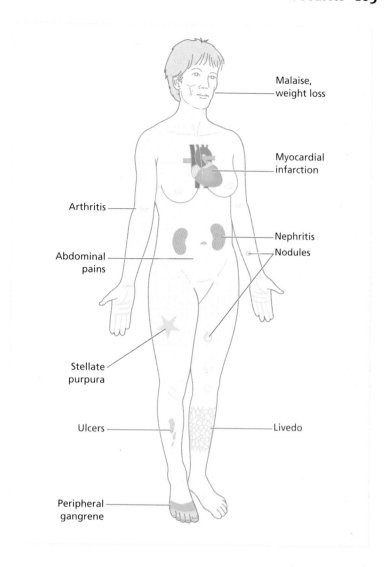

Fig. 8.15 Clinical features of polyarteritis nodosa.

Immune complexes may initiate this vasculitis, and sometimes contain hepatitis B or C virus or antigen. Other known causes are adulterated drugs, B-cell lymphomas and immunotherapy.

Presentation

Tender subcutaneous nodules appear along the line of arteries. The skin over them may ulcerate or develop stellate patches of purpura and necrosis. Splinter haemorrhages and a peculiar net-like vascular pattern (livedo reticularis) aid the clinical diagnosis. The disorder may be of the skin only (cutaneous polyarteritis nodosa), or also affect the kidneys, heart muscle, nerves and joints (Fig. 8.15). Patients may be febrile, lose weight and feel pain in the muscles, joints or abdomen. Some develop peripheral neuropathy, hypertension and ischaemic heart disease. Renal involvement, with or without hypertension, is common.

Course

Untreated, systemic polyarteritis nodosa becomes chronic. Death, often from renal disease, is common, even in treated patients.

Differential diagnosis

Embolism, panniculitis and infarctions can cause a similar clinical picture. Wegener's granulomatosis, allergic granulomatosis, temporal arteritis, and the vasculitis that accompanies systemic lupus erythematosus and rheumatoid arthritis should be considered.

Investigations

The laboratory findings are non-specific. An elevated ESR, neutrophil count, and gammaglobulin level are common. Investigations for cryoglobulins, rheumatoid factor, antinuclear antibody, antineutrophil antibodies and hepatitis C and B surface antigen are worthwhile, as are checks for disease in the kidneys, heart, liver and gut. Low levels of complement suggest active disease. The use of biopsy to confirm the diagnosis of large vessel vasculitis is not always easy as the arterial involvement may be segmental, and surgery itself difficult. Histological confirmation is most likely when biopsies are from a fresh lesion. Affected vessels show aneurysmal dilatation or necrosis, fibrinoid changes in their walls, and an intense neutrophilic infiltrate around and even in the vessel wall.

Treatment

Systemic steroids and cyclophosphamide improve chances of survival. Low-dose systemic steroids alone are usually sufficient for the purely cutaneous form.

Wegener's granulomatosis

In this granulomatous vasculitis of unknown cause, fever, weight loss and fatigue accompany nasorespiratory symptoms such as rhinitis, hearing loss or sinusitis. Only half of the patients have skin lesions, usually symmetrical ulcers or papules on the extremities. Other organs can be affected, including the eye, joints, heart, nerves, lung and kidney. Antineutrophil antibodies are present in most cases and are a useful but non-specific diagnostic marker. Cyclophosphamide is the treatment of choice, used alone or with systemic steroids.

Further reading

Cousin, F., Philips, K., Favier, B., Bienvenu, J. & Nicolas, J.F. (2001) Drug-induced urticaria. *European Journal of Dermatology* 11, 181–187.

Cuellar, M.L. & Espinoza, L.R. (2000) Laboratory testing in the evaluation and diagnosis of vasculitis. *Current Rheumatology Reports* 2, 417–422.

Grattan, C., Powell, S. & Humphreys, F. (2001) Management and diagnostic guidelines for urticaria and angio-oedema. *British Journal of Dermatology* 144, 708–714.

Greaves, M.W. (2001) Antihistamines. *Dermatologic Clinics* 19, 53–62.

Joint Task Force on Practice Parameters (2000) The diagnosis and management of urticaria: a practice parameter. I. Acute urticaria/angioedema. II. Chronic urticaria/angioedema. *Annals of Allergy, Asthma and Immunology* 85, 521–544.

Lotti, T., Ghersetich, I., Comacci, C. & Jorizzo, J.L. (1998) Cutaneous small vessel vasculitis. *Journal of the American Academy of Dermatology* 39, 667–687.

Schachner, L.A. (2000) Erythema multiforme. *Pediatric Dermatology* 17, 75–83.

Sharma, J.K., Miller, R. & Murray, S. (2000) Chronic urticaria: a Canadian perspective on patterns and practical management strategies. *Journal of Cutaneous Medicine and Surgery* 4, 89–93.

Wakelin, S.H. (2001) Contact urticaria. *Clinical and Experimental Dermatology* 26, 132–136.

Bullous diseases

Blisters are accumulations of fluid within or under the epidermis. They have many causes, and a correct clinical diagnosis must be based on a close study of the physical signs.

The appearance of a blister is determined by the level at which it forms. Subepidermal blisters occur between the dermis and the epidermis. Their roofs are relatively thick and so they tend to be tense and intact. They may contain blood. Intraepidermal blisters appear within the prickle cell layer of the epidermis, and so have thin roofs and rupture easily to leave an oozing denuded surface: this tendency is even more marked with subcorneal blisters, which form just beneath the stratum corneum at the outermost edge of the viable epidermis, and therefore have even thinner roofs.

Sometimes the morphology or distribution of a bullous eruption gives the diagnosis away, as in herpes simplex or zoster. Sometimes the history helps too, as in cold or thermal injury, or in an acute contact dermatitis. When the cause is not obvious, a biopsy should be taken to show the level in the skin at which the blister has arisen. A list of differential diagnoses, based on the level at which blisters form, is given in Fig. 9.1.

The bulk of this chapter is taken up by the three most important immunobullous disorders—pemphigus, pemphigoid and dermatitis herpetiformis (Table 9.1) —and by the group of inherited bullous disorders known as epidermolysis bullosa. Our understanding of both groups has advanced in parallel, as several of the skin components targeted by autoantibodies in the immunobullous disorders are the same as those inherited in an abnormal form in epidermolysis bullosa.

Bullous disorders of immunological origin

In pemphigus and pemphigoid, the damage is done by autoantibodies directed at molecules that norm-

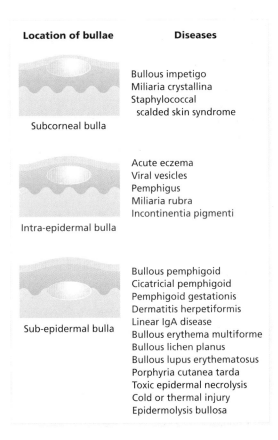

Fig. 9.1 The differential diagnosis of bullous diseases based on the histological location of the blister.

ally bind the skin (p. 11 and p. 15). This type of mechanism has not yet been proven for dermatitis herpetiformis; but the characteristic deposition of immunoglobulin (Ig) A in the papillary dermis, and an association with a variety of autoimmune disorders, both suggest an immunological basis for the disease.

Table 9.1 Distinguishing features of the three main immunobullous diseases.

	Age	Site of blisters	General health	Blisters in mouth	Nature of blisters	Circulating antibodies	Fixed antibodies	Treatment
Pemphigus	Middle age	Trunk, flexures and scalp	Poor	Common	Superficial and flaccid	IgG to intercellular adhesion proteins	IgG in intercellular space	Steroids Immunosuppressives
Pemphigoid	Old	Often flexural	Good	Rare	Tense and blood-filled	IgG to basement membrane region	IgG at basement membrane	Steroids Immunosuppressives
Dermatitis herpetiformis	Primarily adults	Elbows, knees, upper back, buttocks	Itchy	Rare	Small, excoriated and grouped	IgG to the endomysium of muscle	IgA granular deposits in papillary dermis	Gluten-free diet Dapsone Sulphapyridine

Pemphigus

Pemphigus is severe and potentially life-threatening. There are two main types. The most common is pemphigus vulgaris, which accounts for at least three-quarters of all cases, and for most of the deaths. Pemphigus vegetans is a rare variant of pemphigus vulgaris. The other important type of pemphigus, superficial pemphigus, also has two variants: the generalized foliaceus type and localized erythematosus type. A few drugs, led by penicillamine, can trigger a pemphigus-like reaction, but autoantibodies are then seldom found. Finally, a rare type of pemphigus (paraneoplastic pemphigus) has been described in association with a thymoma or an underlying carcinoma; it is characterized by unusually severe mucosal lesions.

Cause

All types of pemphigus are autoimmune diseases in which pathogenic IgG antibodies bind to antigens within the epidermis. The main antigens are desmoglein 3 (in pemphigus vulgaris) and desmoglein 1 (in superficial pemphigus). Both are cell-adhesion molecules of the cadherin family (see Table 2.5), found in desmosomes. The antigen–antibody reaction interferes with adhesion, causing the keratinocytes to fall apart.

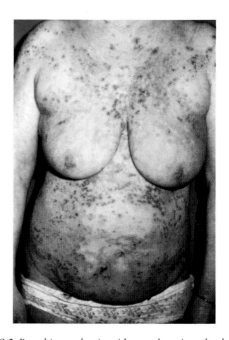

Fig. 9.2 Pemphigus vulgaris: widespread erosions that have followed blisters.

Presentation

Pemphigus vulgaris is characterized by flaccid blisters of the skin (Fig. 9.2) and mouth (Fig. 9.3) and, after the blisters rupture, by widespread painful erosions. Most patients develop the mouth lesions first. Shearing

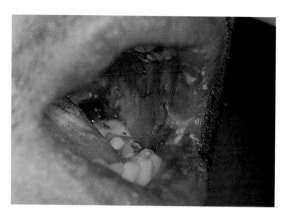

Fig. 9.3 Painful sloughy mouth ulcers in pemphigus vulgaris.

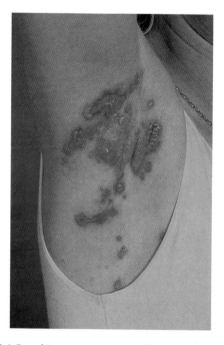

Fig. 9.4 Pemphigus vegetans in the axilla, some intact blisters can be seen.

stresses on normal skin can cause new erosions to form (a positive Nikolsky sign). In the vegetans variant (Fig. 9.4), heaped up cauliflower-like weeping areas are present in the groin and body folds. The blisters in pemphigus foliaceus are so superficial, and rupture so easily, that the clinical picture is dominated more by weeping and crusting erosions than by blisters. In the rarer pemphigus erythematosus, the facial lesions are often pink, dry and scaly.

Course

The course of all forms of pemphigus is prolonged, even with treatment, and the mortality rate of pemphigus vulgaris is still at least 15%. Superficial pemphigus is less severe. With modern treatments, most patients with pemphigus can live relatively normal lives, with occasional exacerbations.

Complications

Complications are inevitable with the high doses of steroids and immunosuppressive drugs that are needed to control the condition. Indeed, side-effects of treatment are now the leading cause of death. Infections of all types are common. The large areas of denudation may become infected and smelly, and severe oral ulcers make eating painful.

Differential diagnosis

Widespread erosions may suggest a pyoderma, impetigo, epidermolysis bullosa or ecthyma. Mouth ulcers can be mistaken for aphthae, Behçet's disease or a herpes simplex infection.

Investigations

Biopsy shows that the vesicles are intraepidermal, with rounded keratinocytes floating freely within the blister cavity (acantholysis). Direct immunofluorescence (p. 39) of adjacent normal skin shows intercellular epidermal deposits of IgG and C3 (Fig. 9.5). The serum from a patient with pemphigus contains antibodies that bind to the desmogleins in the desmosomes of normal epidermis, so that indirect immunofluorescence (p. 39) can also be used to confirm the diagnosis. The titre of these antibodies correlates loosely with clinical activity and may guide changes in the dosage of systemic steroids.

> **LEARNING POINT**
>
> Pemphigus is more attacking than pemphigoid and needs higher doses of steroids to control it.

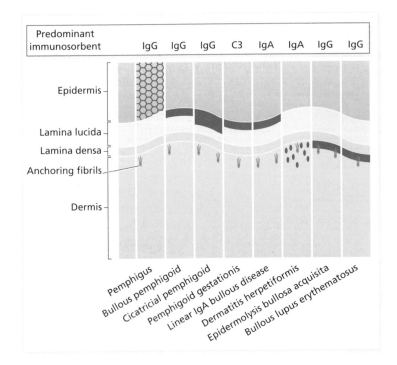

| Predominant immunosorbent | IgG | IgG | IgG | C3 | IgA | IgA | IgG | IgG |

Epidermis

Lamina lucida

Lamina densa

Anchoring fibrils

Dermis

Pemphigus · Bullous pemphigoid · Cicatricial pemphigoid · Pemphigoid gestationis · Linear IgA bullous disease · Dermatitis herpetiformis · Epidermolysis bullosa acquisita · Bullous lupus erythematosus

Fig. 9.5 Immunofluorescence (red) in bullous diseases.

Treatment

Because of the dangers of pemphigus vulgaris, and the difficulty in controlling it, patients should be treated in a specialized unit. Resistant and severe cases need very high doses of systemic steroids, such as prednisolone (Formulary 2, p. 348) 80–320 mg/day, and the dose is dropped only when new blisters stop appearing. Immunosuppressive agents, such as azathioprine or cyclophosphamide and, recently, mycophenylate mofetil, are often used as steroid-sparing agents. New and promising approaches include plasmapheresis and intravenous immunoglobulin as used in other autoimmune diseases. Treatment needs regular follow-up and is usually prolonged. In superficial pemphigus, smaller doses are usually needed, and the use of topical corticosteroids may help too.

Other causes of subcorneal and intraepidermal blistering

Bullous impetigo (p. 190)

This is a common cause of blistering in children. The bullae are flaccid, often contain pus and are frequently grouped or located in body folds. Bullous impetigo is caused by *Staphylococcus aureus*.

Scalded skin syndrome (p. 192)

A toxin elaborated by some strains of *S. aureus* makes the skin painful and red; later it peels like a scald. The staphylococcus is usually hidden (e.g. conjunctiva, throat, wound, furuncle).

Miliaria crystallina (p. 161)

Here sweat accumulates under the stratum corneum leading to the development of multitudes of uniformly spaced vesicles without underlying redness. Often this occurs after a fever or heavy exertion. The vesicles look like droplets of water lying on the surface, but the skin is dry to the touch. The disorder is self-limiting and needs no treatment.

Subcorneal pustular dermatosis

As its name implies, the lesions are small groups of pustules rather than vesicles. However, the pustules pout out of the skin in a way that suggests they were once vesicles (like the vesico-pustules of chickenpox).

The cause of this rare disease is unknown, but oral dapsone (Formulary 2, p. 351) usually suppresses it.

Acute dermatitis (Chapter 7)

Severe acute eczema, especially of the contact allergic type, can be bullous. Plants such as poison ivy, poison oak or primula are common causes. The varied size of the vesicles, their close grouping, their asymmetry, their odd configurations (e.g. linear, square, rectilinear) and a history of contact with plants are helpful guides to the diagnosis.

Pompholyx (p. 89)

In pompholyx, highly itchy small eczematous vesicles occur along the sides of the fingers, and sometimes also on the palms and soles. Some call it 'dyshidrotic eczema', but the vesicles are not related to sweating or sweat ducts. The disorder is very common, but its cause is not known.

Viral infections (Chapter 14)

Some viruses create blisters in the skin by destroying epithelial cells. The vesicles of herpes simplex and zoster are the most common examples.

Transient acantholytic dermatosis (Grover's disease)

Itchy vesicles appear on the sun-damaged skin of the trunk, usually of middle-aged males. The cause is not known and the condition can be persistent—despite its name.

Subepidermal immunobullous disorders

These can be hard to separate on clinical grounds and only the two most important, pemphigoid and dermatitis herpetiformis, are described in detail here. Several others are mentioned briefly.

Pemphigoid

Pemphigoid is an autoimmune disease. Serum from about 70% of patients contains antibodies that bind *in vitro* to normal skin at the basement membrane zone.

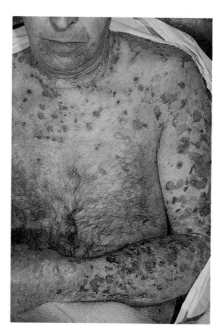

Fig. 9.6 Numerous large tense blisters in an elderly person suggest pemphigoid.

However, their titre does not correlate with clinical disease activity. The IgG antibodies bind to two main antigens: most commonly to BP230 (within the cellular part of the hemidesmosome, p. 15), and less often to BP180 (a transmembrane molecule with one end within the hemidesmosome and the other bound to the lamina lucida). Complement is then activated (p. 24), an inflammatory cascade starts and mast cells degranulate, liberating a variety of inflammatory mediators.

Presentation

Pemphigoid is a chronic, usually itchy, blistering disease, mainly affecting the elderly. The tense bullae can arise from normal skin but usually do so from urticarial plaques (Fig. 9.6). The flexures are often affected; the mucous membranes usually are not. The Nikolsky test is negative.

Course

Pemphigoid is usually self-limiting and treatment can often be stopped after 1–2 years.

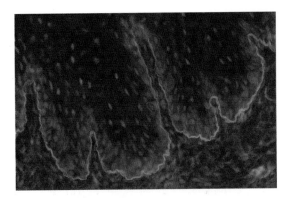

Fig. 9.7 Indirect immunofluorescence using serum from a patient with pemphigoid, showing basement zone immunofluorescence.

Complications

Untreated, the disease causes much discomfort and loss of fluid from ruptured bullae. Systemic steroids and immunosuppressive agents carry their usual complications if used long-term (Formulary 2, p. 348 and p. 346, respectively). The validity of a possible association with internal malignancy is still debated.

Differential diagnosis

Pemphigoid may look like other bullous diseases, especially epidermolysis bullosa acquisita, bullous lupus erythematosus, dermatitis herpetiformis, pemphigoid gestationis, bullous erythema multiforme and linear IgA bullous disease. Immunofluorescence helps to separate it from these (Fig. 9.5).

Investigations

The histology is that of a subepidermal blister, often filled with eosinophils. Direct immunofluorescence shows a linear band of IgG and C3 along the basement membrane zone. Indirect immunofluorescence, using serum from the patient, identifies IgG antibodies that react with the basement membrane zone in some 70% of patients (Fig. 9.7).

Treatment

In the acute phase, prednisolone or prednisone (Formulary 2, p. 348) at a dosage of 40–60 mg/day is usually needed to control the eruption. Immuno-suppressive agents may also be required. The dosage is reduced as soon as possible, and patients end up on a low maintenance regimen of systemic steroids, taken on alternate days until treatment is stopped. For unknown reasons, tetracyclines and niacinamide help some patients.

Pemphigoid gestationis (herpes gestationis)

This is pemphigoid occurring in pregnancy, or in the presence of a hydatidiform mole or a choriocarcinoma. As in pemphigoid, most patients have linear deposits of C3 along the basement membrane zone (Fig. 9.5), although IgG is detected less often. The condition usually remits after the birth but may return in future pregnancies. It is not caused by a herpes virus: the name herpes gestationis should be discarded now so that the disease is not confused with herpes genitalis. Treatment is with systemic steroids. Oral contraceptives should be avoided.

Cicatricial pemphigoid (Fig. 9.8)

Like pemphigoid itself, cicatricial pemphigoid is an autoimmune skin disease showing IgG and C3 deposition at the basement membrane zone (Fig. 9.5). The antigens are often as in pemphigoid, but other antigens are sometimes targeted such as laminin 5 (in anchoring filaments). The condition differs from pemphigoid in that its blisters and ulcers occur mainly on mucous membranes such as the conjunctivae, the mouth and genital tract. Bullae on the skin itself are uncommon. Lesions heal with scarring: around the eyes this may cause blindness, especially when the palpebral conjunctivae are affected (Fig. 9.8). The condition tends to persist and treatment is relatively ineffective, although very potent local steroids, systemic steroids and immunosuppressive agents are

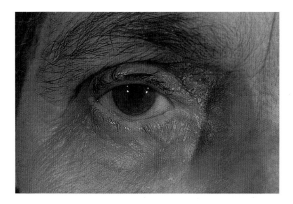

Fig. 9.8 Longstanding cicatricial pemphigoid. Adhesions are now forming between the upper and lower eyelids.

usually tried. Good eye hygiene and the removal of ingrowing eyelashes are important.

Linear IgA bullous disease

This is clinically similar to pemphigoid, but affects children as well as adults. Blisters arise on urticarial plaques, and are more often grouped, and on extensor surfaces, than is the case with pemphigoid. The so-called 'string of pearls sign', seen in some affected children, is the presence of blistering around the rim of polycyclic urticarial lesions. The conjunctivae may be involved. Linear IgA bullous disease is, as its name implies, associated with linear deposits of IgA and C3 at the basement membrane zone (Fig. 9.5). IgG is sometimes also found. The disorder responds well to oral dapsone (Formulary 2, p. 352).

Acquired epidermolysis bullosa

This can also look like pemphigoid, but has two important extra features: many of the blisters are a response to trauma and arise on otherwise normal skin; and milia are a feature of healing lesions. The target of the autoantibodies is type VII collagen in anchoring fibrils (see Fig. 9.5). The antigen lies on the dermal side of the lamina densa, in contrast to the pemphigoid antigens, which lie on the epidermal side—a difference that can be demonstrated when the basement membrane is split by incubating skin in a saline solution (the 'salt-split' technique). The condition responds poorly to systemic corticosteroids or immunosuppressive agents.

Dermatitis herpetiformis

Dermatitis herpetiformis is a very itchy chronic subepidermal vesicular disease, in which the vesicles erupt in groups as in herpes simplex—hence the name 'herpetiformis'.

Cause

Gluten-sensitive enteropathy, demonstrable by small bowel biopsy, is always present, but most patients do not suffer from diarrhoea, constipation or malnutrition as the enteropathy is mild, patchy and involves only the proximal small intestine. Absorption of gluten, or another dietary antigen, may form circulating immune complexes that lodge in the skin. A range of antibodies can be detected, notably directed against reticulin, gliadin and endomysium—a component of smooth muscle. Granular deposits of IgA and C3 in the superficial dermis under the basement membrane zone (Fig. 9.5) induce inflammation, which then separates the epidermis from the dermis. These deposits clear slowly after the introduction of a gluten-free diet.

Presentation

The extremely itchy, grouped vesicles (Fig. 9.9) and urticated papules develop particularly over the elbows (Fig. 9.10) and knees, buttocks and shoulders. They are often broken by scratching before they reach any size. A typical patient therefore shows only grouped excoriations, sometimes with eczema-like changes added by scratching.

Course

The condition typically lasts for decades.

Complications

The complications of gluten-sensitive enteropathy include diarrhoea, abdominal pain, anaemia and, rarely, malabsorption. Small bowel lymphomas have been reported, and the use of a gluten-free diet may reduce this risk. There is a proven association with other autoimmune diseases, most commonly of the thyroid. Treatment, notably with dapsone (Formulary 2, p. 352), can cause side-effects.

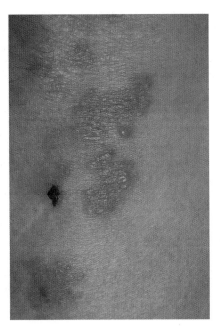

Fig. 9.9 The typical small tense grouped itchy blisters of dermatitis herpetiformis.

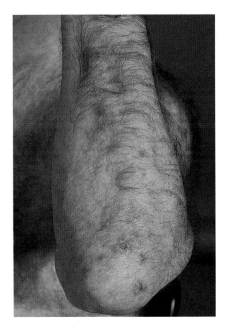

Fig. 9.10 The itchy blisters of dermatitis herpetiformis favour the points of the elbows and knees, where they are quickly destroyed by scratching.

Differential diagnosis

The disorder masquerades as scabies, an excoriated eczema, insect bites or neurodermatitis.

Investigations

If a vesicle can be biopsied before it is scratched away, the histology will be that of a subepidermal blister, with neutrophils packing the adjacent dermal papillae. Direct immunofluorescence of uninvolved skin shows granular deposits of IgA, and usually C3, in the dermal papillae and superficial dermis (Fig. 9.5). Small bowel biopsy is no longer recommended as routine because the changes are often patchy. Tests for malabsorption are seldom needed.

Treatment

The disorder responds to a gluten-free diet, which should be supervised by a dietitian. Adherence to this can be monitored using the titre of antiendomysial antibody, which should fall if gluten is strictly avoided. The bowel changes revert quickly to normal but

IgA deposits remain in the skin, and the skin disease can drag on for many months. Because of this, and because a gluten-free diet is hard to follow and enjoy, some patients prefer to combine the diet with dapsone (Formulary 2, p. 352) or sulphapyridine (sulfapyridine) at the start, although both can cause severe rashes, haemolytic anaemia (especially in those with glucose-6-phosphate dehydrogenase deficiency), leucopenia, thrombocytopenia, methaemoglobinaemia and peri-

> **LEARNING POINTS**
>
> **1** Biopsy non-involved skin to demonstrate the diagnostic granular deposits of IgA in the dermal papillae.
> **2** The gluten enteropathy of dermatitis herpetiformis seldom causes frank malabsorption.
> **3** Dapsone works quickly and a gluten-free diet only very slowly. Combine the two at the start and slowly reduce the dapsone.

pheral neuropathy. Regular blood checks are therefore necessary.

Other causes of subepidermal blisters

Porphyria cutanea tarda (p. 287)

The bullae and erosions occur on the backs of the hands and on other areas exposed to sunlight.

Blisters in diabetes and renal disease

A few diabetics develop unexplained blisters on their legs or feet. The backs of the hands of patients with chronic renal failure may show changes rather like those of porphyria cutanea tarda (pseudoporphyria). Frusemide (furosemide) can contribute to blister formation.

Bullous lupus erythematosus

Vesicles and bullae may be seen in severe active systemic lupus erythematosus (p. 119). This disorder is uncommon and carries a high risk of kidney disease. Non-cutaneous manifestations of systemic lupus erythematosus do not respond to dapsone; however, the bullae do.

Bullous erythema multiforme

Bullous erythema multiforme in the form of the Stevens–Johnson syndrome is discussed in Chapter 8.

Toxic epidermal necrolysis (Lyell's disease)

Cause

Toxic epidermal necrolysis is usually a drug reaction, most commonly to sulphonamides, barbiturates, carbamazepine or allopurinol (Chapter 22), but can also be a manifestation of graft-vs.-host disease. Sometimes it is unexplained.

Presentation

The skin becomes red and intensely painful, and then begins to come off in sheets like a scald. This leaves an eroded painful glistening surface (Fig. 9.11). Nikolsky's

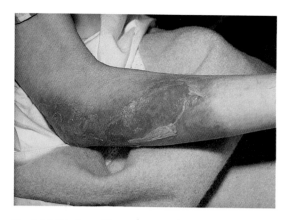

Fig. 9.11 The burn-like appearance of toxic epidermal necrolysis.

sign is positive (p. 109). The mucous membranes may be affected, including the mouth, eyes, and even the bronchial tree.

Course

The condition usually clears if the offending drug is stopped. New epidermis grows out from hair follicles so that skin grafts are not usually needed. The disorder may come back if the drug is taken again.

Complications

Toxic epidermal necrolysis is a skin emergency and can be fatal. Infection, and the loss of fluids and electrolytes, are life-threatening, and the painful denuded skin surfaces make life a misery. Corneal scarring may remain when the acute episode has settled.

Differential diagnosis

The epidermolysis of the staphylococcal scalded skin syndrome (p. 192) looks like toxic epidermal necrolysis clinically, but only the stratum corneum is lost. Whereas toxic epidermal necrolysis affects adults, the staphylococcal scalded skin syndrome is seen in infancy or early childhood. Histology differentiates the two. Pemphigus may also look similar, but starts more slowly and is more localized. Severe graft-vs.-host reactions can also cause this syndrome. Some believe that toxic epidermal necrolysis can evolve from Stevens–Johnson syndrome because some patients have the clinical features of both.

Investigations

Biopsy helps to confirm the diagnosis. The split is subepidermal in toxic epidermal necrolysis, and the entire epidermis may be necrotic. A frozen section provides a quick answer if there is genuine difficulty in separating toxic epidermal necrolysis from the scalded skin syndrome (p. 192). There are no tests to tell which drug, if any, caused the disease.

Treatment

If toxic epidermal necrolysis is caused by a drug, this must be stopped (Chapter 22); otherwise, treatment relies mainly on symptomatic management. Intensive nursing care and medical support are needed, including the use of central venous lines, intravenous fluids and electrolytes. Many patients are treated in units designed to deal with extensive thermal burns. Air suspension beds increase comfort. The weight of opinion has turned against the use of systemic corticosteroids but, if they are given, it should be for short periods only, right at the start. Intravenous IgG seems more promising.

Epidermolysis bullosa

There are many types of epidermolysis bullosa: the five main ones are listed in Table 9.2. All are characterized by an inherited tendency to develop blisters after minimal trauma, although at different levels in the skin (Fig. 9.12). The more severe types have a catastrophic impact on the lives of sufferers. Acquired

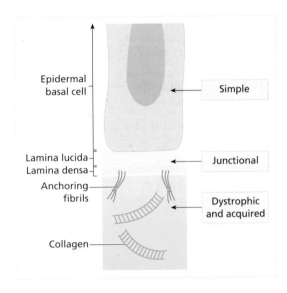

Fig. 9.12 Levels of blister formation in epidermolysis bullosa at the dermo-epidermal junction.

epidermolysis bullosa is not inherited and was discussed earlier in this chapter.

Simple epidermolysis bullosa

Several subtypes are recognized, of which the most common are the Weber–Cockayne (mainly affecting the hands and feet) and the Dowling–Meara (featuring herpetiform blisters on the trunk) types. Most are inherited as autosomal dominant conditions and are caused by abnormalities in genes responsible for production of the paired keratins (K5 and K14) expressed

Table 9.2 Simplified classification of epidermolysis bullosa.

Type	Mode of inheritance	Level of split	Mutations in
Simple epidermolysis bullosa	Usually autosomal dominant	Intraepidermal	Keratins 5 and 14
Junctional epidermolysis bullosa (epidermolysis bullosa letalis)	Autosomal recessive	Lamina lucida	Components of the hemidesmosome-anchoring filaments (e.g. laminins, integrins and bullous pemphigoid 180 molecule)
Dystrophic epidermolysis bullosa	Autosomal dominant	Beneath lamina densa	Type VII collagen
Dystrophic epidermolysis bullosa	Autosomal recessive	Beneath lamina densa	Type VII collagen
Acquired epidermolysis bullosa	Not inherited	Dermal side of lamina densa	Nil

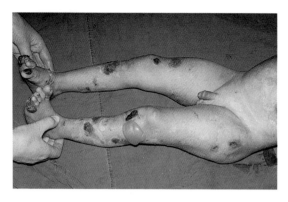

Fig. 9.13 Junctional epidermolysis bullosa: minor trauma has caused large blisters and erosions which will heal slowly or not at all.

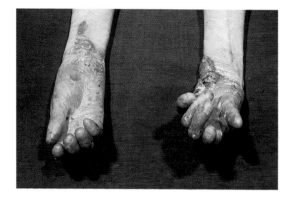

Fig. 9.14 Autosomal recessive dystrophic epidermolysis bullosa: note large blood-filled blister. Scarring has led to fixed deformity of the fingers and loss of nails.

in basal keratinocytes (see Fig. 2.4). Linkage studies show that the genetic defects responsible for the most common types of simple epidermolysis bullosa lie on chromosomes 17 and 12.

Blisters form within or just above the basal cell layers of the epidermis and so tend to heal without scarring. Nails and mucosae are not involved. The problems are made worse by sweating and ill-fitting shoes. Blistering can be minimized by avoiding trauma, wearing soft well-fitting shoes and using foot powder. Large blisters should be pricked with a sterile needle and dressed. Their roofs should not be removed. Local antibiotics may be needed.

Junctional epidermolysis bullosa

The abnormalities in the basal lamina include loss of anchoring filaments and defective laminins (p. 15; see Fig. 2.9). This rare and often lethal condition is evident at birth. The newborn child has large raw areas and flaccid blisters, which are slow to heal (Fig. 9.13). The peri-oral and peri-anal skin is usually involved, as are the nails and oral mucous membrane. There is no effective systemic treatment. Hopes for the future include adding the normal gene to epidermal stem cells, and then layering these onto the denuded skin.

Dystrophic epidermolysis bullosa

There are many subtypes, all of which probably result from abnormalities of collagen VII, the major structural component of anchoring fibrils.

Autosomal dominant dystrophic epidermolysis bullosa

In this type blisters appear in late infancy. They are most common on friction sites (e.g. the knees, elbows and fingers), healing with scarring and milia formation. The nails may be deformed or even lost. The mouth is not affected. The only treatment is to avoid trauma and to dress the blistered areas.

Autosomal recessive dystrophic epidermolysis bullosa

In this tragic form of epidermolysis bullosa, blisters start in infancy. They are subepidermal and may be filled with blood. They heal with scarring, which can be so severe that the nails are lost and webs form between the digits (Fig. 9.14). The hands and feet may become useless balls, having lost all fingers and toes. The teeth, mouth and upper part of the oesophagus are all affected; oesophageal strictures may form. Squamous cell carcinomas of the skin are a late complication. Treatment is unsatisfactory. Phenytoin, which reduces the raised dermal collagenase levels found in this variant, and systemic steroids are disappointing. It is especially important to minimize trauma, to prevent contractures and web formation between the digits, and to combat anaemia and secondary infection. Referral to centres with expertise in management of these patients is strongly recommended.

Further reading

Cotell, S., Robinson, N.D. & Chan, L.S. (2000) Autoimmune blistering skin diseases. *American Journal of Emergency Medicine* 18, 288–299.

Fleming, T.E. & Korman, N.J. (2000) Cicatricial pemphigoid. *Journal of the American Academy of Dermatology* 43, 571–591.

Nousari, H.C. & Anhalt, G.J. (1999) Pemphigus and bullous pemphigoid. *Lancet* 354, 667–672.

Schmidt, E. & Zillikens, D. (2000) Autoimmune and inherited subepidermal blistering diseases: advances in the clinic and the laboratory. *Advances in Dermatology* 16, 113–157.

Connective tissue disorders

The cardinal feature of these conditions is inflammation in the connective tissue which leads to dermal atrophy or sclerosis, to arthritis, and sometimes to abnormalities in other organs. In addition, antibodies form against normal tissues and cellular components; these disorders are therefore classed as autoimmune. Many have difficulty in remembering which antibody features in which condition: Table 10.1 should help here.

The main connective tissue disorders present as a spectrum ranging from the benign cutaneous variants to severe multisystem diseases (Table 10.2).

Lupus erythematosus

Lupus erythematosus (LE) is a good example of such a spectrum, ranging from the purely cutaneous type (discoid LE), through patterns associated with some internal problems (disseminated discoid LE and sub-acute cutaneous LE), to a severe multisystem disease (systemic lupus erythematosus, SLE; Table 10.2).

Systemic lupus erythematosus

Cause

This is unknown, but hereditary factors, e.g. complement deficiency and certain HLA types, increase susceptibility. Particles looking like viruses have been seen in endothelial cells, and in other tissues, but their role is not clear. Patients with LE have autoantibodies to DNA, nuclear proteins and to other normal antigens, and this points to an autoimmune cause. Exposure to sunlight and artificial ultraviolet radiation (UVR), pregnancy and infection may precipitate the disease or lead to flare-ups. Some drugs, such as hydralazine and procainamide trigger SLE in a dose-dependent way, whereas others including oral contraceptives, anticonvulsants, minocycline and captopril, precipitate the disease just occasionally.

Presentation

Typically, but not always, the onset is acute. SLE is an uncommon disorder, affecting women more often than men (in a ratio of about 8 : 1). The classic rash of acute SLE is an erythema of the cheeks and nose in the rough shape of a butterfly (Figs 10.1 and 10.2), with facial swelling. Occasionally, a few blisters may be seen. Some patients develop widespread discoid papulosquamous plaques very like those of discoid LE; others, about 20% of patients, have no skin disease at any stage.

Other dermatological features include peri-ungual telangiectasia (see Fig. 10.7), erythema over the digits, hair fall (especially at the frontal margin of the scalp), and photosensitivity. Ulcers may occur on the palate, tongue or buccal mucosa.

Course

The skin changes may be transient, continuous or recurrent; they correlate well with the activity of the systemic disease. Acute SLE may be associated with fever, arthritis, nephritis, polyarteritis, pleurisy, pneumonitis, pericarditis, myocarditis and involvement of the central nervous system. Internal involvement can be fatal, but the overall prognosis now is for about three-quarters of patients to survive for 15 years. Renal involvement suggests a poorer prognosis.

Complications

The skin disease may cause scarring or hyperpigmentation, but the main dangers lie with damage to other

Table 10.1 Some important associations with non-organ-specific autoantibodies.

	Antibody directed against									
	Nucleoprotein (ANA or ANF)* (IF pattern in brackets)	Double stranded DNA	Ro (SSA) and La (SSB)	Sm (ENA)	Cardiolipin	Nuclear RNP	Centromere	Histones	Jo-1	Topoisomerase (Scl-70)
Discoid LE	+ive in up to 35% (homogenous and speckled)		Rarely +ive							
Subacute LE	+ive in up to 80% (homogenous and speckled)		+ive in 60%							
Systemic LE	+ive in up to 100% (homogenous and speckled)	+ive in 50–70% (esp with nephritis)	May be +ive (e.g. 20%) if ANF –ive	+ive in 30%	+ive in subset with recurrent abortions, thrombosis, livedo and skin necrosis		+ive in 6%	+ive in drug-induced cases		
Dermatomyositis	+ive in up to 80% (speckled)					Occasionally +ive			+ive in 20%	
Systemic sclerosis	+ive in up to 90% (speckled and nucleolar)						+ive in up to 50%			+ive in 20%
Mixed connective tissue disorder	+ive in 100% (speckled)			+ive in high titre—up to 100%		High titre is diagnostic	+ive in 6%			

* Antibodies tested against human substrates (e.g. Human Hep. 2 cells).

Table 10.2 Classification of connective tissue disease.

Localized disease	Intermediate type	Aggressive multisystem disease
Discoid lupus erythematosus	Subacute lupus erythematosus Juvenile dermatomyositis	Systemic lupus erythematosus Adult dermatomyositis
Morphoea	CREST syndrome	Systemic sclerosis

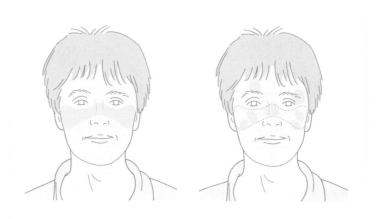

Fig. 10.1 In systemic lupus erythematosus (SLE) (left) the eruption is often just an erythema, sometimes transient, but occupying most of the 'butterfly' area. In discoid LE (right) the fixed scaling and scarring plaques may occur in the butterfly area (dotted line), but can occur outside it too.

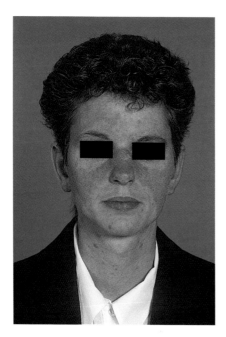

Fig. 10.2 Erythema in the butterfly area, suggestive of SLE.

organs and the side-effects of treatment, especially systemic steroids.

Differential diagnosis

SLE is a great imitator. Its malar rash can be confused with sunburn, polymorphic light eruption (p. 238) and rosacea (p. 156). The discoid lesions are distinctive, but are also seen in discoid LE and in subacute cutaneous LE. Occasionally, they look like psoriasis or lichen planus (p. 64). The hair fall suggests telogen effluvium (p. 168). Plaques on the scalp may cause a scarring alopecia. SLE should be suspected when a characteristic rash is combined with fever, malaise and internal disease (Table 10.3).

Investigations

Conduct a full physical examination, looking for internal disease. Biopsy of skin lesions is worthwhile because the pathology and immunopathology are distinctive. There is usually some thinning of the epidermis,

Table 10.3 Criteria for the diagnosis of SLE (must have at least four).

Malar rash
Discoid plaques
Photosensitivity
Mouth ulcers
Arthritis
Serositis
Renal disorder
Neurological disorder
Haematological disorder
Immunological disorder
Antinuclear antibodies (ANA)

LEARNING POINTS

1 Do not wait for the laboratory to confirm that your patient has severe SLE: use systemic steroids quickly if indicated by clinical findings.
2 A person with aching joints and small amounts of antinuclear antibodies probably does not have SLE.
3 Once committed to systemic steroids, adjust their dosage on clinical rather than laboratory grounds.

liquefaction degeneration of epidermal basal cells, and a mild perivascular mononuclear cell infiltrate. Direct immunofluorescence is helpful: IgG, IgM, IgA and C3 are found individually or together in a band-like pattern at the dermo-epidermal junction of involved skin and often uninvolved skin as well. Relevant laboratory tests are listed in Table 10.4.

Treatment

Systemic steroids are the mainstay of treatment, with bed rest needed during exacerbations. Large doses of prednisolone (Formulary 2, p. 348) are often needed to achieve control, as assessed by symptoms, signs, erythrocyte sedimentation rate (ESR), total complement level and tests of organ function. The dosage is then reduced to the smallest that suppresses the disease. Immunosuppressive agents, such as azathioprine (Formulary 2, p. 346), cyclophosphamide and

other drugs (e.g. antihypertensive therapy or anticonvulsants) may also be needed. Antimalarial drugs may help some patients with marked photosensitivity, as may sunscreens. Intermittent intravenous infusions of gamma globulin show promise. Long-term and regular follow-up is necessary.

Subacute cutaneous lupus erythematosus

This is less severe than acute SLE, but is also often associated with systemic disease. Its cause is unknown, but probably involves an antibody-dependent cellular cytotoxic attack on basal cells by K cells bridged by antibody to Ro (SS-A) antigen.

Presentation

Patients with subacute cutaneous LE are often photosensitive. The skin lesions are sharply marginated

Table 10.4 Investigations in SLE.

Test	Usual findings
Skin biopsy	Degeneration of basal cells, epidermal thinning, inflammation around appendages
Skin immunofluorescence	Fibrillar or granular deposits of IgG, IgM, IgA and/or C3 alone in basement membrane zone
Haematology	Anaemia, raised ESR, thrombocytopenia, decreased white cell count
Immunology	Antinuclear antibody, antibodies to double-stranded DNA, false positive tests for syphilis, low total complement level, lupus anticoagulant factor
Urine analysis	Proteinuria or haematuria, often with casts if kidneys involved
Tests for function of other organs	As indicated by history but always test kidney and liver function

scaling psoriasiform plaques, sometimes annular, lying on the forehead, nose, cheeks, chest, hands and extensor surfaces of the arms. They tend to be symmetrical and are hard to tell from discoid LE, or SLE with widespread discoid lesions.

Course

As in SLE, the course is prolonged. The skin lesions are slow to clear but, in contrast to discoid LE, do so with little or no scarring.

Complications

Systemic disease is frequent, but not usually serious. Children born to mothers who have, or have had, this condition are liable to neonatal LE with transient annular skin lesions and permanent heart block.

Differential diagnosis

The morphology is characteristic, but lesions can be mistaken for psoriasis or widespread discoid LE. Annular lesions may resemble tinea corporis (p. 216) or figurate erythemas (p. 133).

Investigations

Patients with subacute cutaneous LE should be evaluated in the same way as those with acute SLE, although deposits of immunoglobulins in the skin and antinuclear antibodies in serum are present less often. Many have antibodies to the cytoplasmic antigen Ro (SS-A).

Treatment

Subacute cutaneous LE does better with antimalarials, such as hydroxychloroquine (Formulary 2, p. 352), than acute SLE. Oral retinoids (Formulary 2, p. 349) are also effective in some cases. Systemic steroids may be needed too.

Discoid lupus erythematosus

This is the most common form of LE. Patients with discoid LE may have one or two plaques only, or many in several areas. The cause is also unknown but UVR is one factor.

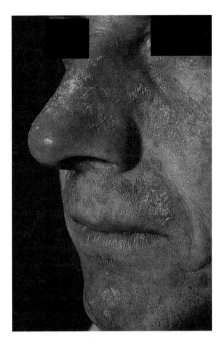

Fig. 10.3 Red scaly fixed plaques of discoid LE. This degree of scaling is not uncommon in the active stage. Follicular plugging is seen on the nose.

Presentation

Plaques show erythema, scaling, follicular plugging (like a nutmeg grater), scarring and atrophy, telangiectasia, hypopigmentation and a peripheral zone of hyperpigmentation. They are well demarcated and lie mostly on sun-exposed skin of the scalp, face and ears (Figs 10.1 and 10.3). In one variant (chilblain LE) dusky lesions appear on the fingers and toes.

Course

The disease may spread relentlessly, but in about half of the cases the disease goes into remission over the course of several years. Scarring is common and hair may be lost permanently if there is scarring in the scalp (Fig. 10.4). Whiteness remains after the inflammation has cleared, and hypopigmentation is common in dark-skinned people. Discoid LE rarely progresses to SLE.

Differential diagnosis

Psoriasis is hard to tell from discoid LE when its plaques first arise but has larger thicker scales, and later it is usually symmetrical and affects sites different from

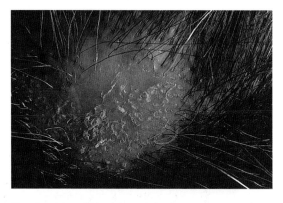

Fig. 10.4 Discoid LE of the scalp leading to permanent hair loss. Note the marked follicular plugging.

those of discoid LE. Discoid LE is more common on the face and ears, and in sun-exposed areas, whereas psoriasis favours the elbows, knees, scalp and sacrum. Discoid LE is far more prone than psoriasis to scar and cause hair loss. Jessner's lymphocytic infiltration is best viewed as a dermal form of discoid LE.

Investigations

Most patients with discoid LE remain well. However, screening for SLE and internal disease is still worthwhile. A skin biopsy is most helpful if taken from an untreated plaque where appendages are still present (Fig. 10.5). Direct immunofluorescence shows deposits of IgG, IgM, IgA and C3 at the basement membrane zone. Biopsies for direct immunofluorescence are best taken from older untreated plaques. Blood tests are usually normal but occasionally serum contains antinuclear antibodies (Table 10.5).

Treatment

Discoid LE needs potent or very potent topical corticosteroids (Formulary 1, p. 333). In this condition, it is justifiable to use them on the face, as the risk of scarring is worse than that of atrophy. Topical steroids should be applied twice daily until the lesions disappear or side-effects, such as atrophy, develop; weaker preparations can then be used for maintenance. If discoid LE does not respond to this, intralesional injections of triamcinolone (2.5 or 10 mg/mL) may help. Stubborn and widespread lesions often do well with oral antimalarials such as hydroxychloroquine (Formulary 2, p. 352), but rarely these cause irreversible eye damage. The eyes should therefore be tested before and at intervals during treatment. Sun avoidance and screens are also important. Oral retinoids (Formulary 2, p. 349) and thalidomide have proved helpful in stubborn cases but a specialist, with experience of their use, should prescribe these controlled treatments and supervise management.

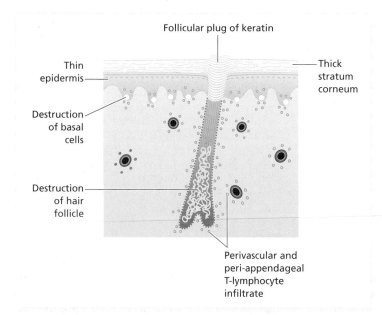

Follicular plug of keratin

Thin epidermis

Thick stratum corneum

Destruction of basal cells

Destruction of hair follicle

Perivascular and peri-appendageal T-lymphocyte infiltrate

Fig. 10.5 The histology of discoid LE.

Table 10.5 Some factors distinguishing the different types of LE.

	Antinuclear antibodies	Sun sensitivity	Internal organ involvement
Systemic LE	++++	+++	++
Subacute LE	+	++++	+
Discoid LE	+/−	+	−

Dermatomyositis

Dermatomyositis is a subset of polymyositis with distinctive skin changes. There are adult and juvenile types (Table 10.2). The cause is unknown but an auto-immune mechanism seems likely. Autoantibodies to striated muscle are found. When starting after the age of 40, dermatomyositis may signal an internal malignancy. Presumably, the epitopes of some tumour antigens are so similar to those of muscle antigens that antibodies directed against the tumour cross-react with muscle cells and initiate the disease in a few adults with internal malignancy. Serological evidence for acute toxoplasmosis in polymyositis-dermatomyositis was found in one series.

Presentation

The skin signs are characteristic. Typical patients have a faint lilac discoloration around their eyes (sometimes called 'heliotrope' because of the colour of the flower). This is associated with malar erythema and oedema (Fig. 10.6) and, sometimes, less striking erythema of the neck and presternal area. Most patients also develop lilac slightly atrophic papules over the knuckles of their fingers (Gottron's papules), streaks of erythema over the extensor tendons of the hand, peri-ungual telangiectasia and ragged cuticles (Fig. 10.7). The skin signs usually appear at the same time as the muscle symptoms but, occasionally, appear months or even years earlier. Sometimes, the skin signs appear in isolation. Many, but not all, patients have weakness of proximal muscles. Climbing stairs, getting up from chairs and combing the hair become difficult.

Course

In children the disorder is often self-limiting, but in adults it may be prolonged and progressive. Raynaud's phenomenon, arthralgia, dysphagia and calcinosis may

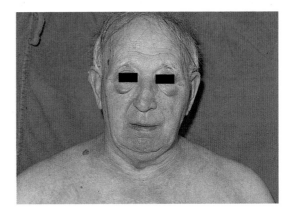

Fig. 10.6 Acute dermatomyositis: oedematous purple face with erythema on presternal area. Severe progressive muscle weakness, but no underlying tumour was found.

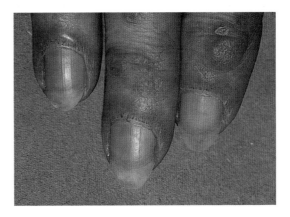

Fig. 10.7 Erythema and telangiectasia of the nail folds are important clues to systemic connective tissue disorders. This patient has dermatomyositis. Note Gottron's papules over the knuckles.

follow. The rash may become scaly and, rarely, itchy; eventually that on the light-exposed areas and overlying involved muscles develops poikiloderma (p. 252). Features of mixed connective disease (see below) may develop. The presence of calcinosis suggests a good prognosis.

Complications

Myositis may lead to permanent weakness and immobility, and inflammation to contractures or cutaneous calcinosis. Some die from progessive and severe myopathy.

Differential diagnosis

Other connective tissue disorders may look similar, particularly mixed connective tissue disease (p. 129) and SLE. In LE, the finger lesions favour the skin between the knuckles whereas in dermatomyositis the knuckles are preferred. Toxoplasmosis may cause a dermatomyositis-like syndrome. Myopathy can be a side-effect of systemic steroids, so weakness is not always caused by the disease itself.

Investigations

About 30% of adults with dermatomyositis also have an underlying malignancy. Their dermatomyositis coincides with the onset of the tumour and may improve if it is removed. Adult dermatomyositis or polymyositis therefore requires a search for such an underlying malignancy. The levels of muscle enzymes such as aldolase and creatinine phosphokinase (CPK) are often elevated. Electromyography (EMG) detects muscle abnormalities, and biopsy of an affected muscle shows inflammation and destruction. Surprisingly, the ESR is often normal and antinuclear antibodies may not be detected. Toxoplasmosis should be excluded by serology.

Treatment

Systemic steroids, often in high doses (e.g. prednisolone 60 mg/day for an average adult; Formulary 2, p. 348), are the cornerstone of treatment and protect the muscles from destruction. A maintenance regimen may be needed for several years. Immunosuppressive agents, such as azathioprine (Formulary 2, p. 346), also help to control the condition and to reduce the high steroid dose. Cyclosporin (Formulary 2, p. 347) and methotrexate (Formulary 2, p. 348) have proved useful alternatives in stubborn cases. Maintenance

LEARNING POINT

Hunt for internal malignancy in the middle aged and elderly, but not in juvenile cases.

treatment is adjusted according to clinical response and CPK level. As in SLE, intravenous gamma globulin infusions seem promising. Long-term and regular follow-up is necessary.

Systemic sclerosis

In this disorder the skin becomes hard as connective tissues thicken. Early in the condition, T-helper cells dominate the inflammatory infiltrate in the dermis and cause fibroblasts to proliferate and produce more hyaluronic acid and type I collagen (p. 16). In addition there is intimal thickening of arterioles and arteries. These processes are not confined to the skin, but involve many other organs, including the gut, lungs, kidneys and heart, leading to their dysfunction and to death.

The cause of systemic sclerosis is unknown but many, apparently unrelated, pieces of the complex jigsaw are now beginning to come together. A systemic sclerosis-like syndrome is a feature of the chronic graft-vs.-host disease sometimes seen after bone marrow transplantation (p. 286) and prolonged, untreated porphyria cutanea torda (p. 287). Similar syndromes have been reported following ingestion of adulterated rapeseed oil in Spain and dimerised L-tryptophan for insomnia and treatment with the antitumour agent, bleomycin. Environmental factors may also be relevant in isolated cases; changes like those of systemic sclerosis have affected workers exposed to polyvinyl chloride monomers, trichlorethylene and epoxy resins and in those subjected for years to severe vibration.

Presentation

Most patients suffer from Raynaud's phenomenon (p. 135) and sclerodactyly. Their fingers become immobile, hard and shiny. Some become hyperpigmented and itchy early in their disease. Peri-ungual telangiectasia is common.

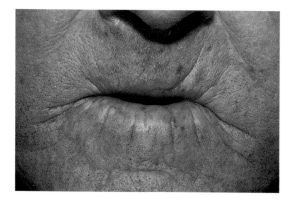

Fig. 10.8 Systemic sclerosis: radial furrowing around the mouth.

Course

As the disease progresses, sclerosis spreads to the face, scalp and trunk. The nose becomes beak-like, and wrinkles radiate around the mouth (Fig. 10.8–10.10). Most have abnormalities of the gut including dysphagia, oesophagitis, constipation, diarrhoea and malabsorption. Fibrosis of the lungs leads to dyspnoea, and fibrosis of the heart to congestive failure. The kidneys are involved late, but this has a grave prognosis from malignant hypertension.

Complications

Most complications are caused by the involvement of organs other than the skin, but ulcers of the fingertips and calcinosis are distressing (Fig. 10.11). Hard skin immobilizes the joints and leads to contractures.

Differential diagnosis

Other causes of Raynaud's phenomenon are given in Table 11.5. The differential diagnosis includes chilblains (p. 132) and erythromelalgia (p. 132). The sclerosis should be distinguished from that of widespread morphoea, porphyria cutanea tarda, mixed connective tissue disease, eosinophilic fasciitis, diabetic sclerodactyly and an acute arthritis with swollen fingers. Rarely the disease is mimicked by progeria, scleromyxoedema, amyloidosis or carcinoid syndrome. Changes like those of progressive systemic sclerosis affect workers exposed to polyvinyl chloride monomers or to severe chronic vibration, and are also seen

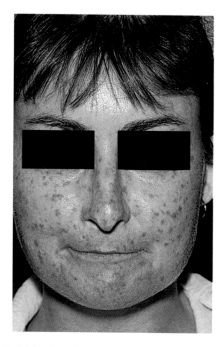

Fig. 10.9 Mat-like telangiectasia seen in a patient with systemic sclerosis.

in chronic graft-vs.-host reactions after bone marrow transplants.

Investigations

The diagnosis is made clinically because histological abnormalities are seldom present until the physical signs are well established. Laboratory tests should include a fluorescent antinuclear antibody test and the evaluation of the heart, kidney, lungs, joints and muscles. Barium studies are best avoided as obstruction may follow poor evacuation. Other contrast media are available. X-rays of the hands, measurement of muscle enzymes and immunoglobulin levels, and a blood count, ESR and test for the scleroderma-associated antibody Scl-70 are also worthwhile.

Treatment

This is unsatisfactory. The calcium channel blocker nifedipine may help Raynaud's phenomenon (p. 135). Systemic steroids, salicylates, antimalarials and long-term penicillin are used, but are not of proven value. D-penicillamine has many side-effects, especially on

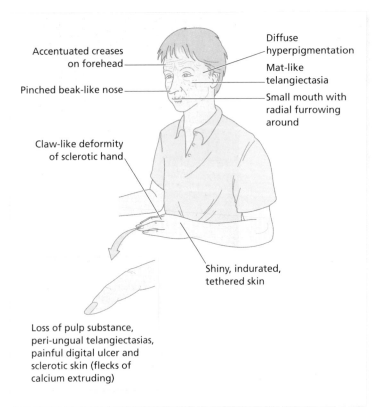

Accentuated creases on forehead

Pinched beak-like nose

Claw-like deformity of sclerotic hand

Diffuse hyperpigmentation

Mat-like telangiectasia

Small mouth with radial furrowing around

Shiny, indurated, tethered skin

Loss of pulp substance, peri-ungual telangiectasias, painful digital ulcer and sclerotic skin (flecks of calcium extruding)

Fig. 10.10 Signs of systemic sclerosis.

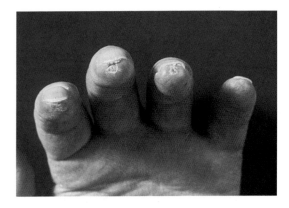

Fig. 10.11 Loss of fingertip pulp, and extrusion of chalky material.

renal function. Physiotherapy is helpful; photopheresis is experimental. Recently, there have been promising reports of the efficacy of ultraviolet A-1 (340–400 nm) phototherapy for affected skin in systemic sclerosis.

CREST syndrome

This is a variant of systemic sclerosis with a relatively good prognosis associated often with serum antibodies to nuclear centromeres. The mnemonic stands for Calcinosis, Raynaud's phenomenon, oEsophageal dysmotility, Sclerodactyly and Telangiectasia. Telangiectasia is peri-ungual on the fingers and flat, mat-like or rectangular on the face. Many patients with this syndrome develop a diffuse progressive systemic sclerosis after months or years.

Eosinophilic fasciitis

Localized areas of skin become indurated, sometimes after an upper respiratory tract infection or prolonged severe exercise. Hypergammaglobulinaemia and eosinophilia are present and a deep skin biopsy, which includes muscle, shows that the fascia overlying the muscle is thickened. Despite its name, and despite a profound eosinophilia in the peripheral blood, the

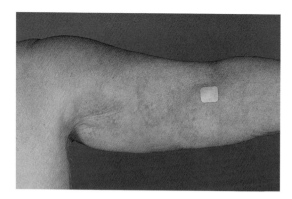

Fig. 10.12 Morphoea. Pale indurated plaques on the arm, showing a purplish rim.

fascia is not eosinophilic or permeated by eosinophils. The disease responds promptly to systemic steroids; the long-term prognosis is good but disability in the short term can be severe.

Morphoea

Morphoea is a localized form of scleroderma with pale indurated plaques on the skin but no internal sclerosis (Figs 10.12 and 10.13). Many plaques are surrounded by a violaceous halo. Its prognosis is usually good, and the fibrosis slowly clears leaving slight depression and hyperpigmentation. A rare type may lead to arrest of growth of the underlying bones causing, for example, facial hemiatrophy or shortening of a limb. Little is known about the cause, except that Lyme borreliosis may be associated with the disease in Europe but not in the Americas. Treatments work slowly, if at all, and include topical steroids, calcipotriene, non-steroidal anti-inflammatory drugs (NSAIDs), psoralen with ultraviolet A (PUVA), UVA and hydroxychloroquine in selected patients.

Lichen sclerosus

Many think that this condition is related to morphoea, with which it may coexist. However, its patches are non-indurated white shiny macules, sometimes with obvious plugging in the follicular openings. Women are affected far more often than men and, although any area of skin can be involved, the classical ivory-coloured lesions often surround the vulva and anus. Intractable itching is common in these areas and the development of vulval carcinoma is a risk. In men the

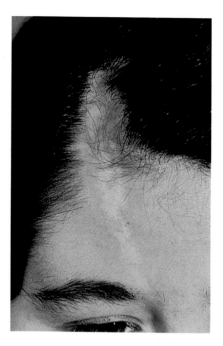

Fig. 10.13 Morphoea (*en coup de sabre* type) on the forehead. In a young child this can lead to facial hemiatrophy.

condition may cause stenosis of the urethral meatus, and adhesions between the foreskin and glans of the penis (see also Chapter 13).

Mixed connective tissue disease

This is an overlap between SLE and either scleroderma or polymyositis.

Presentation

As in LE, women are affected more often than men. Many develop swollen hands and sclerodactyly, and skin lesions like those of cutaneous LE may also be present. Alopecia is mild and the hair fall mimics telogen effluvium. Peri-ungual telangiectasia and pigmentary disturbances are common. About 25% of patients have a small vessel vasculitis with palpable purpura, leg ulcers and painful dermal nodules on the hands or elbows. Many show Raynaud's phenomenon, arthritis, serositis and myositis. Headaches, weakness, fatigue, lymph node enlargement or hoarseness occur in about one in three patients; renal and central nervous system disease are less common.

Course

The disorder is chronic, and usually turns into either SLE or systemic sclerosis.

Differential diagnosis

The disorder can be confused with SLE, dermatomyositis, polymyositis, systemic sclerosis and other sclerosing processes such as porphyria cutanea tarda (p. 287).

Investigations

Patients with mixed connective tissue disease have antibodies in high titre directed against one or more extractable nuclear antigens. These give a speckled pattern when serum is reacted against nuclei and detected by indirect immunofluorescence. Direct immunofluorescence of involved and uninvolved skin shows IgG within the epidermal nuclei, also in a speckled pattern. Only one-third of patients have subepidermal immunoglobulin deposits in involved skin. Most have hypergammaglobulinaemia, a high ESR, oesophageal dysmotility, abnormal pulmonary function tests and a positive rheumatoid factor. Hypocomplementaemia, leucopenia, anaemia, cryoglobulinaemia and false-positive biological tests for syphilis occur in a few patients.

Treatment

Treatment depends upon which organs are involved, but systemic steroids are usually needed, in the same dosage as for SLE. Immunosuppressive agents reduce the dosage of systemic steroids, and NSAIDs help with arthralgia, myalgia and swelling of the hands.

Other connective tissue diseases

Rheumatoid arthritis

Most patients with rheumatoid arthritis have no skin disease, but some have tiny fingertip infarcts, purpura, ulcers, palmar or peri-ungual erythema, or pyoderma gangrenosum. The most common skin manifestations are marble-like nodules near joints. These are always associated with the presence of rheumatoid factor. Some patients with rheumatoid arthritis have a vasculitis of larger blood vessels with deep 'punched out' ulcers on the legs (p. 106).

Reiter's syndrome

Reiter's syndrome, precipitated by non-specific urethritis or dysentery, combines skin lesions, arthropathy, conjunctivitis, balanitis, mucositis and spondylitis. Arthritis is the most severe element. The skin lesions (keratoderma blenorrhagicum) are psoriasis-like red scaling plaques, often studded with vesicles and pustules, seen most often on the feet. The toes are red and swollen, and the nails thicken. Psoriasiform plaques may also occur on the penis and scrotum, with redness near the penile meatus. Topical steroids and systemic NSAIDs help, but many patients need methotrexate (Formulary 2, p. 348) and/or systemic steroids.

Relapsing polychondritis

This process can affect any cartilage as the disorder is apparently caused by autoimmunity to collagen. The ears are the usual target. The overlying skin becomes red, swollen and tender. The cartilage in joints, the nose and the tracheo-bronchial tree may be involved, so that patients develop floppy ears, a saddle nose, hoarseness, stridor and respiratory insufficiency. Aortic aneurysms are also seen. Treatment is with systemic steroids and NSAIDs. Tracheostomy may be necessary.

Behçet's syndrome

Behçet's syndrome is discussed in Chapter 13.

Polyarteritis nodosa

This is discussed in Chapter 8 but is considered by some to be a connective tissue disorder.

Panniculitis

Panniculitis is an inflammation of the subcutaneous fat. It includes a number of diseases with different causes but a similar appearance: some are listed in Table 10.6.

Table 10.6 Causes of panniculitis.

Erythema nodosum (p. 101)
Erythema nodosum leprosum (leprosy)
Nodular vasculitis (p. 102)
Erythema induratum
Weber–Christian type
Polyarteritis nodosa (p. 104)
Associated with pancreatitis
Associated with SLE (lupus profundus)
Cold-induced
Withdrawal of systemic steroids
Superficial and migratory thrombophlebitis
Deficiency of α_1-antitrypsin
Factitial (e.g. from injection of milk)

Presentation

Most patients have tender ill-defined red nodules on the lower legs, thighs and buttocks.

Course

This depends upon the cause. Migratory thrombophlebitis may be associated with underlying malignancy. In lupus profundus, a panniculitis is associated with discoid or SLE. Causes of erythema nodosum are discussed in Chapter 8. Erythema induratum may be caused by tuberculosis. Erythema nodosum leprosum is a reactional state in leprosy. Patients with pancreatitis may liberate enough lipase into the systemic circulation to cause fat in the skin to liquefy and discharge through the overlying skin. The Weber–Christian variant is associated with fever, but its cause is unknown.

Investigations

The type of panniculitis can sometimes be identified by skin biopsy, which must include subcutaneous fat. A complete blood count, ESR, chest X-ray, serum lipase, serum α_1-antitrypsin and tests for antinuclear antibodies are needed.

Treatment

This depends upon the cause. Rest, elevation of affected extremities and local heat often help symptoms. NSAIDs may also bring help in the absence of specific therapy.

Further reading

Callen, J.P. (1998) Collagen-vascular diseases. *Medical Clinics of North America* **82**, 1217–1237.

Callen, J.P. (2000) Dermatomyositis. *Lancet* **355**, 53–57.

Davidson, A. & Diamond, B. (2001) Autoimmune diseases. *New England Journal of Medicine* **345**, 340–350.

McCauliffe, D.P. (2001) Cutaneous lupus erythematosus. *Seminars in Cutaneous Medicine and Surgery* **20**, 14–26.

Patterson, J.W. (1991) Differential diagnosis of panniculitis. *Advances in Dermatology* **6**, 309–329.

Ruiz-Irastorza, G., Khamashta, M.A., Castellino, G. & Hughes, G.R. (2001) Systemic lupus erythematosus. *Lancet* **357**, 1027–1032.

Disorders of blood vessels and lymphatics

In functional diseases of the blood and lymphatic vessels, abnormalities of flow are reversible, and there is no vessel wall damage (e.g. in urticaria; discussed in Chapter 8). The diseases of structure include the many types of vasculitis, some of which, with an immunological basis, are also covered in Chapter 8. For convenience, disorders of the blood vessels are grouped according to the size and type of the vessels affected.

Disorders involving small blood vessels

Acrocyanosis

This type of 'poor circulation', often familial, is more common in females than males. The hands, feet, nose, ears and cheeks become blue-red and cold. The palms are often cold and clammy. The condition is caused by arteriolar constriction and dilatation of the subpapillary venous plexus, and to cold-induced increases in blood viscosity. The best answers are warm clothes and the avoidance of cold.

Erythrocyanosis

This occurs in fat, often young, women. Purple-red mottled discoloration is seen over the buttocks, thighs and lower legs. Cold provokes it and causes an unpleasant burning sensation. An area of acrocyanosis or erythrocyanosis may be the site where other disorders will settle in the future, e.g. perniosis, erythema induratum, lupus erythematosus, sarcoidosis, cutaneous tuberculosis and leprosy.

Perniosis (chilblains)

In this common, sometimes familial, condition, inflamed purple-pink swellings appear on the fingers,

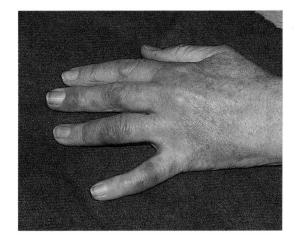

Fig. 11.1 The typical purplish swellings of chilblains.

toes and, rarely, ears (Fig. 11.1). They arrive with winter and are induced by cold. They are painful, and itchy or burning on rewarming. Occasionally they ulcerate. Chilblains are caused by a combination of arteriolar and venular constriction, the latter predominating on rewarming with exudation of fluid into the tissues. Warm housing and clothing help. Topical remedies rarely work, but the oral calcium channel blocker nifedipidine may be useful (p. 136). The blood pressure should be monitored at the start of treatment and at return visits. The vasodilator nicotinamide (500 mg three times daily) may be helpful alone or in addition to calcium channel blockers. Sympathectomy may be advised in severe cases.

Erythromelalgia

This is a rare condition in which the extremities become red, hot and painful when they or their owner are exposed to heat. The condition may be idiopathic,

Table 11.1 Classification of erythemas.

Widespread
Caused by infection (bacterial or viral)
Drug reactions
Connective tissue diseases
Underlying malignancy (e.g. figurate erythema)
Idiopathic ('toxic' or 'reactive')

Localized
Pregnancy, liver disease, rheumatoid arthritis (causing
  palmar erythema)
Drug reaction (fixed drug eruption)
Infection (e.g. erythema chronicum migrans caused by
  Borrelia burgdorferi)

or caused by a myeloproliferative disease (e.g. polycythaemia rubra vera or thrombocythaemia), lupus erythematosus, rheumatoid arthritis, diabetes, degenerative peripheral vascular disease or hypertension. Small doses of aspirin give symptomatic relief. Alternatives include non-steroidal anti-inflammatory drugs (NSAIDs), α blockers and oxpentifylline (pentoxifylline).

Erythemas

Erythema accompanies all inflammatory skin conditions, but the term 'the erythemas' is usually applied to a group of conditions with redness but without primary scaling. Such areas are seen in some bacterial and viral infections such as toxic shock syndrome and measles. Drugs are another common cause (Chapter 22). If no cause is obvious, the rash is often called a 'toxic' or 'reactive' erythema (Table 11.1).

When erythema is associated with oedema ('urticated erythema') it becomes palpable.

Figurate erythemas

These are chronic eruptions, made up of bizarre serpiginous and erythematous rings. In the past most carried Latin labels; happily, these eruptions are now grouped under the general term of 'figurate erythemas'. Underlying malignancy, a connective tissue disorder, a bacterial, fungal or yeast infection, worm infestation, drug sensitivity and rheumatic heart disease should be excluded, but often the cause remains obscure.

Palmar erythema

This may be an isolated finding in a normal person or be familial. Sometimes it is seen in pregnancy, liver disease or rheumatoid arthritis. Often associated with spider telangiectases (see below), it may be caused by increased circulating oestrogens.

Erythema migrans (p. 195)

These annular erythematous areas are usually solitary, and occur most often on exposed skin after a tick bite. They expand slowly and may become very large.

Telangiectases

This term refers to permanently dilatated and visible small vessels in the skin. They appear as linear, punctate or stellate crimson-purple markings. The common causes are given in Table 11.2.

Spider naevi

These stellate telangiectases do look rather like spiders, with legs radiating from a central, often palpable, feeding vessel. If the diagnosis is in doubt, press on the central feeding vessel with the corner of a glass slide and the entire lesion will disappear. Spider naevi are seen frequently on the faces of normal children, and may erupt in pregnancy or be the presenting sign of liver disease, with many lesions on the upper trunk. Liver function should be checked in those with many spider naevi. The central vessel can be destroyed by electrodessication without local anaesthesia or with a pulsed dye laser (p. 327).

Livedo reticularis

This cyanosis of the skin is net-like or marbled and caused by stasis in the capillaries furthest from their arterial supply: at the periphery of the inverted cone supplied by a dermal arteriole (see Fig. 2.1). 'Cutis marmorata' is the name given to the mottling of the skin seen in many normal children. It is physiological and disappears on warming, whereas true livedo reticularis remains.

The causes of livedo reticularis are listed in Table 11.3. Livedo vasculitis and cutaneous polyarteritis are

Table 11.2 Causes of telangiectasia.

Primary telangiectasia	
Hereditary haemorrhagic telangiectasia	Autosomal dominant Nose and gastointestinal bleeds Lesions on face
Ataxia telangiectasia	Autosomal recessive Telangiectases develop between the ages of 3 and 5 years Cerebellar ataxia Recurrent respiratory infections Immunological abnormalities
Generalized essential telangiectasia	Runs benign course No other associations
Unilateral naevoid telangiectasia	May occur in pregnancy or in females on oral contraceptive
Secondary telangiectasia	
Atrophy	Seen on exposed skin of elderly, after topical steroid applications, after X-irradiation and with poikiloderma
Connective tissue disorders	Always worth inspecting nail folds. Mat-like on the face in systemic sclerosis
Prolonged vasodilatation	For example, with rosacea and with venous hypertension
Mastocytosis	Accompanying a rare and diffuse variant
Liver disease	Multiple spider telangiectases are common
Drugs	Nifedipine

Table 11.3 Causes of livedo reticularis.

Physiological	Cutis marmorata
Vessel wall disease	Atherosclerosis Connective tissue disorders (especially polyarteritis, livedo vasculitis and systemic lupus erythematosus) Syphilis Tuberculosis
Hyperviscosity states	Polycythaemia/thrombocythaemia Macroglobulinaemia
Cryopathies	Cryoglobulinaemia Cold agglutininaemia
Autoimmune	Antiphospholipid syndrome
Congenital	
Idiopathic	

forms of vasculitis associated with livedo reticularis (Chapter 8).

Antiphospholipid syndrome

Some patients with an apparently idiopathic livedo reticularis develop progressive disease in their peripheral, cerebral, coronary and renal arteries. Others, usually women, have multiple arterial or venous thrombo-embolic episodes accompanying livedo reticularis. Recurrent spontaneous abortions and intrauterine fetal growth retardation are also features. Prolongation of the activated partial thromboplastin time (APTT) and the presence of antiphospholipid antibodies (either anticardiolipin antibody or lupus anticoagulant, or both) help to identify this syndrome. Systemic lupus erythematosus should be excluded (Chapter 10).

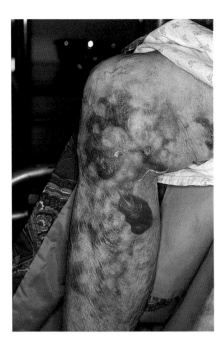

Fig. 11.2 Erythema ab igne: this patient persisted in sitting too close to an open fire and burned herself.

Table 11.4 Causes of flushing.

Physiological	Emotional
	Menopausal
Foods	Hot drinks
	Spicy foods
	Additives (monosodium glutamate)
	Alcohol (especially in Oriental people)
Drugs	Vasodilatators including nicotinic acid
	Bromocriptine
	Calcium channel blockers including nifedipine
	Disulfiram
	Chlorpropamide + alcohol (diabetics)
Pathological	Rosacea (p. 156)
	Carcinoid tumours—with asthma and diarrhoea
	Phaeochromocytoma (type producing adrenaline)—with episodic headaches (caused by transient hypertension) and palpitations

Erythema ab igne

This appearance is also determined by the underlying vascular network. Its reticulate pigmented erythema, with variable scaling, is caused by damage from long-term exposure to local heat—usually from an open fire, hot water bottle or heating pad. If on one side of the leg, it gives a clue to the side of the fire on which granny likes to sit (Fig. 11.2). The condition is common in northern Europe ('tinker's tartan'), but rare in the USA, where central heating is the rule.

Flushing

This transient vasodilatation of the face may spread to the neck, upper chest and, more rarely, other parts of the body. There is no sharp distinction between flushing and blushing apart from the emotional provocation of the latter. The mechanism varies with the many causes that are listed in Table 11.4. Paroxysmal flushing ('hot flushes'), common at the menopause, is associated with the pulsatile release of luteinizing hormone from the pituitary, as a consequence of low circulating oestrogens and failure of normal negative feedback. However, luteinizing hormone itself cannot

be responsible for flushing as this can occur after hypophysectomy. It is possible that menopausal flushing is mediated by central mechanisms involving encephalins. Hot flushes can usually be helped by oestrogen replacement.

Alcohol-induced flushing is most commonly seen in oriental people. Ethanol is broken down to acetaldehyde by alcohol dehydrogenase and acetaldehyde is metabolized to acetic acid by aldehyde dehydrogenase (Fig. 11.3). Acetaldehyde accumulation is in part responsible for flushing. Oriental people not only may have a high-activity variant of alcohol dehydrogenase but also defective aldehyde dehydrogenase. Disulfuram (Antabuse) and, to a lesser extent, chlorpropamide inhibit aldehyde dehydrogenase so that some individuals taking these drugs may flush.

Arterial disease

Raynaud's phenomenon

This is a paroxysmal pallor of the digits provoked by cold or, rarely, emotional stress. At first the top of one or more fingers becomes white. On rewarming, a

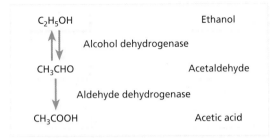

Fig. 11.3 The metabolism of ethanol.

painful cyanosis appears and the area turns red before the hands return to their normal colour. In severe disease the fingers lose pulp substance, ulcerate or become gangrenous (Fig. 11.4). Some causes are listed in Table 11.5. Raynaud's disease, often familial, is the name given when no cause can be found. However, some patients with what seems to be Raynaud's disease will later develop a connective tissue disease, usually scleroderma.

The main treatment is to protect the vulnerable digits from cold. Warm clothing reduces the need for peripheral vasoconstriction to conserve heat. Smoking should be abandoned. Calcium channel blockers (e.g. nifedipine 10–30 mg three times daily) are the most effective agents although they work best in patients with primary Raynaud's disease. Patients should be warned about dizziness caused by postural hypotension. Initially it is worth giving nifedipine as a 5-mg test dose with monitoring of the blood pressure in the clinic. If this is tolerated satisfactorily the starting dosage should be 5 mg daily, increasing by 5 mg every

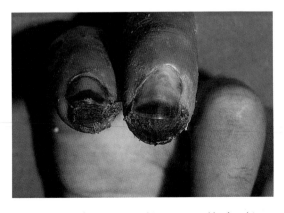

Fig. 11.4 Digital gangrene. In this case caused by frostbite.

Table 11.5 Causes of Raynaud's phenomenon.

Familial	Raynaud's disease
Connective tissue diseases	Systemic sclerosis Lupus erythematosus Mixed connective tissue disease
Arterial occlusion	Thoracic outlet syndrome Atherosclerosis Endarteritis obliterans
Repeated trauma	Pneumatic hammer/drill operators ('vibration white finger')
Hyperviscosity	Polycythaemia Macroglobulinaemia
Cryopathies	Cryoglobulinaemia Cryofibrinogenaemia Cold agglutinaemia
Neurological disease	Peripheral neuropathy Syringomyelia
Toxins	Ergot Vinyl-chloride

5 days until a therapeutic dose is achieved (e.g. 5–20 mg three times daily) or until intolerable side-effects occur. The blood pressure should be monitored before each incremental increase in the dosage. Diltiazem (30–60 mg three times daily) is less effective than nifedipine but has fewer side-effects. Systemic vasodilators such as naftidrofuryl oxalate, nicotinic acid and thymoxamine (moxisylyte) are also worth trying. Glycerol trinitrate ointment, applied once daily may reduce the severity and frequency of attacks and may allow reduction in the dosage of calcium channel blockers and vasodilators. Infusions with reserpine or prostacyclin help some severe cases although occasionally sympathectomy is needed.

Polyarteritis nodosa

This is discussed in Chapter 8.

Temporal arteritis

Here the brunt is borne by the larger vessels of the head and neck. The condition affects elderly people and may be associated with polymyalgia rheumatica. The classical site is the temporal arteries, which become tender and pulseless, in association with severe headaches. Rarely, necrotic ulcers appear on the scalp. Blindness may follow if the ophthalmic arteries are involved, and to reduce this risk systemic steroids should be given as soon as the diagnosis has been made. In active phases the erythrocyte sedimentation rate (ESR) is high and its level can be used to guide treatment, which is often prolonged.

Atherosclerosis

This occlusive disease, most common in developed countries, will not be discussed in detail here, but involvement of the large arteries of the legs is of concern to dermatologists. It may cause intermittent claudication, nocturnal cramp, ulcers or gangrene. These may develop slowly over the years, or within minutes if a thrombus forms on an atheromatous plaque. The feet are cold and pale, the skin is often atrophic, with little hair, and peripheral pulses are diminished or absent.

Investigations should include urine testing to exclude diabetes mellitus. Fasting plasma lipids (cholesterol, triglycerides and lipoproteins) should be checked in the young, especially if there is a family history of vascular disease. Doppler ultrasound measurements help to distinguish atherosclerotic from venous leg ulcers in the elderly (p. 142). Complete assessment is best carried out by a specialist in peripheral vascular disease or a vascular surgeon.

Arterial emboli

Emboli may lodge in arteries supplying the skin and cause gangrene, ulcers or necrotic papules, depending on the size of the vessel obstructed. Causes include dislodged thrombi (usually from areas of atherosclerosis), fat emboli (after major trauma), infected emboli (e.g. gonococcal septicaemia or subacute bacterial endocarditis) and tumour emboli.

Pressure sores (Fig. 11.5)

Sustained or repeated pressure on skin over bony prominences can cause ischaemia and pressure sores. These are common in patients over 70 years old who are confined to hospital, especially those with a fractured neck of femur. The morbidity and mortality of those with deep ulcers is high.

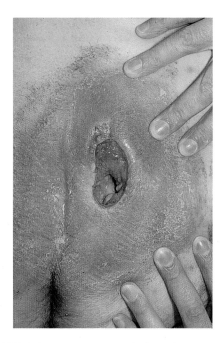

Fig. 11.5 A deep pressure sore on the buttock.

Cause

The main factors responsible for pressure sores are as follows.
1 Prolonged immobility and recumbency (e.g. caused by paraplegia, arthritis or senility).
2 Vascular disease (e.g. atherosclerosis).
3 Neurological disease causing diminished sensation (e.g. in paraplegia).
4 Malnutrition, severe systemic disease and general debility.

Clinical features

The sore begins as an area of erythema which progresses to a superficial blister or erosion. If pressure continues, deeper damage occurs with the development of a black eschar which, when removed or shed, reveals a deep ulcer, often colonized by *Pseudomonas aeruginosa*. The skin overlying the sacrum, greater trochanter, ischial tuberosity, the heel and the lateral malleolus is especially at risk.

Management

The following are important.

1 Prevention: by turning recumbent patients regularly and using antipressure mattresses for susceptible patients.

2 Treatment of malnutrition and the general condition.

3 Debridement. Regular cleansing with normal saline or 0.5% aqueous silver nitrate. Antibacterial preparations locally (Formulary 1, p. 334). Absorbent dressings (Formulary 1, p. 338). Semipermeable dressings such as Opsite, if there is no infection. Appropriate systemic antibiotic if an infection is spreading.

4 Plastic surgical reconstruction may be indicated in the young when the ulcer is clean.

Venous disease

Deep vein thrombosis

The common causes are listed in Table 11.6.

The onset may be 'silent' or heralded by pain in the calf, often about 10 days after immobilization for surgery, parturition or an infection. The leg becomes swollen and cyanotic distal to the thrombus. The calf may hurt when handled or if the foot is dorsiflexed (Homan's sign). Sometimes a pulmonary embolus is the first sign of a silent deep vein thrombosis.

Suitable investigations include venography, Doppler ultrasonography, which can only detect thrombi in large veins at, or above, the popliteal fossa, and ^{125}I-fibrinogen isotope leg scanning.

Treatment is anticoagulation with heparin and later with a coumarin. The value of thrombolytic regimens has yet to be assessed properly. Prevention is important. Deep vein thrombosis after a surgical operation is less frequent now, with early postoperative mobilization, regular leg exercises, the use of elastic stockings over the operative period and prophylaxis with low dose heparin.

Thrombophlebitis

This is thrombosis in an inflamed vein. If the affected vein is varicose or superficial it will be red and feel like a tender cord. The leg may be diffusely inflamed, making a distinction from cellulitis (p. 193) difficult. There may be fever, leucocytosis and a high ESR. Migratory superficial thrombophlebitis should arouse suspicion of an underlying malignancy or pancreatic disease.

Treatment is based on rest, local heat and NSAIDs. Antibiotics or anticoagulants rarely help.

Table 11.6 Some causes of deep vein thrombosis.

Abnormalities of the vein wall	Trauma (operations and injuries)
	Chemicals (intravenous infusions)
	Neighbouring infection (e.g. in leg ulcer)
	Tumour (local invasion)
Abnormalities of blood flow	Stasis (immobility, operations, long aircraft flights, pressure, pregnancy, myocardial infarction, heart failure, incompetent valves)
	Impaired venous return
Abnormalities of clotting	Platelets increased or sticky (thrombocythaemia, polycythaemia vera, leukaemia, trauma, splenectomy)
	Decreased fibrinolysis (postoperative)
	Deficiency of clotting factors (e.g. antithrombin, Proteins C and S, Factor V Leiden)
	Alteration in clotting factors (oral contraceptive, infection, leukaemia, pregnancy, shock and haemorrhage)
	Antiphospholipid antibody
Unknown mechanisms	Malignancy (thrombophlebitis migrans)
	Smoking
	Behçet's syndrome
	Inflammatory bowel disease

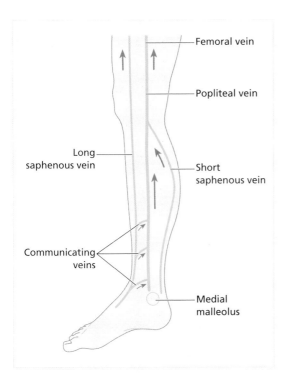

Fig. 11.6 The direction of blood flow in normal leg veins.

Venous hypertension, the gravitational syndrome and venous leg ulceration

Ulcers of the lower leg, secondary to venous hypertension, have an estimated prevalence of around 1%, are more common in women than in men, and account for some 85% of all leg ulcers seen in the UK and USA.

Cause

Satisfactory venous drainage of the leg requires three sets of veins: deep veins surrounded by muscles; superficial veins; and the veins connecting these together—the perforating or communicating veins (Fig. 11.6). When the leg muscles contract, blood in the deep veins is squeezed back, against gravity, to the heart (the calf muscle pump); reflux is prevented by valves. When the muscles relax, with the help of gravity, blood from the superficial veins passes into the deep veins via the communicating vessels. If the valves in the deep and communicating veins are incompetent, the calf muscle pump now pushes blood into the superficial veins, where the pressure remains high ('venous

hypertension') instead of dropping during exercise. This persisting venous hypertension enlarges the capillary bed; white cells accumulate here and are then activated (by hypoxic endothelial cells), releasing oxygen free radicals and other toxic products which cause local tissue destruction and ulceration. The increased venous pressure also forces fibrinogen and α_2-macroglobulin out through the capillary walls; these macromolecules trap growth and repair factors so that minor traumatic wounds cannot be repaired and an ulcer develops. Patients with these changes develop lipodermatosclerosis (see below) and have a high serum fibrinogen and reduced blood fibrinolytic activity. Figure 11.7 shows the factors causing venous ulceration.

Clinical features

Venous hypertension is heralded by a feeling of heaviness in the legs and by pitting oedema. Other signs include:
1 red or bluish discoloration;
2 loss of hair;
3 brown pigmentation (mainly haemosiderin from the breakdown of extravasated red blood cells) and scattered petechiae;
4 atrophie blanche (ivory white scarring with dilatated capillary loops; Fig. 11.8); and
5 induration, caused by fibrosis and oedema of the dermis and subcutis—sometimes called 'lipodermatosclerosis'.

Ulceration is most common near the medial malleolus (Fig. 11.9). In contrast to arterial ulcers, which are usually deep and round, with a punched out appearance, venous ulcers are often large but shallow, with prominent granulation tissue in their bases. Incompetent perforating branches (blowouts) between the superficial and deep veins are best felt with the patient standing. Under favourable conditions the exudative phase gives way to a granulating and healing phase, signalled by a blurring of the ulcer margin, ingrowth of skin from it, and the appearance of scattered small grey epithelial islands over the base. Prolonged ulceration, with lipodermatosclerosis, gives the leg the look of an inverted champagne bottle.

Complications

Bacterial superinfection is inevitable in a longstanding ulcer, but needs systemic antibiotics only if there is

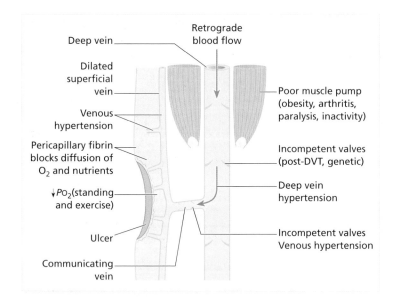

Deep vein

Retrograde blood flow

Dilated superficial vein

Venous hypertension

Pericapillary fibrin blocks diffusion of O_2 and nutrients

$\downarrow PO_2$(standing and exercise)

Ulcer

Communicating vein

Poor muscle pump (obesity, arthritis, paralysis, inactivity)

Incompetent valves (post-DVT, genetic)

Deep vein hypertension

Incompetent valves Venous hypertension

Fig. 11.7 Factors causing venous leg ulceration.

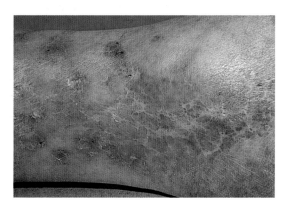

Fig. 11.8 Irregular areas of whitish scarring and dilatated capillary loops—the changes of atrophic blanche.

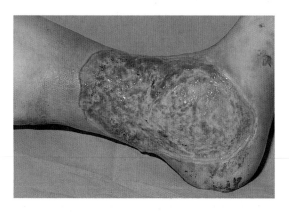

Fig. 11.9 Large venous ulcer overlying the medial malleolus.

pyrexia, a purulent discharge, rapid extension or an increase in pain, cellulitis, lymphangitis or septicaemia.

Eczema (p. 90) is common around venous ulcers. Allergic contact dermatitis (p. 80) is a common complication and should be suspected if the rash worsens, itches or fails to improve with local treatment. Lanolin, parabens (a preservative) and neomycin are the most common culprits.

Malignant change can occur. If an ulcer has a hyperplastic base or a rolled edge, biopsy may be needed to rule out a squamous cell carcinoma (Fig. 11.10).

Differential diagnosis

The main causes of leg ulceration are given in Table 11.7. The most important differences between venous and other leg ulcers are the following.

Atherosclerotic. These ulcers are more common on the toes, dorsum of foot, heel, calf and shin, and are unrelated to perforating veins. Their edges are often sharply defined, their outline may be polycyclic and the ulcers may be deep and gangrenous. Islands of intact skin are characteristically seen within the ulcer. Claudication may be present and peripheral pulses absent.

Vasculitic. These ulcers start as painful palpable purpuric lesions, turning into small punched-out ulcers.

Elevation of the affected limb

Preferably above the hips, this aids venous drainage, decreases oedema and raises oxygen tension in the limb. Patients should rest with their bodies horizontal and their legs up for at least 2 h every afternoon. The foot of the bed should be raised by at least 15 cm; it is not enough just to put a pillow under the feet.

Walking

Walking, in moderation, is beneficial, but prolonged standing or sitting with dependent legs is not.

Physiotherapy

Some physiotherapists are good at persuading venous ulcers to heal. Their secret lies in a combination of the following: leg exercises, elevation, gentle massage, ultrasound treatment to the skin around the ulcers, oedema pumps and graduated compression bandaging.

Diet

Many patients are obese and should lose weight.

Local therapy

Remember that many ulcers will heal with no treatment at all but, if their blood flow is compromised, they will not heal despite meticulous care.

Local therapy should be chosen to:
- control or absorb the exudates;
- reduce the pain;
- control the odour;
- protect the surrounding skin;
- remove surface debris;
- promote re-epithelialization; and
- make optimal use of nursing time.

There are many preparations to choose from; those we have found most useful are listed in Formulary 1 (p. 338).

Clean ulcers (Fig. 11.13)

Dressings need be changed only once or twice a week, keeping the ulcer moist. Paraffin tulle dressings, plain or impregnated with 0.5% chlorhexidine, 0.25%

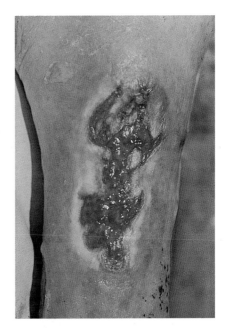

Fig. 11.13 Clean healing ulcer. Weekly dressing would be suitable.

silver proteinate in compound calamine cream spread on a non-stick dressing, 1% silver sulphadiazine cream, and simple zinc and castor oil ointment, are all helpful and easy to apply. The area should be cleaned gently with arachis oil, 5% hydrogen peroxide or saline before the next dressing is applied. Sometimes immersing the whole ulcer in a tub of warm water helps to loosen or dissolve adherent crusts. The prolonged use of antiseptics may be harmful.

Many dressings have absorbent and protective properties (Formulary 1, p. 338). These include Granuflex and DuoDERM Extra Thin (which have the advantage of sticking to the surrounding skin), Geliperm, Kaltostat and Sorbsan in the UK and Duoderm, Opsite and Tegaderm in the USA. Actisorb (UK) is a useful charcoal dressing that absorbs exudate and minimizes odour. Ointments containing recombinant human platelet growth factor may aid revascularization.

Medicated bandages (Formulary 1, p. 338) based on zinc paste, with ichthammol, or with calamine and clioquinol, are useful when there is much surrounding eczema, and can be used for all types of ulcers, even infected exuding ones. The bandage is applied in strips from the foot to below the knee. Worsening of eczema under a medicated bandage may signal

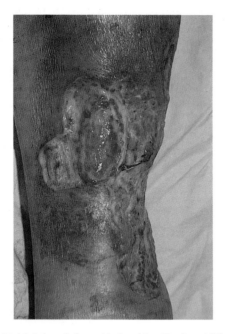

Fig. 11.14 Infected ulcer with sloughing. Tendon visible at bottom of figure. Hospital admission and frequent dressings needed to save leg.

the development of allergic contact dermatitis to a component of the paste, most often parabens (a preservative) or cetostearyl alcohols.

Infected ulcers (Fig. 11.14)

These have to be cleaned and dressed more often than clean ones, sometimes even twice daily. Useful preparations include 0.5% silver nitrate, 0.25% sodium hypochlorite, 0.25% acetic acid, potassium permanganate (1 in 10 000 dilution) and 5% hydrogen peroxide, all made up in aqueous solution, and applied as compresses with or without occlusion. Helpful creams and lotions include 1.5% hydrogen peroxide, 20% benzoyl peroxide, 1% silver sulphadiazine, 10% povidone-iodine (Formulary 1, p. 338). The main function of dextran polymer beads, and starch polymer beads within cadexomer iodine, is to absorb exudate. Although antibiotic tulles are easy to apply and are well tolerated, they should not be used for long periods as they can induce bacterial resistance and sensitize. Resistance is not such a problem with povidone-iodine, and a readily applied non-adherent dressing impregnated with this antiseptic may be useful. Surrounding eczema is helped by weak or moderate strength local steroids, which must never be put on the ulcer itself. Lassar's paste, zinc cream or paste bandages (see above) are suitable alternatives.

Oral treatment

The following may be helpful.

Diuretics. Pressure bandaging is more important as the oedema associated with venous ulceration is largely mechanical. Diuretics will combat the oedema of cardiac failure.

Analgesics. Adequate analgesia is important. Aspirin may not be well tolerated by the elderly. Paracetamol (not available in the USA), or acetaminophen is often adequate but dihydrocodeine may be required. Analgesia may be needed only when the dressing is changed.

Antibiotics. Ulcers need not be 'sterilized' by local or systemic antibiotics. Short courses of systemic antibiotics should be reserved for spreading infections (see under Complications above) but are sometimes tried for pain or even odour. Bacteriological guidance is needed and the drugs used include erythromycin and flucloxacillin (streptococcal or staphylococcal cellulitis), metronidazole (*Bacteroides* infection) and ciprofloxacin (*Pseudomonas aeruginosa* infection). Bacterial infection may prejudice the outcome of skin grafting.

Ferrous sulphate and folic acid. For anaemia.

Zinc sulphate. May help to promote healing, especially if the plasma zinc level is low.

Oxypentifylline (pentoxyfylline) is fibrinolytic, increases the deformability of red and white blood cells, decreases blood viscosity and diminishes platelet adhesiveness. It may speed the healing of venous ulcers if used with compression bandages.

Stanozolol. This anabolic steroid may not heal an existing ulcer more quickly, but may prevent ulceration in lipodermatosclerosis and may protect against recurrences. The manufacturer's advice on contraindications, e.g. prostatic cancer and abnormal liver function, and on monitoring treatment must not be overlooked.

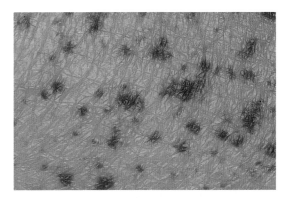

Fig. 11.15 Typical purpura, which is not abolished by pressure.

Oxerutins. These may help the oedema and symptoms of venous hypertension and are said to reduce leakage from capillaries by acting on the endothelial cells.

Surgery

Autologous pinch, split-thickness or mesh grafts have a place. Lyophilized pig dermis, and synthetic films similar to skin, may also be tried. Sheets of human epidermis grown in tissue culture can be purchased and placed on granulating wound beds. Even if grafts do not take, they may stimulate wound healing and relieve pain. In general, grafts work best on clean ulcers.

Venous surgery on younger patients with varicose veins may prevent recurrences, if the deep veins are competent. Patients with atherosclerotic ulcers should see a vascular surgeon for assessment. Some blockages are surgically remediable.

Purpura

Purpura (Fig. 11.15), petechiae and ecchymoses may be caused by a coagulation or platelet disorder, or by an abnormality of the vessel wall or the surrounding dermis. Some common causes are listed in Table 11.8. In general, coagulation defects give rise to ecchymoses and external bleeding. Platelet defects present more often as purpura, although bleeding and ecchymoses can still occur. Vasculitis of small vessels causes purpura, often palpable and painful, but not bleeding;

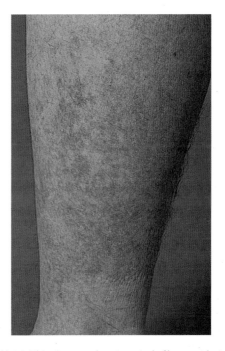

Fig. 11.16 This gingery colour is typical of haemosiderin rather than melanin. It is caused by capillary fragility.

this is discussed in Chapter 8. Purpura from vasodilatation and gravity is seen in many diseases of the legs, especially in the elderly (defective dermis around the blood vessels), and seldom requires extensive investigation.

Cryoglobulinaemia is a rare cause of purpura, which is most prominent on exposed parts. It may also cause cold urticaria (p. 95) and livedo reticularis (p. 133).

Coagulation defects
Inherited defects (e.g. haemophilia, Christmas disease)
Connective tissue disorders
Disseminated intravascular coagulation
Paraproteinaemias (e.g. macroglobulinaemia)
Acquired defects (e.g. liver disease, anticoagulant therapy, vitamin K deficiency, drugs)

Platelet defects
Thrombocytopenia
  Idiopathic
  Connective tissue disorders, especially lupus erythematosus
  Disseminated intravascular coagulation
  Haemolytic anaemia
  Hypersplenism
  Giant haemangiomas (Kasabach–Merritt syndrome)
  Bone marrow damage (cytostatic drugs, leukaemia, carcinoma)
  Drugs (quinine, aspirin, thiazides and sulphonamides)
Abnormal function
  von Willebrand's disease
Drugs (e.g aspirin)

Vascular defect
Raised intravascular pressure (coughing, vomiting, venous hypertension, gravitational)
Vasculitis (including Henoch–Schönlein purpura)
Infections (e.g. meningococcal septicaemia, Rocky Mountain spotted fever)
Drugs (carbromal, aspirin, sulphonamides, quinine, phenylbutazone and gold salts)
Painful bruising syndrome

Idiopathic
Progressive pigmented dermatoses (Fig. 11.16)

Lack of support from surrounding dermis
Senile purpura
Topical or systemic corticosteroid therapy
Scurvy (perifollicular purpura)
Lichen sclerosus et atrophicus
Systemic amyloidosis

Table 11.8 Causes of intracutaneous bleeding.

The condition may be idiopathic, or secondary to myeloma, leukaemia, a previous hepatitis C infection or an autoimmune disease.

Investigations

The most common cause of purpura is trauma, especially to the thin sun-damaged skin of elderly forearms. When purpura has no obvious cause, investigations should include a platelet count, prothrombin time, activated partial thromboplastin time (APTT), a full blood count and biochemical screen. Electrophoresis is needed to exclude hypergammaglobulinaemia and paraproteinaemia. Cryoglobulinaemia should also be excluded. To help detect a consumptive coagulopathy, a coagulation screen, including measurement of fibrinogen and fibrin degradation products, may be necessary. The bleeding time, and a Hess tourniquet test for capillary fragility, help less often. Skin biopsy will confirm a small vessel vasculitis, if the purpura is palpable.

Table 11.9 Causes of secondary lymphoedema.

Recurrent lymphangitis	Erysipelas
	Infected pompholyx
Lymphatic obstruction	Filariasis
	Granuloma inguinale
	Tuberculosis
	Tumour
Lymphatic destruction	Surgery
	Radiation therapy
	Tumour
Uncertain aetiology	Rosacea
	Melkersson–Rosenthal syndrome (facial nerve palsy, fissuring of tongue and lymphoedema of lip)
	Yellow nail syndrome

Treatment

Treat the underlying condition. Replacement of relevant blood constituents may be needed initially. Systemic steroids are usually effective in vasculitis (Chapter 8).

Disorders of the lymphatics

Lymphoedema

The skin overlying chronic lymphoedema is firm and pits poorly. Longstanding lymphoedema may lead to gross, almost furry, hyperkeratosis, as in the so-called 'mossy foot'.

Cause

Lymphoedema may be primary or secondary. The primary forms are developmental defects, although signs may only appear in early puberty or even in adulthood. Sometimes lymphoedema involves only one leg. Secondary causes are listed in Table 11.9.

Treatment

Elevation, graduated compression bandages and stockings (p. 142), diuretics and the early treatment of lymphangitis or erysipelas are the cornerstones of treatment. If erysipelas recurs, long-term penicillin should be given. Surgery occasionally helps to remove an obstruction or restore drainage.

Lymphangitis

This streptococcal infection of the lymphatics may occur without any lymphoedema. A tender red line extends proximally. Penicillin flucloxacillin, cephalexin and erythromycin are usually effective.

Further reading

Douglas, W.S. & Simpson, N.B. (1995) Guidelines for the management of chronic venous ulceration: report of a multidisciplinary workshop. *British Journal of Dermatology* **132**, 446–452.
Valencia, I.C., Falabella, A., Kirsner, R.S. & Eaglstein, W.H. (2001) Chronic venous insufficiency and venous leg ulceration. *Journal of the American Academy of Dermatology* **44**, 401–421.

Sebaceous glands

Most sebaceous glands develop embryologically from hair germs, but a few free glands arise from the epidermis. Those associated with hairs lie in the obtuse angle between the follicle and the epidermis (Fig. 13.1). The glands themselves are multilobed and contain cells full of lipid, which are shed whole (holocrine secretion) during secretion so that sebum contains their remnants in a complex mixture of triglycerides, fatty acids, wax esters, squalene and cholesterol. Sebum is discharged into the upper part of the hair follicle. It lubricates and waterproofs the skin, and protects it from drying; it is also mildly bacteriocidal and fungistatic. Free sebaceous glands may be found in the eyelid (meibomian glands), mucous membranes (Fordyce spots), nipple, peri-anal region and genitalia.

Androgenic hormones, especially dihydrotestosterone, stimulate sebaceous gland activity. Human sebaceous glands contain 5α-reductase, 3α- and 17α-hydroxysteroid dehydrogenase, which convert weaker androgens to dihydrotestosterone, which in turn binds to specific receptors in sebaceous glands, increasing sebum secretion. The sebaceous glands react to maternal androgens for a short time after birth, and then lie dormant until puberty when a surge of androgens produces a sudden increase in sebum excretion and sets the stage for acne.

Acne

Acne is a disorder of the pilosebaceous apparatus characterized by comedones, papules, pustules, cysts and scars.

Prevalence

Nearly all teenagers have some acne (acne vulgaris).

It affects the sexes equally, starting usually between the ages of 12 and 14 years, tending to be earlier in females. The peak age for severity in females is 16–17 and in males 17–19 years. Variants of acne are much less common.

Cause

Acne vulgaris

Many factors combine to cause acne (Fig. 12.1), characterized by chronic inflammation around pilosebaceous follicles.

• *Sebum.* Sebum excretion is increased. However, this alone need not cause acne; patients with acromegaly, or with Parkinson's disease, have high sebum excretion rates but no acne. Furthermore, sebum excretion often remains high long after the acne has gone away.

• *Hormonal.* Androgens (from the testes, ovaries and adrenals) are the main stimulants of sebum excretion, although other hormones (e.g. thyroid hormones and growth hormone) have minor effects too. Those castrated before puberty never develop acne. In acne, the sebaceous glands respond excessively to what are usually normal levels of these hormones (increased target organ sensitivity). This may be caused by 5α-reductase activity being higher in the target sebaceous glands than in other parts of the body. Fifty per cent of females with acne have slightly raised free testosterone levels—usually because of a low level of sex hormone binding globulin rather than a high total testosterone—but this is still only a fraction of the concentration in males, and its relevance is debatable.

• *Poral occlusion.* Both genetic and environmental factors (e.g. some cosmetics) cause the epithelium to overgrow the follicular surface. Follicles then retain sebum that has an increased concentration of bacteria

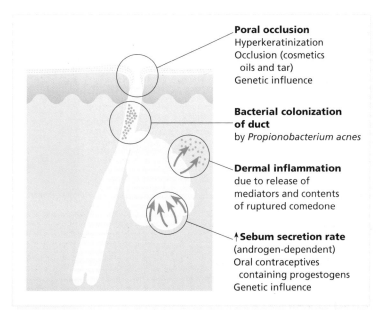

Poral occlusion
Hyperkeratinization
Occlusion (cosmetics
  oils and tar)
Genetic influence

**Bacterial colonization
of duct**
by *Propionobacterium acnes*

Dermal inflammation
due to release of
mediators and contents
of ruptured comedone

↑**Sebum secretion rate**
(androgen-dependent)
Oral contraceptives
  containing progestogens
Genetic influence

Fig. 12.1 Factors causing acne.

and free fatty acids. Rupture of these follicles is associated with intense inflammation and tissue damage, mediated by oxygen free radicals and enzymes such as elastase, released by white cells.

• *Bacterial. Propionibacterium acnes*, a normal skin commensal, plays a pathogenic part. It colonizes the pilosebaceous ducts, breaks down triglycerides releasing free fatty acids, produces substances chemotactic for inflammatory cells and induces the ductal epithelium to secrete pro-inflammatory cytokines. The inflammatory reaction is kept going by a type IV immune reaction (p. 26) to one or more antigens in the follicle.

• *Genetic*. The condition is familial in about half of those with acne. There is a high concordance of the sebum excretion rate and acne in monozygotic, but not dizygotic, twins. Further studies are required to determine the precise mode of inheritance.

Variants of acne

• *Infantile acne* may follow transplacental stimulation of a child's sebaceous glands by maternal androgens.

• *Mechanical*. Excessive scrubbing, picking, or the rubbing of chin straps or a fiddle (see Fig. 12.2) can rupture occluded follicles.

• *Acne associated with virilization*, including clitoromegaly, may be caused by an androgen-secreting

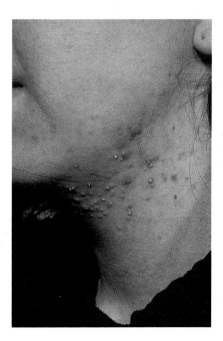

Fig. 12.2 Papulopustular lesions in an odd distribution. The patient played the violin ('fiddler's neck').

tumour of the adrenals, ovaries or testes or, rarely, to congenital adrenal hyperplasia caused by mild 21-hydroxylase deficiency. The gene frequency for this autosomal recessive disorder is high in Ashkenazi

Jews (19%), inhabitants of the former Yugoslavia (12%) and Italians (6%).
• *Acne accompanying the polycystic ovarian syndrome* is caused by modestly raised circulating androgen levels.
• *Drug-induced*. Corticosteroids, androgenic and anabolic steroids, gonadotrophins, oral contraceptives, lithium, iodides, bromides, antituberculosis and anticonvulsant therapy can all cause an acneiform rash.
• *Tropical*. Heat and humidity are responsible for this variant, which affects Caucasoids with a tendency to acne.
• *Acne cosmetica* (see p. 151).

Presentation

Common type

Lesions are confined to the face, shoulders, upper chest and back. Seborrhoea (a greasy skin; Fig. 12.3) is often present. Open comedones (blackheads), because of the plugging by keratin and sebum of the pilosebaceous orifice, or closed comedones (whiteheads), caused by overgrowth of the follicle openings by surrounding epithelium, are always seen. Inflammatory papules, nodules and cysts (Figs 12.4 and 12.5) occur, with one or two types of lesion predominating. Depressed or hypertrophic scarring and postinflammatory hyperpigmentation can follow.

Conglobate (gathered into balls; from the Latin *globus* meaning 'ball') is the name given to a severe

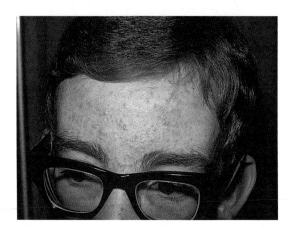

Fig. 12.3 The seborrhoea, comedones and scattered inflammatory papules of teenage acne.

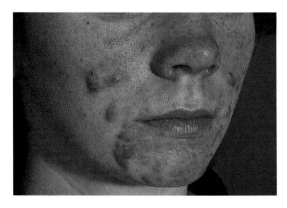

Fig. 12.4 Prominent and inflamed cysts are the main features here.

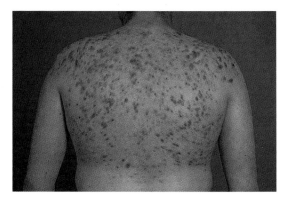

Fig. 12.5 Conglobate acne with inflammatory nodules, pustulocystic lesions and depressed scars.

form of acne with all of the above features as well as abscesses or cysts with intercommunicating sinuses that contain thick serosanguinous fluid or pus. On resolution, it leaves deeply pitted or hypertrophic scars, sometimes joined by keloidal bridges. Although hyperpigmentation is usually transient, it can persist, particularly in those with an already dark skin.

Psychological depression is common in persistent acne, which need not necessarily be severe.

Variants

• *Infantile*. This rare type of acne is present at, or appears soon after birth. It is more common in males and may last up to 3 years. Its morphology is like that of common acne (Fig. 12.6) and it may be the forerunner of severe acne in adolescence.

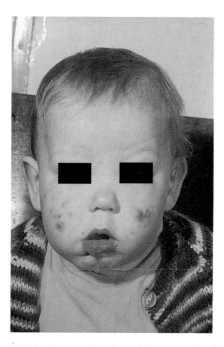

Fig. 12.6 Infantile acne. Pustulocystic lesions on the cheeks.

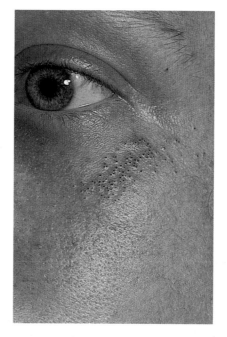

Fig. 12.7 A group of open comedones (blackheads) following the use of a greasy cosmetic.

- *Fulminans*. Acne fulminans is a rare variant in which conglobate acne is accompanied by fever, joint pains and a high erythrocyte sedimentation rate (ESR).
- *Exogenous*. Tars, chlorinated hydrocarbons, oils, and oily cosmetics can cause or exacerbate acne. Suspicion should be raised if the distribution is odd or if comedones predominate (Fig. 12.7).
- *Excoriated*. This is most common in young girls. Obsessional picking or rubbing leaves discrete denuded areas.
- *Late onset*. This too occurs mainly in women and is often limited to the chin (Fig. 12.8). Nodular and cystic lesions predominate. It is stubborn and persistent.
- *Acne associated with suppurative hidradenitis and perifolliculitis of scalp* (see below).
- *Tropical*. This occurs mainly on the trunk and may be conglobate.
- *Drug-induced* (Fig. 12.9). Suspicion should be raised when acne, dominated by papulo-pustules rather than comedones, appears suddenly in a non-teenager and coincides with the prescription of a drug known to cause acneiform lesions (see above). Some athletes still use anabolic steroids to enhance their performance.

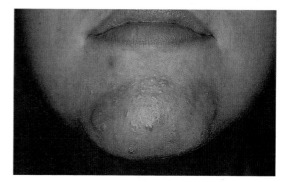

Fig. 12.8 Late-onset acne in a woman. Often localized to the chin.

- *Polycystic ovarian syndrome*. Consider this in obese females with oligomenorrhoea or secondary amenorrhoea or infertility. Glucose intolerance, dyslipidaemia and hypertension may be other features.
- *Congenital adrenal hyperplasia*. Hyperpigmentation, ambiguous genitalia, history of salt-wasting in childhood, and a Jewish background, are all clues to this rare diagnosis.

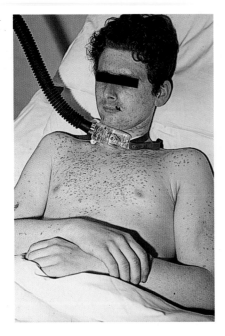

Fig. 12.9 Steroid-induced acne in a seriously ill patient.

• *Androgen-secreting tumours.* These cause the rapid onset of virilization (clitoromegaly, deepening of voice, breast atrophy, male pattern balding and hirsutism) as well as acne.

Course

Acne vulgaris clears by the age of 23–25 years in 90% of patients, but some 5% of women and 1% of men still need treatment in their thirties or even forties.

Investigations

None are usually necessary. Cultures are occasionally needed to exclude a pyogenic infection, an anaerobic infection or Gram-negative folliculitis. Only a few laboratories routinely culture *P. acnes* and test its sensitivity to antibiotics.

Any acne, including infantile acne, which is associated with virilization, needs investigation to exclude an androgen-secreting tumour of the adrenals, ovaries or testes, and to rule out congenital adrenal hyperplasia caused by 21-hydroxylase deficiency. Tests should then include the measurement of plasma testosterone, sex hormone-binding globulin, luteinizing hormone (LH), follicle-stimulating hormone (FSH), dehydroepiandros-terone sulphate, androstenedione,

17-hydroxyprogesterone, urinary free cortisol and, depending on the results, ultrasound examination or computed tomography scan of the ovaries and adrenals. Congenital adrenal hyperplasia is associated with high levels of 17-hydroxyprogesterone, and androgensecreting tumours with high androgen levels.

Polycystic ovarian syndrome is characterized by modestly elevated testosterone, androstenedione and dehydroepiandrosterone sulphate levels, a reduced sex hormone-binding level and a LH : FSH ratio of greater than 2.5 : 1. Pelvic ultrasound may reveal multiple small ovarian cysts, although some acne patients have ovarian cysts without biochemical evidence of the polycystic ovarian syndrome.

Differential diagnosis

Rosacea (see below) affects older individuals; comedones are absent; the papules and pustules occur only on the face; and the rash has an erythematous background. Pyogenic folliculitis can be excluded by culture. Hidradenitis suppurativa (see below) is associated with acne conglobata, but attacks the axillae and groin. Pseudofolliculitis barbae, caused by ingrowing hairs, occurs on the necks of men with curly facial hair and clears up if shaving is stopped.

Treatment

Acne frequently has marked psychological effects. Even those with mild acne need sympathy. An optimistic approach is essential, and regular encouragement worthwhile.

Occasionally an underlying cause (see above) is found; this should be removed or treated.

At some time most teenagers try antiacne preparations bought from their pharmacist; local treatment is enough for most patients with comedo-papular acne, although both local and systemic treatment are needed for pustulocystic scarring acne (Fig. 12.10).

Local treatment (Formulary 1, p. 336)

1 *Regular gentle cleansing* with soap and water should be encouraged, to remove surface sebum. Antibacterial cleansers are also useful, e.g. chlorhexidine.
2 *Benzoyl peroxide.* This antibacterial agent is applied only at night initially, but can be used twice daily if this does not cause too much dryness and irritation. It is most effective for inflammatory lesions.

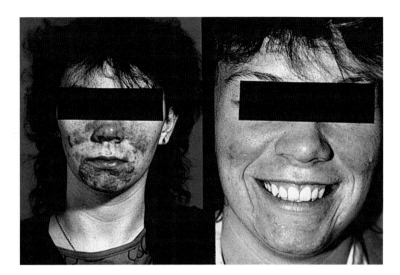

Fig. 12.10 A successful systemic treatment of acne—the picture tells its own story.

It is wise to start with a 2.5 or 5% preparation, moving up to 10% if necessary. Benzoyl peroxide bleaches coloured materials, particularly towels and flannels.

3 *Retinoids.* The vitamin A (retinol) analogues (tretinoin, adapalene, tazarotene) normalize follicular keratinization, and are especially effective against comedones. Patients should be warned about skin irritation (start with small amounts) and photosensitivity. Concomitant eczema is usually a contraindication to its use. Tretinoin can be prescribed as a lotion, cream or gel. New preparations use microspheres (Retin-A micro) or specially formulated bases (Aveta) that minimize irritation. The weakest preparation should be used first, and applied overnight on alternate nights. Sometimes, after a week or two, it will have to be stopped temporarily because of irritation. As with benzoyl peroxide, it may be worth increasing the strength of tretinoin after 6 weeks if it has been well tolerated. The combination of benzoyl peroxide in the morning and tretinoin at night has many advocates.

- Isotretinoin 0.05% is made up in a gel base (not available in USA) and applied once or twice daily. It irritates less than the same concentration of tretinoin.
- Adapalene (0.1% gel) is a retinoid-like drug indicated for mild to moderate acne. It appears to work quicker and to be tolerated better than tretinoin.
- Tazarotene (0.1% gel), applied once daily, was found in one study to be more effective than tretinoin (0.1% microsponge).

Topical retinoids should not be prescribed for pregnant woman with acne.

4 *Azelaic acid* is bacteriocidal for *P. acnes*: it is also anti-inflammatory and inhibits the formation of comedones by reducing the proliferation of keratinocytes. It should be applied twice daily, but not used for more than 6 months at a time.

5 *Abrasive pastes* containing aluminium oxide have largely been replaced by topical retinoids as aggressive scrubbing can rupture comedones.

6 *Sulphur.* A number of time-honoured preparations containing sulphur are available on both sides of the Atlantic. Some are included in Formulary 1 (p. 336).

7 *Local antibiotics.* These include topical clindamycin, erythromycin and sulfacetamide (Formulary 1, p. 336).

8 *Combinations.* Some combinations work better than either of the drugs used separately. Erythromycin combined with a zinc acetate complex (Formulary 1, p. 336) is popular and effective. It works as an antimicrobial, an inhibitor of 5α-reductase (see above), an antioxidant and as an immunomodulator. Erythromycin and clindamycin, in mixtures with benzoyl peroxide, reduce *P. acnes* numbers and the likelihood of resistant strains emerging (Formulary 1, p. 336).

9 *Aluminium chloride.* Alcoholic solutions of aluminium chloride, used as antiperspirants, may help tropical acne.

10 *Cosmetic camouflage.* Cover-ups help some patients, especially females, whose scarring is unsightly. They also obscure postinflammatory pigmentation. A range of make-ups is available in the UK and USA (Formulary 1, p. 330).

Systemic treatment (Formulary 2, p. 340)

Antibiotics: tetracyclines

• *Oxytetracycline and tetracycline.* An average starting dosage for an adult is 250 mg up to four times daily, but up to 1.5 g/day may be needed in resistant cases. The antibiotic should not be used for less than 3 months and may be needed for a year or two, or even longer. It should be taken on an empty stomach, 1 h before meals, or 4 h after food, as the absorption of these tetracyclines is decreased by milk, antacids and calcium, iron and magnesium salts. The dosage should be tapered in line with clinical improvement, an average maintenance dosage being 250–500 mg/day. Even with long courses, serious side-effects are rare, although candidal vulvovaginitis may force a change to a narrower spectrum antibiotic such as erythromycin.

• *Minocycline,* 50 mg twice daily or 100 mg once or twice daily (in a modified release preparation) is now preferred by many dermatologists, although it is much more expensive. Absorption is not significantly affected by food or drink. Minocycline is much more lipophilic than oxytetracycline and so probably concentrates better in the sebaceous glands. It is bacteriologically more effective than oxytetracycline and tetracycline and, unlike erythromycin, little resistance to it by *Proprionibacteria* has been recorded. It can be effective even when oxytetracycline has failed, but can cause abnormalities of liver function and a lupus-like syndrome.

• *Doxycycline,* 100 mg once or twice daily is a cheaper alternative to minocycline, but more frequently associated with phototoxic skin reactions.

Tetracyclines should not be taken in pregnancy or by children under 12 years as they are deposited in growing bone and developing teeth, causing stained teeth and dental hypoplasia. Rarely, the long-term administration of minocycline causes a greyish pigmentation, like a bruise, especially on the faces of those with actinic damage and over the shins.

Erythromycin (dosage as for oxytetracycline) is the next antibiotic of choice but is preferable to tetracyclines in women who might become pregnant. Its major drawback is the development of resistant *Proprionibacteria,* now present in at least one in four patients with acne, which leads to therapeutic failure.

Trimethoprim is used by some as a third-line antibiotic for acne, when a tetracycline and erythromycin have not helped. White blood cell counts should be monitored. *Ampicillin* is another alternative.

Hormonal. A combined antiandrogen–oestrogen treatment (Dianette: 2 mg cyproterone acetate and 0.035 mg ethinylestradiol) is available in many countries and may help persistent acne in women. Monitoring is as for any patient on an oral contraceptive, and further contraceptive measures are unnecessary. Courses last for 8–12 months and the drug is then replaced by a low oestrogen/low progestogen oral contraceptive. These drugs are not for males.

A triphasic pill, or a pill with a high oestrogen content, is best for women with acne who also require oral contraception. Those on antibiotics should be warned of their possible interaction with oral contraceptives and should use other contraceptive precautions, especially if the antibiotics induce diarrhoea.

Isotretinoin (13-*cis*-retinoic acid, Formulary 2, p. 350). This is an oral retinoid, which inhibits sebum excretion, the growth of *P. acnes,* and acute inflammatory processes. The drug is reserved for severe nodulocystic acne, unresponsive to the measures outlined above. It is routinely given for 4–6 months only, in a dosage of 0.5–1 mg/kg body weight/day; young men with truncal acne usually require the higher dosage. A full blood count, liver function tests and fasting lipid levels should be checked, and routine urine analysis performed before the start of the course, and then at 4 weeks after starting the drug. Some physicians also monitor at 10 and 16 weeks and perform a final check 1 month after completing the course. The drug seldom has to be stopped, although rarely abnormalities of liver function limit treatment.

Isotretinoin is highly teratogenic: before starting treatment women should sign a form confirming that, as far as they know, they are not pregnant and that they have been warned about this risk. They should take an oral contraceptive or Dianette for 2 months before starting isotretinoin, throughout treatment and for 1 month thereafter. Tests for pregnancy, preferably performed on a blood sample, should be carried out twice before starting treatment and at follow-up visits. Contraception and teratogenicity of the drug must be discussed at all visits. The recommendations in the USA are especially stringent. Before receiving

Table 12.1 Avoidance list for patients taking isotretinoin.

Avoid	Reason
Pregnancy	Teratogenicity
Breast feeding	Unknown effect on baby
Giving blood	Teratogenicity in recipient
Uncontrolled hyperlipidaemia	Additive side-effects
Taking vitamin A and hypervitaminosis A	Additive side-effects
Cosmetic procedures	Increased scarring
Excessive natural or artificial UVR	Photosensitivity
Oral contraceptive with low dose of progesterone—'minipills'	Ineffective contraception
Concomitant antibiotics, unless with permission of prescribing doctor	Intracranial hypertension

the drug the patient must sign that 'I understand that I cannot receive a prescription for Accutane unless I have two negative pregnancy test results. The first pregnancy test should be during the office visit when my prescriber decides to prescribe Accutane. The second test should be on the second day of my next menstrual cycle or 11 days after the last time I had unprotected sexual intercourse, whichever is later. I understand that I will have additional pregnancy testing, monthly, throughout my Accutane therapy.' Furthermore, the manufacturer's medication guide recommends that 'you must use two separate effective forms of birth control at the same time for at least 1 month before starting Accutane, while you take it, and for 1 month after you stop taking it'. Treatment should start on day 3 of the patient's next menstrual cycle following a negative pregnancy test.

Depression, sometimes leading to suicide, is a rare accompaniment of treatment. A causal relationship seems likely in a few patients, although this has yet to be confirmed in a large controlled study. Nevertheless, patients and their family doctors should be warned about the appearance or worsening of depression before starting a course of isotretinoin and patients should be asked to sign a document that indicates that the issue of adverse psychiatric events has been discussed. The drug should be stopped immediately if there is any concern on this score. The possibility of adverse psychiatric events should be discussed at all visits. This potentially severe accompaniment of isotretinoin treatment has to be balanced against its remarkable efficacy in severe acne. The lives of most patients with conglobate acne have been transformed after successful treatment with isotretinoin.

Other side-effects of isotretinoin include a dry skin, dry and inflamed lips and eyes, nosebleeds, facial erythema, muscle aches, hyperlipidaemia and hair loss; these are reversible and often tolerable, especially if the acne is doing well. Rarer and potentially more serious side-effects include changes in night-time vision and hearing loss. Occasionally, isotretinoin flares acne at first, but this effect is usually short lived and the drug can be continued. It is because of its early side-effects that some dermatologists start isotretinoin in a low dose (e.g. 20 mg/day) and then work up to the target dose if no significant side-effects are reported at review during the first month of treatment. Early review appointments (e.g. at 1 and 2 weeks into treatment) are comforting to both patient and doctor. A useful 'avoidance list' for patients taking isotretinoin is given in Table 12.1.

Diet

It is sensible for patients to avoid foods (e.g. nuts, chocolates, dairy products and wine) that they think make their acne worse, but there is little evidence that any dietary constituent, except iodine, causes acne.

Physical

Ultraviolet B radiation therapy often helps with exacerbations. Two-month courses, during which the patient attends two or three times weekly, are usually adequate.

Cysts can be incised and drained with or without a local anaesthetic.

Intralesional injections of 0.1 mL of triamcinolone acetonide (2.5–10 mg/mL) hasten the resolution of stubborn cysts, but can leave atrophy.

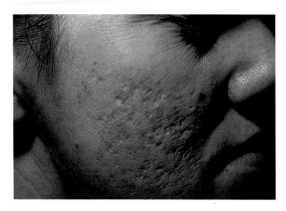

Fig. 12.11 Acne scarring: worth treating a test area with a resurfacing laser.

Dermabrasion. This helps to smooth out facial scars. A high-speed rotating wire brush planes down to a bleeding dermis. Dermabrasion should not be carried out if there are any active lesions and does not help depressed 'ice-pick' scars, which may best be excised. Unsightly hyperpigmentation may follow in darker skins. Microdermabrasion is well tolerated but its effects are usually transient.

Lasers. Skin resurfacing with CO_2 and erbium lasers is rapidly replacing dermabrasion and chemical peeling as the best treatment for postacne scarring. The procedure, which should be delayed until the acne is quiescent, is usually performed under local anaesthesia. Initially a small test area is treated and then assessed (Fig. 12.11). If the result is satisfactory, the

---

LEARNING POINTS

1 Never prescribe short courses of many different antibiotics.
2 Avoid tetracyclines in children and pregnant women.
3 Make sure that females with acne are not pregnant before you prescribe isotretinoin, and that they do not become pregnant during the course of treatment and for 3 months after it.
4 Look out for depression in patients taking isotretinoin. If it occurs, stop the drug immediately, seek specialist advice and review your therapeutic options.

---

treatment is extended. In expert hands the results can be dramatic.

Collagen injections. Bovine collagen can be injected into depressed scars to improve their appearance. Patients with a history of any autoimmune disorder are excluded from this treatment. Shallow atrophic lesions do better than discrete 'ice-pick' scars. The procedure is expensive and has to be repeated every 6 months as the collagen is resorbed.

Rosacea

Rosacea affects the face of adults, usually women. Although its peak incidence is in the thirties and forties, it can also be seen in the young or old. It may coexist with acne but is distinct from it.

Cause and histopathology

The cause is still unknown. Rosacea is often seen in those who flush easily in response to warmth, spicy food, alcohol or embarrassment. Any psychological abnormalities, including neuroticism and depression, are secondary to the skin condition. No pharmacological defect has been found which explains these flushing attacks. Sebum excretion rate and skin microbiology are normal. A pathogenic role for the hair follicle mite, *Demodex folliculorum*, has not been proved.

Clinical course and complications

The cheeks, nose, centre of forehead, and chin are most commonly affected; the peri-orbital and peri-oral areas are spared (Fig. 12.12). Intermittent flushing is followed by a fixed erythema and telangiectases. Discrete domed inflamed papules, papulopustules and, rarely, nodules develop later. Rosacea, unlike acne, has no comedones or seborrhoea. It is usually symmetrical. Its course is prolonged, with exacerbations and remissions. Complications include blepharitis, conjunctivitis and, occasionally, keratitis. Rhinophyma, caused by hyperplasia of the sebaceous glands and connective tissue on the nose, is a striking complication (Fig. 12.13) that is more common in males. Lymphoedema, below the eyes and on the forehead, is a tiresome feature in a few cases. Some patients treated with potent topical steroids develop a rebound flare of pustules, worse than the original rosacea, when this treatment is stopped.

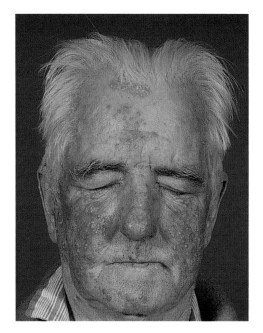

Fig. 12.12 Typical rosacea with papules and pustules on a background of erythema. Note he also has a patch of scaly seborrhoeic eczema on his brow.

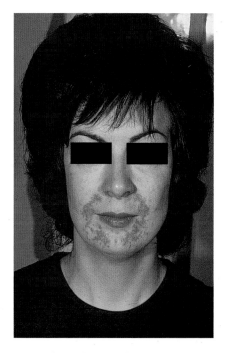

Fig. 12.14 A perioral dermatitis following withdrawal of the potent topical steroid that had been wrongly used to treat seborrhoeic eczema.

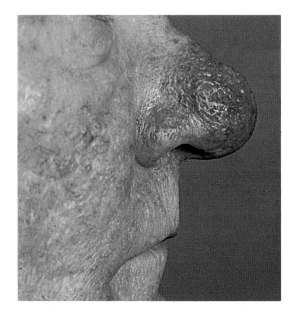

Fig. 12.13 Marked rhinophyma.

Differential diagnosis

Acne has already been mentioned. Rosacea differs from it by its background of erythema and telangiectases, and by the absence of comedones. The distribution of the lesions is different too, as rosacea affects the central face but not the trunk. Also rosacea usually appears after adolescence. Seborrhoeic eczema, perioral dermatitis (Fig. 12.14), systemic lupus erythematosus (p. 119) and photodermatitis should be considered, but do not show the papulopustules of rosacea. The flushing of rosacea can be confused with menopausal symptoms and, rarely, with the carcinoid syndrome. Superior vena caval obstruction has occasionally been mistaken for lymphoedematous rosacea.

Treatment

Tetracyclines, prescribed as for acne (p. 154), are the traditional treatment and are usually effective. Erythromycin is the antibiotic of second choice. Courses should last for at least 10 weeks and, after gaining control with 500–1000 mg daily, the dosage can be

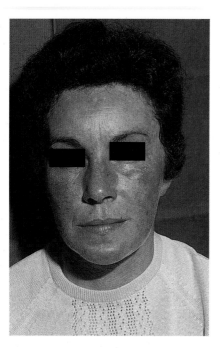

Fig. 12.15 The result of the prolonged use of potent topical steroids for rosacea. Note the extreme telangiectasia.

cut to 250 mg daily. The condition recurs in about half of the patients within 2 years, but repeated antibiotic courses, rather than prolonged maintenance ones, are generally recommended. Topical 0.75% metronidazole gel (Formulary 1, p. 336), applied sparingly once daily, is nearly as effective as oral tetracycline and often prolongs remission. It can be tried before systemic treatment and is especially useful in treating 'stuttering' recurrent lesions that do not then need repeated systemic courses of antibiotics. Rarely systemic metronidazole or isotretinoin (p. 154) is needed for stubborn rosacea. Rosacea and topical steroids go badly together (Fig. 12.15); if possible patients should use traditional applications such as 2% sulphur in aqueous cream or 1% ichthammol in

LEARNING POINT

Never put strong topical steroids on rosacea. If you do, red faces, skin addiction, rebound flares, and a cross dermatologist will all figure in your nightmares.

zinc cream. Sunscreens may help if sun exposure is an aggravating factor, but changes in diet or drinking habits are seldom of value.

Sweat glands

Eccrine sweat glands

There are 2–3 million sweat glands distributed all over the body surface but they are most numerous on the palms, soles and axillae. The tightly coiled glands lie deep in the dermis, and the emerging duct passes to the surface by penetrating the epidermis in a corkscrew fashion. Sweat is formed in the coiled gland by active secretion, involving the sodium pump. Some damage occurs to the membrane of the secretory cells during sweating. Initially sweat is isotonic with plasma but, under normal conditions, it becomes hypotonic by the time it is discharged at the surface, after the tubular resorption of electrolytes and water under the influence of aldosterone and antidiuretic hormone.

In some ways the eccrine sweat duct is like a renal tubule. The pH of sweat is between 4.0 and 6.8; it contains sodium, potassium chloride, lactate, urea and ammonia. The concentration of sodium chloride in sweat is increased in cystic fibrosis, and sweat can be analysed when this is suspected.

Sweat glands have an important role in temperature control, the skin surface being cooled by evaporation. Up to 10 L/day of sweat can be excreted. Three stimuli induce sweating.

1 *Thermal sweating* is a reflex response to a raised environmental temperature and occurs all over the body, especially the chest, back, forehead, scalp and axillae.

2 *Emotional sweating* is provoked by fear or anxiety and is seen mainly on the palms, soles and axillae.

3 *Gustatory sweating* is provoked by hot spicy foods and affects the face.

The eccrine sweat glands are innervated by cholinergic fibres of the sympathetic nervous system. Sweating can therefore be induced by cholinergic, and blocked by anticholinergic drugs. Central control of sweating resides in the preoptic hypothalamic sweat centre.

Clinical disorders can follow increased or decreased sweating, or blockage of sweat gland ducts.

Generalized hyperhidrosis

Thermal hyperhidrosis

The 'thermostat' for sweating lies in the preoptic area of the hypothalamus. Sweating follows any rise in body temperature, whether this is caused by exercise, environmental heat or an illness. The sweating in acute infections, and in some chronic illnesses (e.g. Hodgkin's disease), may be a result of a lowering of the 'set' of this thermostat.

Other causes of general hyperhidrosis

• Emotional stimuli, hypoglycaemia, opiate with-drawal, and shock cause sweating by a direct or reflex stimulation of the sympathetic system at hypothalamic or higher centres. Sweating accompanied by a general sympathetic discharge occurs on a cold pale skin.
• Lesions of the central nervous system (e.g. a cerebral tumour or cerebrovascular accident) can cause gener-alized sweating, presumably by interfering directly with the hypothalamic centre.
• Phaeochromocytoma, the carcinoid syndrome, dia-betes mellitus, thyrotoxicosis, Cushing's syndrome and the hot flushes of menopausal women have all been associated with general sweating. The mechan-isms are not clear.

Local hyperhidrosis (Fig. 12.16)

Local hyperhidrosis plagues many young adults. The most common areas to be affected are the palms, soles and axillae. Too much sweating there is embarrassing,

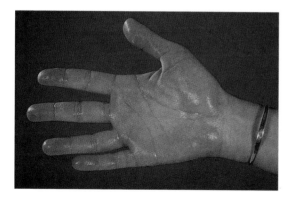

Fig. 12.16 Severe palmar hyperhidrosis demanding treatment.

if not socially crippling. A sodden shirt in contact with a dripping armpit, a wet handshake and stinking feet are hard crosses to bear. Seldom is any cause found, but organic disease, especially thyrotoxicosis, acromegaly, tuberculosis and Hodgkin's disease should be considered. A blatant anxiety state is occasionally present, but more often an otherwise normal person is understandably concerned about his or her antisocial condition. A vicious circle emerges, in which increased anxiety drives further sweating.

These problems may be no more than one end of the normal physiological range. How many students sitting examinations have to dry their hands before putting pen to paper? It is only when the sweating is gross, or continuous, that medical advice is sought. Such sweating is often precipitated by emotional stimuli and stops during sleep.

Treatment

Topical applications. The most useful preparation for axillary hyperhidrosis is 20% aluminium chloride hexahydrate in an alcohol base (Formulary 1, p. 331). At first it is applied to the dry axillae every night. Soon the interval can be increased, and many need the preparation only once or twice a week. The frequency may have to be cut down if the preparation irritates the skin, which is most likely if it is applied after shav-ing or when the skin is wet. Aluminium chloride also helps hyperhidrosis of the palms and soles, but it is less effective there.

Potassium permanganate soaks (1 : 10 000 aqueous solution) combat the bacterial superinfection of sweaty feet that is responsible for their foul smell. Patients should soak their feet for 15 min twice a day until the smell has improved and be warned that potassium permanganate stains the skin and everything else brown. Occasionally glutaraldehyde solutions are used instead, but allergy and yellow-stained skin are potential com-plications. Topical clindamycin is also effective.

Iontophoresis. This is the passage of a low-voltage direct current across the skin. Iontophoresis with tap water or with the anticholinergic drug glycopyrro-nium bromide (glycopyrolate, USA) may help palmar or plantar hyperhidrosis. Patients attend two or three times a week for treatment until the condition improves. Repeated courses or maintenance therapy may be required.

Botulinum toxin. This binds to presynaptic nerve
membranes and then inhibits the release of acetylcholine. It is now the treatment of choice for severe
axillary or plantar hyperhidrosis, unresponsive to
medical measures. Subdermal aliquots of the toxin
are injected into the hyperhidrotic area of the axilla
or sole, one region at a single session. Sweating is
abolished after a delay of 2–3 days. Repeat injections
(about every eighth month) are necessary as the
sweating returns when the toxin has gone. Antibodies
may form against the toxin and diminish its long-term
effectiveness. Botulinum toxin is used less often for
palmar hyperhidrosis because of the risk of paralys-
ing the intrinsic muscles of the hand.

Systemic treatment. Oral anticholinergic agents such
as Pro-Banthine and glycopyronium bromide (USA) are
sometimes tried but their side-effects limit their value.

Surgery. This is used less nowadays as the above
measures are usually effective. However, recalcitrant
axillary hyperhidrosis can be treated by removing the
vault of the axilla, which bears most of the sweat
glands. These can be identified preoperatively by applying starch and iodine, which interact with sweat to
colour the sweat gland openings blue. Thoracoscopic
sympathetic trunkotomy (between the first and second thoracic ganglia) is effective for severe palmar
hyperhidrosis alone but is a last resort.

Hypohidrosis and anhidrosis

*Anhidrosis caused by abnormality of the
sweat glands*

Heat stroke. Caused by sweat gland exhaustion, this
is a medical emergency seen most often in elderly
people moving to a hot climate. It can also occur in the
young, during or after prolonged exercise, especially
in hot climates. Patients present with hyperthermia,
dry skin, weakness, headache, cramps and confusion,
leading to vomiting, hypotension, oliguria, metabolic
acidosis, hyperkalaemia, delirium and death. They
should be cooled down immediately with cold water,
and fluids and electrolytes must be replaced.

Hypohidrotic ectodermal dysplasia. This rare disorder is inherited as an X-linked recessive trait, in which
the sweat glands are either absent or decreased.
Affected boys have a characteristic facial appearance,
with poor hair and teeth (Figs 13.13 and 13.14), and
are intolerant of heat.

Prematurity. The sweat glands function poorly in
premature babies nursed in incubators and hot
nurseries.

*Anhidrosis caused by abnormalities of the
nervous system*

Anhidrosis may follow abnormalities anywhere in
the sympathetic system, from the hypothalamus to
the peripheral nerves. It can therefore be a feature of
multiple sclerosis, a cerebral tumour, trauma, Horner's
syndrome or peripheral neuropathy (e.g. leprosy,
alcoholic neuropathy and diabetes). Patients with
widespread anhidrosis are heat-intolerant, developing nausea, dizziness, tachycardia and hyperthermia
in hot surroundings.

Anhidrosis or hypohidrosis caused by skin disease

Local hypohidrosis has been reported in many skin
diseases, especially those that scar (e.g. lupus erythematosus and morphoea). It may be a feature of
Sjogren's syndrome, ichthyosis, psoriasis and miliaria
profunda (see below).

Interference with sweat delivery

Miliaria. This is the result of plugging or rupture of
sweat ducts. It occurs in hot humid climates, at any
age, and is common in over-clothed infants in hot
nurseries. The physical signs depend on where the
ducts are blocked.

Miliaria crystallina. This presents as tiny clear non-inflamed vesicles that look like dew. This is the most superficial type.

Miliaria rubra (prickly heat). Tiny erythematous and very itchy papules.

Miliaria profunda. These consist of larger erythematous papules or pustules. This is the deepest type.

Treatment. The best treatment is to move to a cooler climate or into air conditioning. Clothing that prevents the evaporation of sweat (e.g. nylon shirts) should be avoided; cotton is best. Claims have been made for ascorbic acid by mouth, but in our hands it rarely if ever helps. Topical steroids reduce irritation but should only be used briefly. Calamine lotion cools and soothes.

Apocrine sweat glands

Apocrine glands are limited to the axillae, nipples, peri-umbilical area, perineum and genitalia. The coiled tubular glands (larger than eccrine glands) lie deep in the dermis, and during sweating the luminal part of their cells is lost (decapitation secretion). Apocrine sweat passes via the duct into the mid-portion of the hair follicle. The action of bacteria on apocrine sweat is responsible for body odour. The glands are innervated by adrenergic fibres of the sympathetic nervous system.

Suppurative hidradenitis (apocrine acne)

This is a severe chronic suppurative disorder of the apocrine glands. Many papules, pustules, cysts, sinuses and scars occur in the axillae, groin and perianal areas. The condition may coexist with conglobate acne. Its cause is unknown, but an underlying follicular abnormality seems likely. Slightly raised androgen levels are found in some affected females. It is probably not an immunodeficiency or a primary infection of the apocrine glands, although *Staphylococcus aureus*, anaerobic streptococci and *Bacterioides* spp. are frequently present. One group of workers has implicated *Streptococcus milleri* as the main pathogen. Treatment is unsatisfactory but should be as for acne vulgaris in the first instance. Systemic antibiotics help early lesions to resolve but are ineffective for chronic draining abscesses and sinuses. Incision and drainage of abscesses, and injections of intralesional triamcinolone (5–10 mg/mL) may reduce the incidence of deforming scars and sinus formation. Topical clindamycin has been shown to prevent new lesions from forming. Systemic antiandrogens help some women. Severe cases need plastic surgery to remove large areas of affected skin.

Fox–Fordyce disease

This rare disease of the apocrine ducts is comparable to miliaria rubra of the eccrine duct. It occurs in women after puberty. Itchy skin-coloured or light brown papules appear in the axillae and other areas where apocrine glands are found, such as the breasts and vulva. Treatment is not usually necessary but removal of the affected skin, or electrodessication of the most irritable lesions can be considered.

Further reading

Collin, J. & Whatling, P. (2000) Treating hyperhidrosis. *British Medical Journal* 320, 1221–1222.

Kreyden, O.P., Böni, R. and Burg, G. (2001) *Hyperhidrosis and Botulinum Toxin in Dermatology*. Karger, Basel.

Mortimer, P.S. & Lunniss, P.J. (2000) Hidradenitis suppurativa. *Journal of The Royal Society of Medicine* 93, 420–422.

Plewig, G. & Kligman, A.M. (1992) *Acne and Rosacea*. Springer, Berlin.

Regional dermatology

The hair

Hair is human plumage: we need just the right amount, in the right places. The twin torments of having too much or too little hair can be understood only when seen against the background of the formation and activity of normal hair follicles.

Hair follicles form before the ninth week of fetal life when the hair germ, a solid cylinder of cells, grows obliquely down into the dermis. Here it is met by a cluster of mesenchymal cells (the placode) bulging into the lower part of the hair germ to form the hair papilla. Eventually the papilla contains blood vessels bringing nutrients to the hair matrix. The sebaceous gland is an outgrowth at the side of the hair germ, establishing early the two parts of the pilosebaceous unit. The hair matrix, the germinative part of the follicle, is equivalent to the basal cells of the epidermis.

Melanocytes migrate into the matrix and are responsible for the different colours of hair (eumelanin, brown/black; phaeomelanin and trichochromes, red). Grey or white hair is caused by low pigment production, and the filling of the cells in the hair medulla with minute air bubbles that reflect light.

The structure of a typical hair follicle is shown in Fig. 13.1.

Classification

Hairs are classified into three main types.
1 *Lanugo hairs.* Fine long hairs covering the fetus, but shed about 1 month before birth.
2 *Vellus hairs.* Fine short unmedullated hairs covering much of the body surface. They replace the lanugo hairs just before birth.

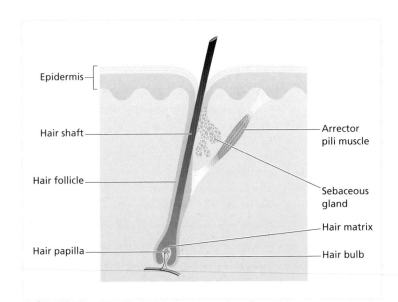

Fig. 13.1 Anatomy of the hair follicle.

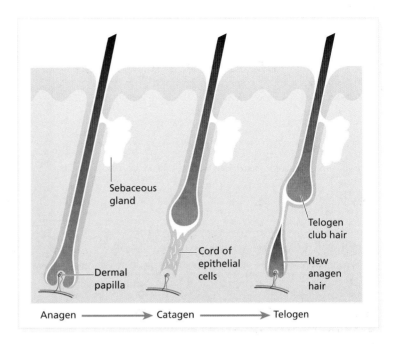

Fig. 13.2 The hair cycle.

3 *Terminal hairs.* Long coarse medullated hairs seen, for example, in the scalp or pubic regions. Their growth is often influenced by circulating androgen levels.

Terminal hairs convert to vellus hairs in male pattern alopecia, and vellus to terminal hairs in hirsutism. The lips, glans penis, labia minora, palms and soles remain free of hair follicles.

The hair cycle

Each follicle passes, independently of its neighbours, through regular cycles of growth and shedding. There are three phases of follicular activity (Fig. 13.2).
1 *Anagen.* The active phase of hair production.
2 *Catagen.* A short phase of conversion from active growth to the resting phase. Growth stops, and the end of the hair becomes club-shaped.
3 *Telogen.* A resting phase at the end of which the club hair is shed.

The duration of each of these stages varies from region to region. On the scalp (Fig. 13.3), said to contain an average of 100 000 hairs, anagen lasts for up to 5 years, catagen for about 2 weeks, and telogen for about 3 months. As many as 100 hairs may be shed from the normal scalp every day as a normal consequence of cycling. The proportion of hairs in the growing and resting stages can be estimated by

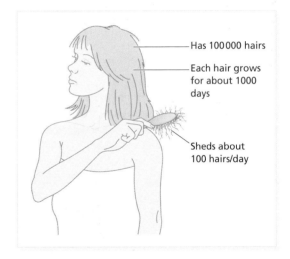

Fig. 13.3 An average scalp.

looking at plucked hairs (a trichogram). On the scalp, about 85% are normally in anagen and 15% in the telogen phase. The length of hair is determined by the duration of anagen; e.g. the hairs of the eyebrows have shorter cycles than those of the scalp.

Each hair follicle goes through its growth cycles out of phase with its neighbours, so there is no moulting period. However, if many pass into the resting phase

Table 13.1 Some causes of localized alopecia.

Non-scarring	Scarring
Alopecia areata	Burns, radiodermatitis
Androgenetic	Aplasia cutis
Hair-pulling habit	Kerion, carbuncle
Traction alopecia	Cicatricial basal cell carcinoma
	Lichen planus, lupus erythematosus
Scalp ringworm (human)	Necrobiosis, sarcoidosis, pseudopelade

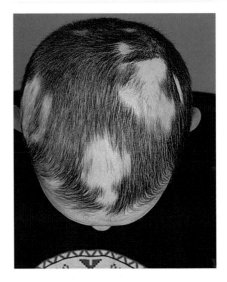

Fig. 13.4 The characteristic uninflamed patches of alopecia areata.

(telogen) at the same time, then a correspondingly large number will be shed 2–3 months later (see Telogen effluvium, below).

There are important racial differences in hair. Asians tend to have straight hair, Negroids woolly hair and Europeans wavy hair. These differences are associated with different cross-sectional shapes (round, flattened, etc.). Mongoloids have less facial and body hair than Mediterranean people who also have more hair than northern Europeans.

Alopecia

The term means loss of hair and alopecia has many causes and patterns. One convenient division is into localized and diffuse types. It is also important to decide whether or not the hair follicles have been replaced by scar tissue; if they have, regrowth cannot occur. The presence of any disease of the skin itself should also be noted.

Localized alopecia

Some of the most common types are listed in Table 13.1; only a few can be dealt with in detail.

Alopecia areata

This affects about 2% of the patients seen at our skin clinics.

Cause

An immunological basis is suspected because of an association with thyroid disease, vitiligo and atopy.

Histologically, T lymphocytes cluster like a swarm of bees around affected hair bulbs, having been attracted and made to divide by cytokines from the dermal papilla. Alopecia areata is probably inherited as a complex genetic trait, with an increased occurrence in the first-degree relatives of affected subjects and twin concordance. The existence of trigger factors, such as stress, fits with this idea.

Presentation

A typical patch is uninflamed, with no scaling, but with easily seen empty hair follicles (Fig. 13.4). Pathognomonic 'exclamation-mark' hairs may be seen around the edge of enlarging areas. They are broken off about 4 mm from the scalp, and are narrowed and less pigmented proximally (Figs 13.5 and 13.6). Patches are most common in the scalp and beard but other areas, especially the eyelashes and eyebrows, can be affected too. An uncommon diffuse pattern is recognized, with exclamation-mark hairs scattered widely over a diffusely thinned scalp. Up to 50% of patients show fine pitting or wrinkling of the nails.

Course

The outcome is unpredictable. In a first attack, regrowth is usual within a few months. New hairs

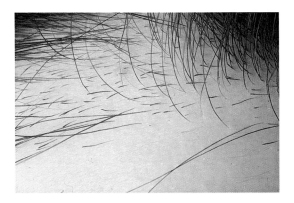

Fig. 13.5 Exclamation-mark hairs: pathognomonic of alopecia areata.

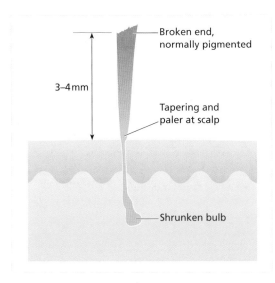

Broken end, normally pigmented

3–4 mm

Tapering and paler at scalp

Shrunken bulb

Fig. 13.6 An exclamation-mark hair.

appear in the centre of patches as fine pale down, and gradually regain their normal thickness and colour, although the new hair may remain white in older patients. Subsequent episodes tend to be more extensive and regrowth is slower. Hair loss in some areas may coexist with regrowth in others. A few patients lose all the hair from their heads (alopecia totalis) or from the whole skin surface (alopecia universalis).

Regrowth is tiresomely erratic but the following suggest a poor prognosis.
1 Onset before puberty.
2 Association with atopy or Down's syndrome.
3 Unusually widespread alopecia.

4 Involvement of the scalp margin (ophiasiform type), especially at the nape of the neck.

Differential diagnosis

Patches are not scaly, in contrast to ringworm, and are usually uninflamed, in contrast to lupus erythematosus and lichen planus. In the hair-pulling habit of children, and in traction alopecia, broken hairs may be seen but true exclamation-mark hairs are absent. Secondary syphilis can also cause a 'moth-eaten' patchy hair loss.

Investigations

None are usually needed. Syphilis can be excluded with serological tests if necessary. Organ-specific auto-antibody screens provide interesting information but do not affect management.

Treatment

A patient with a first or minor attack can be reassured about the prospects for regrowth. Tranquillizers may be helpful at the start. The use of systemic steroids should be avoided in most cases, but the intradermal injection of 0.2 mL of intralesional triamcinolone acetonide (10 mg/mL), raising a small bleb within an affected patch, leads to localized tufts of regrowth (Fig. 13.7) while not affecting the overall outcome. This may be useful to re-establish eyebrows or to stimulate hope. Spirit-based steroid lotions and mild irritants, such as 0.1–0.25% dithranol, are often used but with limited success. Ultraviolet radiation or even psoralen

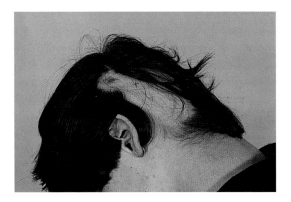

Fig. 13.7 Regrowth within a patch of alopecia areata after a triamcinolone injection.

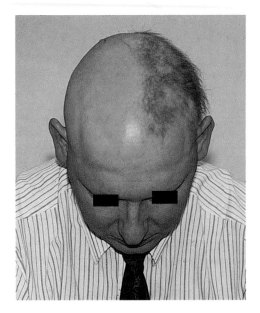

Fig. 13.8 A trial of diphencyprone to one side of the scalp caused some regrowth.

with ultraviolet A (PUVA) therapy may help extensive cases, but hair fall often returns when treatment stops. Contact sensitizers (e.g. diphencyprone) seemed promising (Figs 13.8) but the long-term effect of persistent antigen stimulation is worrying; they are still being used only in a few centres under trial conditions. The efficacy of topical immunosuppressive agents (e.g. tacrolimus) has yet to be proved in a randomized clinical trial. Wigs are necessary for extensive cases.

Androgenetic alopecia (male-pattern baldness)

Cause

Although clearly familial, the exact mode of inheritance has not yet been clarified. The idea of a single autosomal dominant gene, with reduced penetrance in women, now seems less likely than a polygenic type of inheritance. Male-pattern baldness is androgen-dependent; in females, androgenetic alopecia, with circulating levels of androgen within normal limits, is seen only in those who are strongly predisposed genetically.

Presentation

The common pattern in men (Fig. 13.9) is the loss of hair first from the temples, and then from the crown.

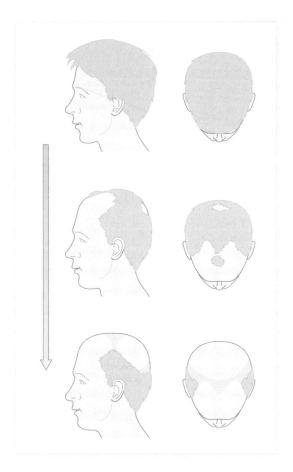

Fig. 13.9 Variations on male-pattern baldness.

However, in women the hair loss may be much more diffuse (Fig. 13.10), particularly over the crown. In bald areas, terminal hairs are replaced by finer vellus ones.

Clinical course

Hair loss is relentless, tending to follow the family pattern with some losing hair quickly and others more slowly. The diffuse pattern seen in women tends to progress slowly.

Complications

Even minor hair loss may lead to great anxiety and rarely to a monosymptomatic hypochondriasis (p. 295). Bald scalps burn easily in the sun, and may develop multiple actinic keratoses. It has been suggested recently that bald men are more likely to have a heart attack than those with a full head of hair.

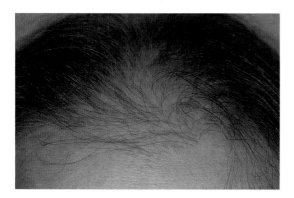

Fig. 13.10 Androgenetic alopecia beginning in the frontal area.

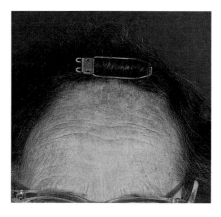

Fig. 13.11 Traction alopecia. The rollers she thought would help to disguise her thin hair actually made it worse.

Differential diagnosis

The diagnosis is usually obvious in men, but other causes of diffuse hair loss have to be considered in women (p. 168).

Investigations

None are usually needed. In women virilization may have to be excluded.

Treatment

Scalp surgery, hair transplants and wigs are welcomed by some. Topical application of minoxidil lotion may slow early hair loss and even stimulate new growth of hair in a few cases (Formulary 1, p. 339). Small and recently acquired patches respond best. When minoxidil treatment stops, the new hairs fall out after about 3 months. Anti-androgens help some women with the diffuse type of androgenetic alopecia.

Finasteride (Propecia), an inhibitor of human type II 5α-reductase, reduces serum and scalp skin levels of dihydrotestosterone in balding men. At the dosage of 1 mg/day, it may increase hair counts and so lead to a noticeable improvement in scalp hair. However, the beneficial effects slowly reverse once treatment has stopped. This treatment is not indicated in women or children. Side-effects are rare, but include decreased libido, erectile dysfunction and altered prostate-specific antigen levels.

Trichotillomania

This is dealt with on p. 298.

Traction alopecia

Cause

Hair can be pulled out by several procedures intended to beautify, including hot-combing to straighten kinky hair, tight hairstyles such as a pony tail or 'corn rows', and using hair rollers too often or too tightly.

Presentation

The changes are usually seen in girls and young women, particularly those whose hair has always tended to be thin anyway. The pattern of hair loss is determined by the cosmetic procedure in use, hair being lost where there is maximal tug. The term 'marginal' alopecia is applied to one common pattern in which hair loss is mainly around the edge of the scalp—at the sides or at the front (Fig. 13.11). The bald areas show short broken hairs, folliculitis and sometimes scarring.

Clinical course

Patients are often slow to accept that they are responsible for the hair loss, and notoriously slow to alter their cosmetic practices. Even if they do, regrowth is often disappointingly incomplete.

Differential diagnosis

The pattern of hair loss provides the main clue to the diagnosis and, if the possibility of traction alopecia is kept in mind, there is usually no difficulty. The absence of exclamation-mark hairs distinguishes it from alopecia areata, and of scaling from tinea capitis.

Treatment

Patients have to stop doing whatever is causing their hair loss. Rollers that tug can be replaced by those that only heat.

Patchy hair loss caused by skin disease

Scalp ringworm

Inflammation, often with pustulation, is a feature of animal ringworm, and the resultant scarring can be severe. The classical scalp ringworm derived from human sources causes areas of scaling with broken hairs. The subject is covered in more detail on p. 216.

Psoriasis

The rough removal of adherent scales can also remove hairs, but regrowth is the rule.

Scarring alopecia

Hair follicles can be damaged in many ways. If the follicular openings can no longer be seen with a lens, regrowth of hair cannot be expected.

Sometimes the cause is obvious: a severe burn, trauma, a carbuncle or an episode of inflammatory scalp ringworm. Discoid lupus erythematosus (p. 123), lichen planus (p. 64) and morphoea (p. 129) can also lead to scarring alopecia. The term 'pseudopelade' is applied to a slowly progressive non-inflamed type of scarring which leads to irregular areas of hair loss without any apparent preceding skin disease. If inflammation is present, a biopsy may help to establish the diagnosis.

Diffuse hair loss

Hair is lost evenly from the whole scalp; this may, or may not, be accompanied by a thinning visible to others (Fig. 13.12). Some of the most common causes are listed in Table 13.2, but often a simple explanation cannot be found.

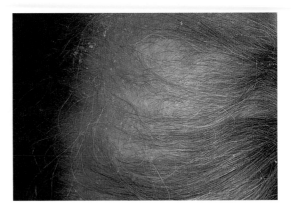

Fig. 13.12 Diffuse hair loss causing much anxiety.

Table 13.2 Some causes of diffuse hair loss.

Telogen effluvium
Endocrine
  hypopituitarism
  hypo- or hyperthyroidism
  hypoparathyroidism
Drug-induced
  antimitotic agents (anagen effluvium)
  anticoagulants
  vitamin A excess
  oral contraceptives
Androgenetic
Iron deficiency
Severe chronic illness
Malnutrition
Diffuse type of alopecia areata

Telogen effluvium

Cause

Telogen effluvium can be triggered by any severe illness, particularly those with bouts of fever or haemorrhage, by childbirth and by severe dieting. All of these synchronize catagen so that, later on, large numbers of hairs are lost at the same time.

Presentation and course

The diffuse hair fall, 2–3 months after the provoking illness, can be mild or severe. In the latter case Beau's lines (p. 175) may be seen on the nails. Regrowth, not always complete, usually occurs within a few months.

Differential diagnosis

This is from other types of diffuse hair loss (Table 13.2).

Treatment

This condition is unaffected by therapy, but patients can be reassured that their hair fall will be temporary.

Other causes of diffuse hair loss

The causes mentioned in Table 13.2 should be considered, and the exclamation-mark hairs of the diffuse type of alopecia areata should be looked for. If no cause is obvious, it is worth checking the haemoglobin, erythrocyte sedimentation rate (ESR), ANF, serum iron, thyroxine and thyroid-stimulating hormone (TSH) levels. Also consider checking the serum free testosterone and dihydroepiandrosterone sulphate levels in women with menstrual irregularities or hirsutism. However, it is true to say that often no cause for diffuse alopecia can be found.

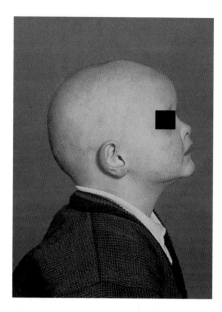

Fig. 13.13 Hypohidrotic ectodermal dysplasia: minimal scalp hair and characteristic facies.

LEARNING POINTS

1 Be sympathetic even if the hair loss seems trivial to you.
2 Reassure your patient that total baldness is not imminent.

Rare genetic causes of hypotrichosis

More than 300 genetic conditions exist that have hair abnormalities as one component. The *hypohidrotic ectodermal dysplasias* are a group of rare inherited disorders characterized by sparse hair, scanty sweat glands, and poor development of the nails and teeth. (Figs 13.13 and 13.14). Heat stroke may follow inadequate sweat production. One type is inherited as an X-linked recessive. The responsible gene for this type (on chromosome Xq12) has recently been shown to encode for a protein (ectodysplasin) involved in the regulation of ectodermal appendage formation. The genes responsible for the dominant/recessive types encode for the ectodysplasin receptor.

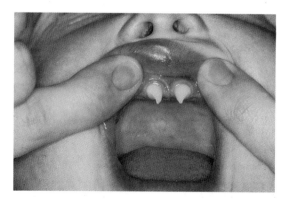

Fig. 13.14 The cone-shaped incisors of hypohidrotic ectodermal dysplasia.

In other inherited disorders the hair may be beaded and brittle (*monilethrix*); flattened and twisted (*pili torti*); kinky (*Menkes' syndrome* caused by mutations in a gene encoding for a copper transporting membrane protein); like bamboo (*Netherton's syndrome*, caused by a gene on chromosome 5q32 encoding a serine protease inhibitor); partly broken in many places (*trichorrhexis nodosa*); 'woolly' or 'uncombable'.

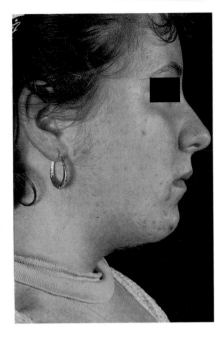

Fig. 13.15 Moderate hirsutism caused by polycystic ovaries.

Hirsutism and hypertrichosis

Hirsutism is the growth of terminal hair in a female (Fig. 13.15), which is distributed in the pattern normally seen in a male. Hypertrichosis is an excessive growth of terminal hair that does not follow an androgen-induced pattern (Fig. 13.16).

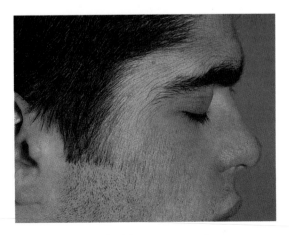

Fig. 13.16 Hypertrichosis in a young man of Mediterranean extraction.

Hirsutism

Cause

Some degree of hirsutism may be a racial or familial trait, and minor facial hirsutism is common after the menopause. In addition, some patients without a family background of hirsutism become hirsute in the absence of any demonstrable hormonal cause (idiopathic hirsutism). Finally, some patients with hirsutism will have one of the disorders shown in Fig. 13.17.

Presentation

An excessive growth of hair appears in the beard area, on the chest and shoulder-tips, around the nipples and in the male pattern of pubic hair. Androgenetic alopecia may complete the picture.

Course

Familial, racial or idiopathic hirsutism tends to start at puberty and to worsen with age.

Complications

Virilization causes infertility; psychological disturbances are common.

Investigations

Significant hormonal abnormalities are not usually found in patients with a normal menstrual cycle.
Investigations are needed:
• if hirsutism occurs in childhood;
• if there are other features of virilization, such as clitoromegaly;
• if the hirsutism is of sudden or recent onset; or
• if there is menstrual irregularity or cessation.
The tests used will include measurement of the serum testosterone, sex-hormone-binding globulin, dehydroepiandrosterone sulphate, androstenedione and prolactin. Ovarian ultrasound is useful if polycystic ovaries are suspected.

Treatment (Fig. 13.17)

Any underlying disorder must be treated on its merits. Home remedies for minor hirsutism include commer-

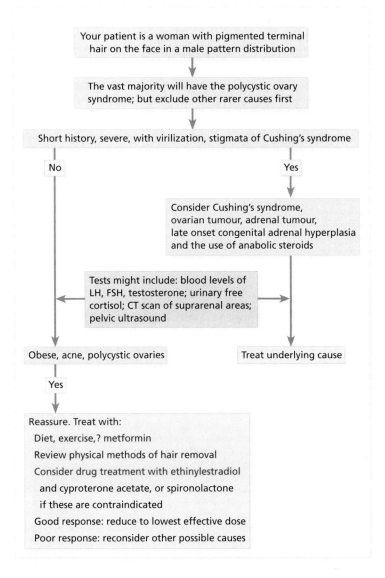

Your patient is a woman with pigmented terminal hair on the face in a male pattern distribution

↓

The vast majority will have the polycystic ovary syndrome; but exclude other rarer causes first

↓

Short history, severe, with virilization, stigmata of Cushing's syndrome

No ← → Yes

Consider Cushing's syndrome, ovarian tumour, adrenal tumour, late onset congenital adrenal hyperplasia and the use of anabolic steroids

Tests might include: blood levels of LH, FSH, testosterone; urinary free cortisol; CT scan of suprarenal areas; pelvic ultrasound

Obese, acne, polycystic ovaries   Treat underlying cause

Yes

↓

Reassure. Treat with:
  Diet, exercise,? metformin
  Review physical methods of hair removal
  Consider drug treatment with ethinylestradiol
    and cyproterone acetate, or spironolactone
    if these are contraindicated
  Good response: reduce to lowest effective dose
  Poor response: reconsider other possible causes

Fig. 13.17 An approach to hirsutism.

cial depilatory creams (often containing a thioglycollate, p. 172), waxing or shaving, or making the appearance less obvious by bleaching; none remove the hair permamently. Plucking should probably be avoided as it can stimulate hair roots into anagen. The abnormally active follicles, if relatively few, can be destroyed by electrolysis. If the hairs are too numerous for this, the excess can be removed by laser (p. 326). Topical therapy with eflornithine, an inhibitor of ornithine decarboxylase, can slow regrowth. Oral antiandrogens (e.g. cyproterone acetate; Dianette, Formulary 2, p. 346) may sometimes be helpful, but will be needed long-term. Pregnancy must be avoided during such

treatment as it carries the risk of feminizing a male fetus. Spironolactone is used less often now.

LEARNING POINTS

1 Full endocrinological assessment is needed for hirsutism plus virilization.
2 Significant hormonal abnormalities are rarely found in patients with a normal menstrual cycle.

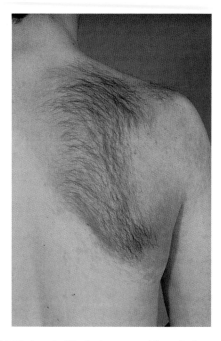

Fig. 13.18 A typical Becker's naevus with marked localized hypertrichosis within a patch of hyperpigmentation.

Hypertrichosis

The localized type is most commonly seen over melanocytic naevi including Becker's naevi (Fig. 13.18). It can also affect the sacral area—as a 'satyr's tuft'—in some patients with spina bifida. Excessive amounts of hair may grow near chronically inflamed joints or under plaster casts. Repeated shaving does not bring on hypertrichosis although occupational pressure may do so, e.g. from carrying weights on the shoulder.

Generalized hypertrichosis is much less common. Some causes are listed in Table 13.3.

Hair cosmetics

Hair can be made more attractive by dyeing, bleaching and waving, but there is often a price to be paid for beauty. Some hair dyes based on paraphenylenediamine are allergens (p. 78). Bleaches can weaken the hair shafts, and hair damaged in this way is especially susceptible to further damage by permanent waving.

Table 13.3 Some causes of generalized hypertrichosis.

Anorexia nervosa, starvation
Drug-induced (minoxidil, diazoxide, cyclosporin)
Hepatic cutaneous porphyria (p. 287)
Fetal alcohol and fetal phenytoin syndromes
Hypertrichosis lanuginosa (both congenital type and acquired types are very rare—the latter signals an internal malignancy)
Some rare syndromes, e.g. Cornelia de Lange syndrome (hypertrichosis, microcephaly and mental deficiency) and Hurler's syndrome

Permanent waving solutions reduce disulphide bonds within hair keratin and so allow the hair to be deformed before being reset in a new position. The thioglycollates in use to dissolve disulphide bonds are also popular as chemical hair removers. If used incorrectly, either too strong or for too long, or on hair already damaged by excessive bleaching or waving, thioglycollate waving lotions can cause hairs to break off flush with the scalp. This hair loss, which can be severe although temporary, may be accompanied by an irritant dermatitis of the scalp.

The nails

The structure of the nail and nail bed is shown in Fig. 13.19. The hard keratin of the nail plate is formed in the nail matrix, which lies in an invagination of the epidermis (the nail fold) on the back of the terminal phalanx of each digit. The matrix runs from the proximal end of the floor of the nail fold to the distal margin of the lunule. From this area the nail plate grows forward over the nail bed, ending in a free margin at the tip of the digit. Longitudinal ridges and grooves on the under surface of the nail plate dovetail with similar ones on the upper surface of the nail bed. The nail bed is capable of producing small amounts of keratin which contribute to the nail and which are responsible for the 'false nail' formed when the nail matrix is obliterated by surgery or injury. The cuticle acts as a seal to protect the potential space of the nail fold from chemicals and from infection. The nails provide strength and protection for the terminal phalanx. Their presence helps with fine touch and with the handling of small objects.

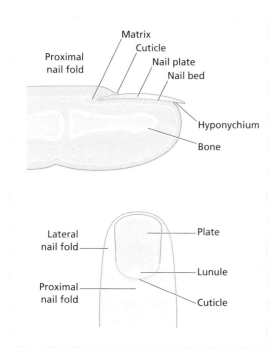

Fig. 13.19 The nail and nail bed.

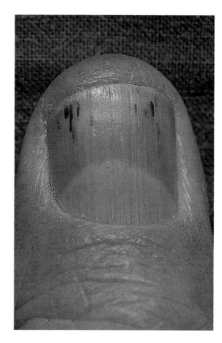

Fig. 13.20 Gross splinter haemorrhages caused by trauma.

The rate at which nails grow varies from person to person: fingernails average between 0.5 and 1.2 mm per week, while toenails grow more slowly. Nails grow faster in the summer, if they are bitten, and in youth. They change with ageing from the thin, occasionally spooned nails of early childhood to the duller, paler and more opaque nails of the very old. Longitudinal ridging and beading are particularly common in the elderly.

Effects of trauma

Permanent ridges or splits in the nail plate can follow damage to the nail matrix. Splinter haemorrhages (Fig. 13.20), the linear nature of which is determined by longitudinal ridges and grooves in the nail bed, are most commonly seen under the nails of manual workers and are caused by minor trauma. They may also be a feature of psoriasis of the nail and of subacute bacterial endocarditis. Larger subungual haematomas (Fig. 13.21) are usually easy to identify but the trauma that caused them may have escaped notice and dark areas of altered blood can raise worries about the presence of a subungual melanoma.

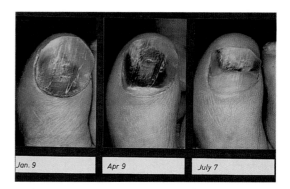

Fig. 13.21 A subungual haematoma of the big toe. Although there was no history of trauma we were happy to watch this grow out over 6 months as the appearance was sudden, the colour was right and the nail folds showed no pigment.

Chronic trauma from sport and from ill-fitting shoes contributes to haemorrhage under the nails of the big toes, to the gross thickening of toenails known as *onychogryphosis* (Fig. 13.22), and to ingrowing nails. *Onycholysis*, a separation of the nail plate from the nail bed (Fig. 13.23), may be a result of minor trauma although it is also seen in nail psoriasis (Fig. 5.8), and possibly in thyroid disease. Usually no cause for it is

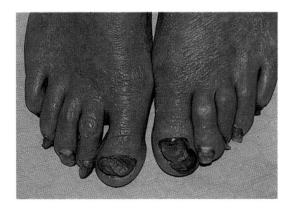

Fig. 13.22 Onychogryphosis.

found. The space created may be colonized by yeasts, or by bacteria such as *Pseudomonas aeruginosa*, which turns it an ugly green colour.

Some nervous habits damage the nails. Bitten nails are short and irregular; some people also bite their cuticles and the skin around the nails. Viral warts can be seeded rapidly in this way. In the common habit tic nail dystrophy, the cuticle of the thumbnail is the target for picking or rubbing. This repetitive trauma causes a ladder pattern of transverse ridges and grooves to run up the centre of the nail plate (Fig. 13.23).

Lamellar splitting of the distal part of the fingernails, so commonly seen in housewives, has been attributed to repeated wetting and drying (Fig. 13.23).

Attempts to beautify nails can lead to contact allergy. Culprits include the acrylate adhesive used with artificial nails and formaldehyde in nail hardeners. In contrast, contact dermatitis caused by allergens in nail polish itself seldom affects the fingers but presents as small itchy eczematous areas where the nail plates rest against the skin during sleep. The eyelids, face and neck are favourite sites.

The nail in systemic disease

The nails can provide useful clues for general physicians.

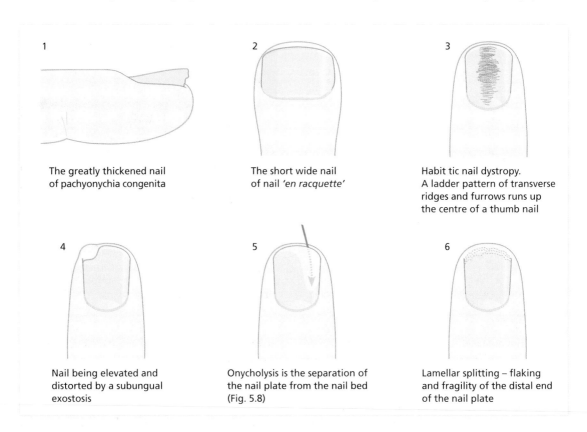

1 The greatly thickened nail of pachyonychia congenita

2 The short wide nail of nail *'en racquette'*

3 Habit tic nail dystropy. A ladder pattern of transverse ridges and furrows runs up the centre of a thumb nail

4 Nail being elevated and distorted by a subungual exostosis

5 Onycholysis is the separation of the nail plate from the nail bed (Fig. 5.8)

6 Lamellar splitting – flaking and fragility of the distal end of the nail plate

Fig. 13.23 Some nail plate abnormalities.

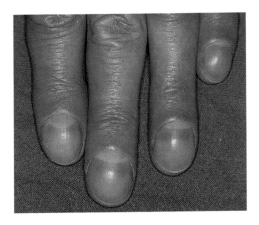

Fig. 13.24 In this case severe clubbing was accompanied by hypertrophic pulmonary osteoarthropathy.

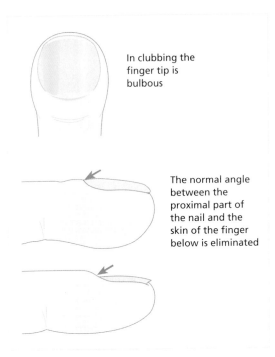

In clubbing the finger tip is bulbous

The normal angle between the proximal part of the nail and the skin of the finger below is eliminated

Fig. 13.25 Clubbing.

Clubbing (Fig. 13.24) is a bulbous enlargement of the terminal phalanx with an increase in the angle between the nail plate and the proximal fold to over 180° (Fig. 13.25). Its association with chronic lung disease and with cyanotic heart disease is well known. Rarely clubbing may be familial with no underlying cause. The mechanisms involved in its formation are still not known.

Koilonychia, a spooning and thinning of the nail plate, indicates iron deficiency (Fig. 13.26).

Colour changes: the 'half-and-half' nail, with a white proximal and red or brown distal half, is seen in a minority of patients with chronic renal failure. Whitening of the nail plates may be related to hypo-albuminaemia, as in cirrhosis of the liver. Some drugs, notably antimalarials, antibiotics and phenothiazines, can discolour the nails.

Beau's lines are transverse grooves which appear synchronously on all nails a few weeks after an acute illness, and which grow steadily out to the free margin (Fig. 13.26).

Connective tissue disorders: nail fold telangiectasia or erythema is a useful physical sign in dermatomyositis, systemic sclerosis and systemic lupus erythematosus (Fig. 13.27). In dermatomyositis the cuticles become shaggy, and in systemic sclerosis loss of finger pulp leads to overcurvature of the nail plates. Thin nails, with longitudinal ridging and sometimes partial onycholysis, are seen when the peripheral circulation is impaired, as in Raynaud's phenomenon.

Nail changes in the common dermatoses

Psoriasis

Most patients with psoriasis have nail changes at some stage; severe nail involvement is more likely in the presence of arthritis. The best-known nail change is pitting of the surface of the nail plate (Fig. 5.7). Almost as common is psoriasis under the nail plate, showing up as red or brown areas, often with ony-cholysis bordered by obvious discoloration (Fig. 5.8). There is no effective treatment for psoriasis of the nails.

Eczema

Some patients with itchy chronic eczema bring their nails to a high state of polish by scratching. In addition, eczema of the nail folds may lead to a coarse irregularity with transverse ridging of the adjacent nail plates.

Lichen planus

Some 10% of patients with lichen planus have nail changes. Most often this is a reversible thinning of the

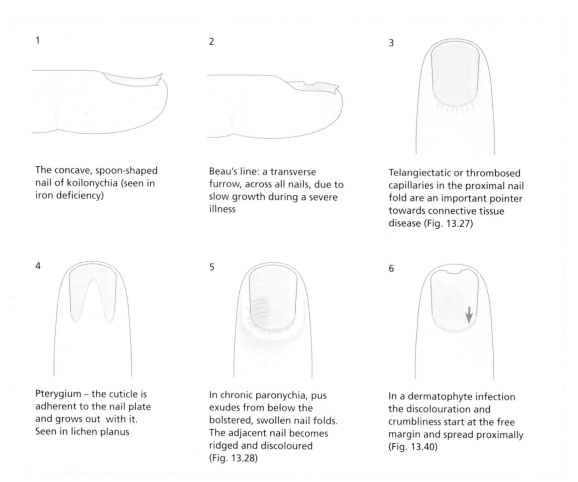

1

The concave, spoon-shaped nail of koilonychia (seen in iron deficiency)

2

Beau's line: a transverse furrow, across all nails, due to slow growth during a severe illness

3

Telangiectatic or thrombosed capillaries in the proximal nail fold are an important pointer towards connective tissue disease (Fig. 13.27)

4

Pterygium – the cuticle is adherent to the nail plate and grows out with it. Seen in lichen planus

5

In chronic paronychia, pus exudes from below the bolstered, swollen nail folds. The adjacent nail becomes ridged and discoloured (Fig. 13.28)

6

In a dermatophyte infection the discolouration and crumbliness start at the free margin and spread proximally (Fig. 13.40)

Fig. 13.26 Some other nail changes.

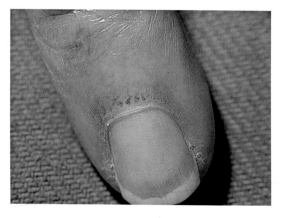

Fig. 13.27 Large tortuous capillary loops of the proximal nail fold signal the presence of a connective tissue disorder.

nail plate with irregular longitudinal grooves and ridges. More severe involvement may lead to pterygium in which the cuticle grows forward over the base of the nail and attaches itself to the nail plate (Fig. 13.26). The threat of severe and permanent nail changes can sometimes justify treatment with systemic steroids.

Alopecia areata

The more severe the hair loss, the more likely there is to be nail involvement. A roughness or fine pitting is seen on the surface of the nail plates and the lunulae may appear mottled.

Infections

Acute paronychia

The portal of entry for the organisms concerned, usually staphylococci, is a break in the skin or cuticle as a result of minor trauma. The subsequent acute inflammation, often with the formation of pus in the nail fold or under the nail, requires systemic treatment with flucloxacillin or erythromycin (Formulary 2, p. 341) and appropriate surgical drainage.

Chronic paronychia

Cause

A combination of circumstances can allow a mixture of opportunistic pathogens (yeasts, Gram-positive cocci and Gram-negative rods) to colonize the space between the nail fold and nail plate. Predisposing factors include a poor peripheral circulation, wet work, working with flour, diabetes, vaginal candidosis and overvigorous cutting back of the cuticles.

Presentation and course

The nail folds become tender and swollen (Figs 13.26 and 13.28) and small amounts of pus are discharged at intervals. The cuticular seal is damaged and the adjacent nail plate becomes ridged and discoloured. The condition may last for years.

Differential diagnosis

In atypical cases, consider the outside chance of an amelanotic melanoma. Paronychia should not be confused with a dermatophyte infection in which the nail folds are not primarily affected.

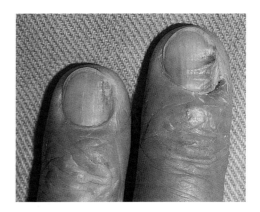

Fig. 13.28 Paronychia with secondary nail ridging.

Investigations

Test the urine for sugar, check for vaginal candidosis. Pus should be cultured.

Treatment

Manicuring of the cuticle should cease. The hands should be kept as warm and as dry as possible, and the damaged nail folds packed several times a day with an imidazole cream (Formulary 1, p. 335). If there is no response, and swabs confirm that candida is present, a 2-week course of itraconazole should be considered (Formulary 2, p. 343).

Dermatophyte infections (Figs 13.26 and 14.40)

Cause

The common dermatophytes that cause tinea pedis can also invade the nails (p. 215).

Presentation

Toenail infection is common and associated with tinea pedis. The early changes occur at the free edge of the nail and spread proximally. The nail plate becomes yellow, crumbly and thickened. Usually only a few nails are infected but occasionally all are. The fingernails are involved less often and the changes, in contrast to those of psoriasis, are usually confined to one hand.

Clinical course

The condition seldom clears spontaneously.

Differential diagnosis

Psoriasis has been mentioned. Yeast infections of the nail plate, much more rare than dermatophyte infections, can look similar. Coexisting tinea pedis favours dermatophyte infection of the nail.

Investigations

Microscopic examination of a nail clipping is a simple procedure (p. 35). Cultures should be carried out in a mycology laboratory.

Treatment

This is given on p. 217. Remember that most symptom-free fungal infections of the toenails need no treatment at all.

Tumours

Peri-ungual warts are common and stubborn. Cryotherapy must be used carefully to avoid damage to the nail matrix. It is painful but effective.

Peri-ungual fibromas (see Fig. 21.5) arise from the nail folds, usually in late childhood, in patients with tuberous sclerosis.

Glomus tumours can occur beneath the nail plate. The small red or bluish lesions are exquisitely painful if touched and when the temperature changes. Treatment is surgical.

Subungual exostoses (Fig. 13.22) protrude painfully under the nail plate. Usually secondary to trauma to the terminal phalanx, the bony abnormality can be seen on X-ray and treatment is surgical.

Myxoid cysts (Fig. 13.29) occur on the proximal nail folds, usually of the fingers. The smooth domed swelling contains a clear jelly-like material that transilluminates well. A groove may form on the adjacent nail plate. Cryotherapy, injections of triamcinolone and surgical excision all have their advocates.

Malignant melanoma should be suspected in any subungual pigmented lesion, particularly if the pigment spreads to the surrounding skin. Subungual haematomas may cause confusion but 'grow out' with

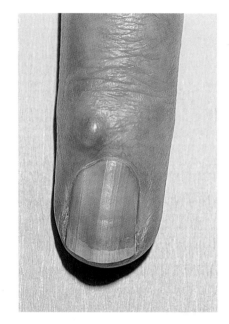

Fig. 13.29 Myxoid cyst creating a groove in the nail.

the nail (Fig. 13.21). The risk of misdiagnosis is highest with an amelanotic melanoma, which may mimic chronic paronychia or a pyogenic granuloma.

Some other nail abnormalities

A few people are born with one or more nails missing. In addition there are many conditions, either inherited or associated with chromosomal abnormalities and usually rare, in which nail changes form a minor part of the clinical picture. Most cannot be dealt with here.

In the rare *nail–patella syndrome*, the thumbnails, and to a lesser extent those of the fingers, are smaller than normal. Rudimentary patellae, and renal disease iliac spines complete the syndrome, which is inherited as an autosomal dominant trait linked with the locus controlling ABO blood groups.

Pachyonychia congenita is also rare and inherited as an autosomal dominant trait. The nails are grossly thickened, especially peripherally, and have a curious triangular profile (Fig. 13.22). Hyperkeratosis may occur on areas of friction on the legs and feet.

Permanent loss of the nails may be seen with the dystrophic types of *epidermolysis bullosa* (p. 117).

In the *yellow nail syndrome* (Fig. 13.30) the nail changes begin in adult life, against a background of

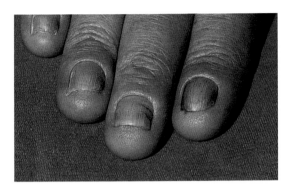

Fig. 13.30 The curved slow-growing greenish-yellow nails of the yellow nail syndrome.

hypoplasia of the lymphatic system. Peripheral oedema is usually present and pleural effusions may occur. The nails grow very slowly and become thickened and greenish-yellow; their surface is smooth but they are overcurved from side to side.

The nail 'en racquette' is a short broad nail (Fig. 13.16), usually a thumbnail, which is seen in some 1–2% of the population and inherited as an autosomal dominant trait. The basic abnormality is shortness of the underlying terminal phalanx.

The mouth and genitals

Mucous membranes are covered with a modified stratified squamous epithelium that lacks a stratum corneum. This makes them moist and susceptible to infection, and to conditions not seen elsewhere. In contrast, the skin around them is like that on other body sites, and develops the standard range of skin disorders. It follows that the diagnosis of puzzling mouth or genital changes is often made easier by looking for skin disease elsewhere.

The mouth

The mouth can harbour an enormous range of diseases, affecting each of its component structures. Inflammatory and infectious disorders of the mouth are usually either red or white—leading to the terms erythroplakia and leukoplakia, respectively. These are descriptive terms but not diagnoses. A biopsy will help sort out the non-dysplastic causes, such as lichen planus and candida infections, from the dysplastic ones that are the precursors of carcinoma.

Some skin diseases cause ulceration in the mouth. These ulcers are accompanied by skin diseases elsewhere on the body, and making a diagnosis there is easier than in the mouth. In other patients with mouth ulcers, the course of the ulcers or erosions, and their size and location in the mouth, provide diagnostic clues. Table 13.4 lists some common tongue troubles.

Lichen planus

Cause

The cause of oral lichen planus is unknown (see also Chapter 6). However, some 40% of patients with symptomatic lichen planus of the mouth have relevant allergies, diagnosable by patch testing. These are usually to metals (especially gold and mercury) and flavourings such as cinnamon, peppermint and spearmint. Lichen planus also results from drug reactions, liver disease and bone marrow transplantation.

Presentation

When a lichen planus-like cutaneous eruption is present, finding lichen planus in the mouth confirms the diagnosis, and vice versa. In the mouth, typically, there is a lace-like whitening of the buccal mucosae (Fig. 6.4), but sometimes this laciness is not present. Oral lichen planus can also be red, and can ulcerate. A 'desquamative gingivitis' may occur, in which the mucosa shears off with friction, such as that from brushing the teeth or eating an apple. Desquamative gingivitis can also result from pemphigus or pemphigoid (see below). Often oral lichen planus is asymptomatic and more of a curiosity than a problem for the patient.

Course

Oral lichen planus can last for years—even for a lifetime. Asymptomatic lichen planus does not usually progress to the symptomatic form.

Differential diagnosis

In its classic lace-like state, the appearance of oral lichen

Table 13.4 Some common tongue problems.

Condition	Cause	Treatment
Furred tongue	Hypertrophy of the filiform papillae	Brush the tongue
Black hairy tongue (Fig. 13.31)	Pigmentation and hypertrophy of filiform papillae caused due to bacterial overgrowth	Brush the tongue
Smooth tongue	Nutritional deficiency, sprue, malabsorption	Vitamins, nutrition
Fissured tongue	Congenital, Down's syndrome, ageing changes	No treatment needed
Median rhomboid glossitis	Developmental defect and candidosis. Smoking and dentures worsen	No treatment needed
Geographic tongue (Fig. 13.32)	Familial, atopic, psoriasis	Topical steroids
Varices	Blue compressible blebs of veins	No treatment needed
Hairy leukoplakia (Fig. 14.36)	Epstein–Barr virus infection in patients with HIV/AIDS	Highly active retroviral therapies (HAART)
Herpetic glossitis	Painful fissures without vesicles	Aciclovir group (p. 344)
Macroglossia	Developmental, tumours, infections, amyloidosis, thyroid	Treat the cause
Glossodynia	Trauma, candida, menopause, diabetes, nutritional, dry mouth	Treat the cause, use tricyclic antidepressants

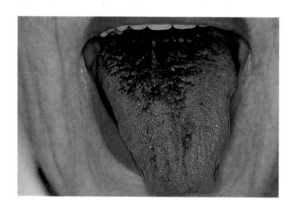

Fig. 13.31 Black hairy tongue.

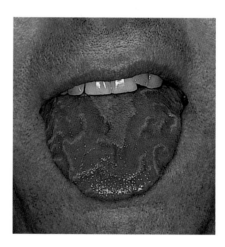

Fig. 13.32 Geographic tongue.

planus is diagnostic. Dysplastic leukoplakias are more likely to be focal, appearing on only a portion of the mucosae, gingivae or lips. They are also more likely to be red and symptomatic, and shown by those who have smoked cigarettes or chewed tobacco. *Candida albicans* infections may occasionally be considered, but their white patches scrape off.

Investigations

A potassium hydroxide (KOH) examination and a culture will rule out candidasis. Biopsy will determine if a white patch is dysplastic or not. The histology of lichen planus, as seen in the skin, may be less typical in the mouth, and may even suggest a dermatitis. Patch testing may be useful as allergic causes can be cured by allergen elimination. Liver function tests, and tests for hepatitis B, hepatitis C and antimitochondrial antibodies, are often recommended.

Treatment

If asymptomatic, no treatment is necessary. High potency topical steroids, in gel or ointment bases, are worth a try if the lesions are painful or ulcerated. Failing that, a few patients require oral prednisone; they should be referred to a dermatologist or specialist in oral medicine. Topical tacrolimus ointment may help, but treatment with this new agent is experimental.

Complications

Watch out for carcinoma, even if previous biopsies have shown no dysplasia. The risk is highest in the ulcerative forms, and the overall risk for development of squamous cell carcinoma in oral lichen planus is probably 1–5%. It should be suspected if an area becomes thickened, nodular or ulcerates.

Candidiasis

Cause and presentation

Infections with *Candida albicans* appear suddenly, on the tongue, lips or other mucosae, in the 'pseudomembranous form' (also called thrush; Fig. 14.47). Small lesions are more common than large ones. About 15% of infants get thrush on the tongue, lips or buccal mucosa, often from an infection acquired while passing through the birth canal. Sometimes candidiasis appears as red sore patches under dentures, or as angular chelitis (perlèche).

Course

If the candidiasis is a complication of systemic antibiotic therapy, treatment will be curative. Immunosuppressed and denture-wearing patients often have recurrent disease.

Differential diagnosis

Many tongues are coated with desquamated epithelial

Table 13.5 Some possible causes underlying oral candidiasis in adults.

Antibiotic treatment ✓
HIV infection
Myelodysplastic syndromes
leukaemia
lymphoma
thymoma
Chemotherapy
Inhalation of corticosteroids for asthma
Widespread metastatic malignancy
Vitamin deficiency ✓
Inflammatory bowel disease ✓
Xerostomia
Previous radiation therapy to mouth
Diabetes ✓
Addison's disease
Myasthenia gravis
Dentures
Chronic mucocutaneous candidiasis (on skin and nails too; p. 219)

cells that create a yellow wet powder on their surface. This scapes off easily, and shows no inflammation underneath. Lichen planus, oral hairy leukoplakia and dysplastic leukoplakia may cause confusion.

Investigations

Thrush does not normally occur in healthy adults, in whom the appearance of candidiasis needs more investigation than just a simple diagnosis by appearance, KOH examination or culture. Table 13.5 lists some possible underlying causes.

Treatment

Topical and systemic imidazoles are the treatments of choice. Creams and solutions can be used, but sucking on a clotrimazole troche (Formulary 1, p. 335) three times daily is better. Some patients are best treated with fluconazole, 150 mg once daily for 1–3 days. If an underlying condition is present, this should be identified and treated. Patients with 'denture sore mouth' should scrub their dentures each night with toothpaste and a toothbrush, sleep without dentures, and swish a teaspoonful of nystatin solution around the dentureless mouth three times a day.

Contact stomatitis

This underdiagnosed problem usually causes a transient soreness, associated with a diffuse redness of the lips and buccal gingivae. Mouthwashes, hard sweets (candies) and hot pizzas are common causes of the irritant type, whereas cinnamon, vanilla, peppermint, spearmint and dentifrices are the most common causes of allergic contact stomatitis. When local stomatitis or ulcers occur near a gold tooth filling, gold allergy should be suspected, but patch testing is needed before recommending that the filling should be removed.

Ulcers

One problem with oral ulcers (as with ulcers elsewhere) is the usual lack of a primary lesion, such as a bulla, papule or plaque. Ulcers are often secondary reactions which rob the clinician of the chance to make a morphological diagnosis. The history, the location of the ulcers within the mouth, their duration and the presence of coexisting non-oral signs or symptoms, especially of the skin, are then all-important clues to the underlying diagnosis.

Bullous diseases

Pemphigus and pemphigoid are most likely (see also Chapter 9).

Pemphigus causes large painful long-lasting erosions (Fig. 9.3). The whole mouth can be involved, but more often it affects just the lips and buccal mucosa. Desquamative gingivitis can occur. The ulcers are large, appear without warning and last months. A biopsy may show an intraepithelial acantholysis and should not be taken from an ulcer, but from normal-appearing mucosa in an active area. Direct immunofluorescence (biopsy normal mucosa) shows antibody rimming each keratinocyte.

Cicatricial (scarring) pemphigoid affects the mucous membranes predominantly, but occasionally affects the skin too. The eyelid conjunctiva and other mucosae can also be affected; scarring often results (see Fig. 9.8). Cicatricial pemphigoid is also a cause of desquamative gingivitis. Biopsy shows a subepidermal bulla, and direct immunofluorescence a linear band of IgG and C3 at the dermal–mucosal junction.

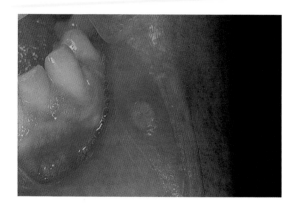

Fig. 13.33 Aphthous ulcer of the labial mucosa.

Aphthae

Presentation

These common small oval painful mouth ulcers arise, usually without an obvious cause, most often in 'movable mucosae' such as the gutters of the mouth, tongue or cheek (Fig. 13.33). An area of tenderness changes into a small red papule that quickly turns into a grey 2–5 mm painful ulcer with a red areola. Herpetiform aphthae occur in groups of 2–5 tiny painful ulcers. Major aphthae (periadenitis mucosa necrotica) are usually larger than 1 cm across and tend to appear in the back of the mouth.

Course

Small ulcers heal in a week or two; the pain stops within days. Major aphthae may persist for months.

Differential diagnosis

Recurrent herpes simplex infections mimic herpetiform apthae but, in the latter, cultures are negative and blisters are not seen. Behçet's disease causes confusion in patients with major aphthae. In fact, a diagnosis of Behçet's is often wrongly made in patients with recurrent aphthae of all sorts, when the patient has some other skin disease or joint pain. Patients with true Behçet's disease should have at least two of these other findings: genital ulcers, pustular vasculitis of skin, synovitis, uveitis or meningoencephalitis.

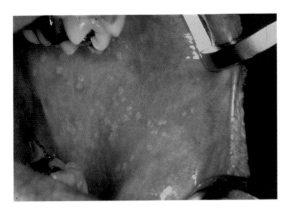

Fig. 13.34 Fordyce spots are ectopic sebaceous glands.

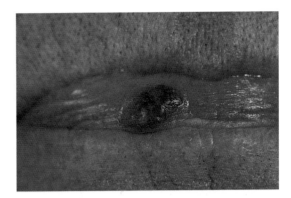

Fig. 13.35 Venous lake.

Investigations

Usually none are needed. Occasional associations include Crohn's disease, ulcerative colitis, gluten-sensitive enteropathy, cyclical neutropenia, other neutropenias, HIV infection, and deficiencies of iron, vitamin B_{12} or folate.

Treatment

Prevention is best. Trauma, such as aggressive tooth brushing, hard or aggravating foods and stress should be avoided if relevant. The application of a topical corticosteroid gel, such as fluocinonide, to new lesions may shorten their course. In severe or complex cases, consider referral.

Some other oral lumps, bumps and colour changes

• Mucocoeles are collections of mucin following the rupture of a minor salivary gland duct. They are blue-tinted soft translucent nodules, usually of the lips, and arise suddenly without pain.
• Fordyce spots are ectopic sebaceous glands, appearing as pinhead-sized whitish-yellow papules on the labial mucosa (Fig. 13.34).
• Yellow patches in the mouth may suggest pseudoxanthoma elasticum.
• Brown macules on the lips should trigger thoughts about the dominantly inherited Peutz–Jehgers syndrome (Fig. 17.12) and its bowel polyps and tumours.
• Neurofibromas may occur, especially in patients with widespread cutaneous neurofibromatosis.

• Telangiectases may suggest hereditary haemorrhagic telangiectasia. These patients may also have telangiectases in their intestinal tract leading to gastrointestinal bleeding, and arteriovenous fistulae especially in the lungs that may lead to cerebral embolism.
• Venous lakes are blue or black papules on the lips (Fig. 13.35). These melanoma-like lesions worry patients and doctors alike, but pressure with a diascope or glass slide causes them to blanch.
• Multiple, somewhat translucent, papules may suggest Cowden's syndrome. These are fibromas. Patients with Cowden's syndrome have facial papules and nodules (tricholemmomas and fibromas), fibrocystic disease of the breasts and a great propensity to develop malignant tumours of the breast, thyroid and other organs.
• Patients with the multiple mucosal neuroma syndrome have neuromas in their mouths, and 75% of those with this autosomal dominantly inherited disorder also have medulary carcinoma of the thyroid. Many also develop pheochromocytomas. Many small bumps appear along the lips, tongue and buccal mucosae.
• Pyogenic granulomas of the gingiva appear as quick-growing red bleeding papules. They are reactive proliferations of blood vessels, and often develop in pregnancy ('pregnancy tumours').
• Fibromas may result from dentures, or from resolving or indolent pyogenic granulomas, but can also appear without reason, usually on the gingiva of adults. Tooth bites may cause fibromas to appear on the tongue and on the buccal mucosae. Cowden's disease (see above) should be considered if multiple lesions are present.
• Warts in the mouth are not uncommon.

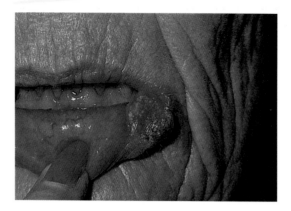

Fig. 13.36 Squamous cell carcinoma in a heavy smoker.

• The differential diagnosis of oral papules and nodules also includes lipomas, keloids, giant cell granulomas, granular cell tumours, myxomas, xanthomas, haemangiomas, myomas, neural tumours and a host of uncommon benign growths.

Squamous cell carcinoma (Fig. 13.36)

Cause

Predisposing factors include smoking or chewing tobacco products, and the 'straight-shot' drinking of alcohol. Cancer can also occur in the plaques and ulcers of lichen planus. Lip cancers may be sun-induced.

Presentation

A thickening or nodule develops, usually on the lower lip, and often in a field of actinic chelitis (rough scaling mucosa from sun damage). Inside the mouth, the tongue is the most common site to be affected, often on its undersurface. The cancer itself appears either as an indurated ulcer with steep edges, or as a diffuse hardness or nodule. Red or white thickened plaques are common precursors, and the cancer may be surrounded by these changes.

Course

Unfortunately, cancer of the mouth often goes undetected. Its symptoms are excused by the patient as aphthous ulcers or denture sores, and its signs are not seen by the physicians who scan the skin. Cancers grow, and squamous cell carcinomas of the mouth are no exception. Plaques and hard areas may ulcerate.

Differential diagnosis

Confusion occurs with ulcerative lichen planus and other causes of white and red patches. Biopsy will differentiate a squamous cell carcinoma from these other conditions.

Treatment

Dermatologists often treat lip cancers by a wedge excision through all layers of the lip, with primary repair. Oral surgeons or otolaryngologists usually remove intraoral cancers. Metastatic disease may require radiotherapy or chemotherapy.

Complications

Squamous cell carcinomas of the lip caused by sun exposure carry a much better prognosis than the others. Left untreated, squamous cell carcinomas are prone to metastasize to regional lymph nodes and elsewhere. The overall 5-year survival for intraoral squamous cell carcinoma is about 40–50%.

The genitals

The genital area is richly supplied with cutaneous nerves. This means that skin disease there makes life more miserable than might be expected from its extent or apparent severity. In addition, patients often feel a special shame when their genitals harbour skin

Table 13.6 Some benign genital problems.

Pearly penile papules	Pinhead-sized angiofibromas of the glans penis
Fordyce spots	Ectopic sebaceous glands of the glans penis
Angiokeratomas	Black papules of scrotum
Balanitis	Many types, but poor hygiene is common
Warts (condyloma accuminata)	Cauliflower-like growths of moist genital skin (see Chapter 14)
Fixed drug eruptions	Red plaques or ulcers can be localized to the penis (see Chapter 22)
Lichen planus (Fig. 13.37)	Look for lesions in the mouth or on the skin to confirm the diagnosis
Psoriasis	Often favours the glans penis
Paget's disease	Intraepithelial adenocarcinoma appearing as a marginated red plaque
Infections	Syphilis, herpes simplex, chancroid, lymphogranuloma venereum

diseases. Skin diseases seen elsewhere may afflict this area, but the patient will often hide them from the examining physician. Many never seek treatment.

Benign conditions

An array of problems can plague the genitals; Table 13.6 lists some of them.

Vulvovaginitis

Inflammatory diseases of the vagina often also affect the vulva, but the vagina alone can be affected. Vaginitis causes discharge, odour, painful intercourse and itching or burning sensations. The differential diagnosis includes candidiasis, trichomoniasis, bacterial vaginosis, cytolytic vaginosis and atrophic vaginitis. The diagnosis can be made by the appearance of the discharge both grossly and under the microscope. Most patients with vaginitis get their care from gynaecologists. Swabs for microbiological examination are essential.

Lichen sclerosus (see also Chapter 10)

Cause

This is unknown but local conditions have a role: not only does skin develop the disease after being

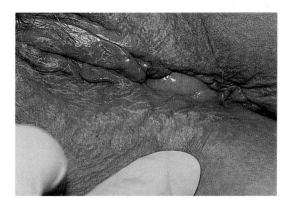

Fig. 13.37 White lace-like appearance of vulval lichen planus.

transplanted into affected areas, but the disease goes away when the grafted skin is returned to a distant site.

Presentation

The affected areas on the vulva, penis (Fig. 13.38), perineum and/or perianal skin show well-marginated white thin fragile patches with a crinkled surface. Itching can be severe, especially in women. The fragility of the atrophic areas may lead to purpura and erosions. Scratching can cause lichenification, and diagnostic confusion.

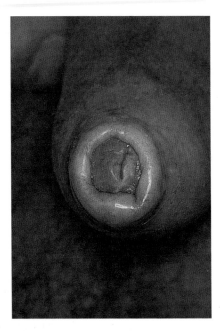

Fig. 13.38 Lichen sclerosus of the foreskin, carrying the risk of causing phimosis.

Women are more commonly afflicted than men, but pre-adolescent girls and boys also can develop this problem. In girls, the white patches circling the vulva and anus take on an hourglass shape around the orifices.

Course

As time goes on, scarring occurs. In adult women, the clitoral prepuce may scar over the clitoris, and the vaginal introitus may narrow, preventing enjoyable sexual intercourse. Scarring is rare in girls and boys; treatment may prevent it occurring in adults.

Differential diagnosis

The sharply marginated white patches of vitiligo can afflict the vulva and penis but lack atrophy, and typical vitiligo may be found elsewhere on the body. Neurodermatitis may be superimposed upon lichen sclerosus after incessant scratching.

Investigations

Biopsy is often unnecessary but the appearances are distinctive. The epidermis is thin, the basal layer shows

damage, and the papillary dermis contains a homogeneous pink-staining material and lymphocytes.

Treatment

At first sight it might seem unwise to rub potent topical steroids onto atrophic thin occluded skin. Yet, treatment with potent topical steroids not only reduces itch, pain and misery, but also reverses hypopigmentation and atrophy by shutting down its cause. However, atrophy, striae and other complications can develop on untreated adjacent skin, if the medication spreads there. Ointments are preferable to creams. Only small amounts (15 g) should be dispensed. After a course of 8–12 weeks, weaker topical steroids can be used to maintain a remission.

Complications

As mentioned earlier, scarring can destroy anatomical structures and narrow the vaginal opening. Squamous cell carcinomas may develop in men as well as women. Any focal thickening needs a biopsy.

Vulval and scrotal pruritus

Cause

Itching of the genital skin is usually caused by skin disease, or by rubbing, sweating, irritation or occlusion. Once started, genital itching seems able to continue on its own.

Presentation

The vulva and scrotum contain nerves that normally transmit pleasurable sensations. However, itching itself is not pleasurable, although scratching is. A torturing itch may be present all day, but more frequently appears or worsens at night. Once scratching has started, it perpetuates itself. The history is of an incessant and embarrassed scratching. Examination may show normal skin, or the tell-tale signs of excoriations and lichenification.

Differential diagnosis

Itch is part of many inflammatory skin diseases. In the groin its most common causes are tinea, candida, erythrasma, atopic dermatitis, psoriasis, pubic lice, intertrigo and irritant or allergic contact dermatitis. However, patients with 'essential' pruritus show no skin changes other than those elicited by scratching. Sometimes the cause is psychogenic, but one should be reluctant to assume that this is the cause. Biopsy rarely helps. Look for clues by hunting for skin disease at other body sites.

Treatment

Low potency topical corticosteroids sometimes help by suppressing secondary inflammation; however, atrophy sometimes quickly occurs, and then the itch is replaced by a burning sensation. A better approach is to eliminate the trigger factors for itch—such as hot baths, tight clothing, rough fabrics, sweating, cool air, the chronic wetness of vaginal secretions, menstrual pads and soaps. Antipruritic creams, such as doxepin cream, pramoxine cream or menthol in a light emollient base, help to abort the itch–scratch–itch cycles. Many patients benefit from systemic antihistamines or tricyclic drugs such as amitriptyline or doxepin.

Complications

Atrophy is common but hard to see. Lichenification creates leathery thickenings, marked with grooves resembling fissures.

Dermatoses

The skin of the groins and genitalia is susceptible to many inflammatory skin diseases. They are listed here (Table 13.7), but discussed in other chapters.

LEARNING POINT

'Jock itch' (tinea) affects the thighs and inguinal folds. Consider other diagnoses for rashes of the groin in other sites.

Malignant conditions

Squamous cell carcinoma

Cause

Human papilloma viruses, especially HPV types 6, 11, 16 and 18, often play a part. These are sexually transmitted, so the risk of carcinoma of the vulva or penis is greatest in those who have had many sexual partners. Squamous cell carcinoma of the glans penis is especially common in the uncircumcised. Smegma can incite inflammation leading to both phimosis and carcinoma. Exposure to tar also predisposes to scrotal carcinoma. Other predisposing factors are immunosuppression, lichen sclerosus and, possibly, lichen planus. Cancer can also develop from bowenoid papulosis—growths on the penis that resemble dark seborrhoeic keratoses clinically, and Bowen's disease histologically. The female equivalent is vulvar intraepithelial neoplasia.

Presentation

In men, a glistening irregular red moist patch (Fig. 13.39; Bowen's disease/erythroplasia of Queyrat) develops on an uncircumcised penis, either on the glans or on

Table 13.7 Nine common groin dermatoses.

Condition	Clinical comments
Tinea cruris	Involves the groin but seldom the scrotum
Candidiasis	Beefy red with satellite papules and pustules
Erythrasma	Brown patches of the upper thighs
Irritant contact dermatitis	Burning sensations may predominate
Allergic contact dermatitis	The scrotum may be oedematous
Inverse psoriasis	Beefy red marginated plaques extend up the gluteal fold
Seborrhoeic dermatitis	Look at the scalp for disease there, to confirm the diagnosis
Neurodermatitis	It feels wonderful to scratch an itchy groin
Intertrigo	Skin breaks down from maceration

the inner prepuce. Maceration may make it look white until evaporation reveals its true colour. It enlarges slowly, and invasion and tumour formation may not occur for years in immunocompetent men. In women, the precursor lesion is often Bowen's disease presenting as a sharply marginated, very slowly growing, mildly hyperkeratotic or slightly scaling, oddly shaped red patch or plaque that is usually a single lesion on one labia or in the perineum. This may become huge (up to 10 cm diameter). Sometimes cancer of the penis or labia resembles a large wart destroying the underlying tissue. Biopsy confirms the diagnosis.

Course

Eventually the precursor lesions become frankly invasive and capable of metastasizing. Invasive carcinomas present either as bleeding ulcerated indurated plaques, or as tumorous nodules.

Treatment

Mohs' micrographic excision (p. 323) is probably the best treatment for small and minimally invasive carcinomas, but partial penectomy is indicated if the tumour is large. Precursor lesions such as warts, bowenoid papulosis, vulvar intraepithelial neoplasia and Bowen's disease can be destroyed with laser surgery (p. 326) or cryotherapy (p. 324). In some patients, topical applications of the cytokine-inducer imiquimod cream or the chemotherapeutic 5-fluorouracil cream can be curative.

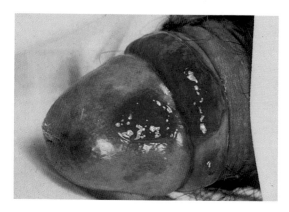

Fig. 13.39 Erythroplasia of Queyrat.

Further reading

Baran, R., Dawber, R.P.R., de Berker, D.A.R., Haneke, E. and Tosti, A. (2001) *Baran and Dawber's Diseases of the Nails and their Management*, 3rd edn. Blackwell Science, Oxford.

Bork, K., Hoede, N., Korting, G.W., Burgdorf, W.H.C. & Young, S.H. (1996) *Diseases of the Oral Mucosa and Lips*. W.B. Saunders, Philadelphia, PA.

Dawber, R. (1997) *Diseases of the Hair and Scalp*. Blackwell Science, Oxford.

Lynch, P.J. & Edwards, L. (1994) *Genital Dermatology*. Churchill Livingstone, Edinburgh.

Ridley, C.M., Oriel, J.D. & Robinson, A. (2000) *Vulval Disease*. Arnold, London.

Infections

Bacterial infections

The resident flora of the skin

The surface of the skin teems with micro-organisms, which are most numerous in moist hairy areas, rich in sebaceous glands. Organisms are found, in clusters, in irregularities in the stratum corneum and within the hair follicles. The resident flora is a mixture of harmless and poorly classified staphylococci, micrococci and diphtheroids. *Staphylococcus epidermidis* and aerobic diphtheroids predominate on the surface, and anaerobic diphtheroids (proprionibacteria sp.) deep in the hair follicles. Several species of lipophilic yeasts also exist on the skin. The proportion of the different organisms varies from person to person but, once established, an individual's skin flora tends to remain stable and helps to defend the skin against outside pathogens by bacterial interference or antibiotic production. Nevertheless, overgrowth of skin diphtheroids can itself lead to clinical problems. The role of Proprionibacteria in the pathogenesis of acne is discussed on p. 149. Overgrowth of aerobic diphtheroids causes the following conditions.

Trichomycosis axillaris

This is a common condition, seen, if looked for, in up to one-quarter of adult males. The axillary hairs become beaded with concretions, usually yellow, made up of colonies of commensal diphtheroids. Clothing becomes stained in the armpits. Topical antibiotic ointments, or shaving, will clear the condition.

Pitted keratolysis

The combination of unusually sweaty feet and occlusive shoes encourages the growth of diphtheroid

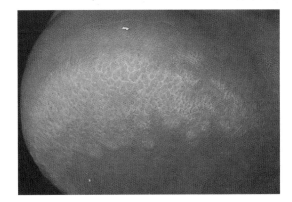

Fig. 14.1 Pitted keratolysis of the heel.

organisms that can digest keratin. The result is a cribriform pattern of fine punched-out depressions on the plantar surface (Fig. 14.1), coupled with an unpleasant smell (of methane-thiol). Fusidic acid or mupirocin ointment is usually effective. Occlusive footwear should be replaced by sandals and cotton socks if possible.

Erythrasma

Some diphtheroid members of the skin flora produce porphyrins when grown in a suitable medium; as a result their colonies fluoresce coral pink under Wood's light. Overgrowth of these strains is sometimes the cause of symptom-free macular wrinkled slightly scaly pink, brown or macerated white areas, most often found in the armpits or groins, or between the toes. In diabetics, larger areas of the trunk may be involved. Diagnosis is helped by the fact that these areas also fluoresce coral pink with Wood's light. Topical fusidic acid or miconazole will clear the condition.

Staphylococcal infections

Staphylococcus aureus is not part of the resident flora of the skin other than in a minority who carry it in their nostrils, perineum or armpits. Carriage rates vary with age. Nasal carriage is almost invariable in babies born in hospital, becomes less frequent during infancy, and rises again during the school years to the adult level of roughly 30%. Rather fewer carry the organism in the armpits or groin. Staphylococci can also multiply on areas of diseased skin such as eczema, often without causing obvious sepsis. A minor breach in the skin's defences is probably necessary for a frank staphylococcal infection to establish itself; some strains are particularly likely to cause skin sepsis.

Impetigo

Cause

Impetigo may be caused by staphylococci, streptococci, or by both together. As a useful rule of thumb, the bullous type is usually caused by *Staphylococcus aureus*, whereas the crusted ulcerated type is caused by β-haemolytic strains of streptococci. Both are highly contagious.

Presentation

A thin-walled flaccid clear blister forms, and may become pustular before rupturing to leave an extending area of exudation and yellowish crusting (Fig. 14.2). Lesions are often multiple, particularly around the face. The lesions may be more obviously bullous in infants. A follicular type of impetigo (superficial folliculitis) is also common.

Course

The condition can spread rapidly through a family or class. It tends to clear slowly even without treatment.

Complications

Streptococcal impetigo can trigger an acute glomerulonephritis.

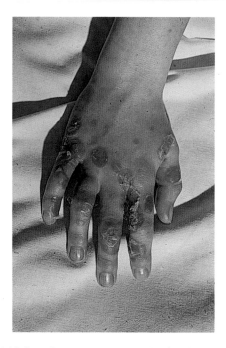

Fig. 14.2 Impetigo on an uncommon site showing erosions, crusting and rupture blisters.

Differential diagnosis

Herpes simplex may become impetiginized, as may eczema. Always think of a possible underlying cause such as this. Recurrent impetigo of the head and neck, for example, should prompt a search for scalp lice.

Investigation and treatment

The diagnosis is usually made on clinical grounds. Swabs should be taken and sent to the laboratory for culture, but treatment must not be held up until the results are available. Systemic antibiotics (such as flucloxacillin, erythromycin or cephalexin (cefalexin)) are needed for severe cases or if a nephritogenic strain of streptococcus is suspected (penicillin V). For minor cases the removal of crusts and a topical antibiotic such as neomycin, fusidic acid (not available in the USA), mupirocin or bacitracin will suffice (Formulary 1, p. 334).

Ecthyma

This term describes ulcers forming under a crusted surface infection. The site may have been that of an insect bite or of neglected minor trauma. The bacterial pathogens and their treatment are similar to those of impetigo; however, in contrast to impetigo, ecthyma heals with scarring.

Furunculosis (boils)

Cause

A boil is an acute pustular infection of a hair follicle, usually with *Staphylococcus aureus*. Adolescent boys are especially susceptible to them.

Presentation and course

A tender red nodule enlarges, and later may discharge pus and its central 'core' before healing to leave a scar. Fever and enlarged draining nodes complete the picture. Most patients have one or two boils only, and then clear; a few suffer from a tiresome sequence of boils (chronic furunculosis).

Complications

Cavernous sinus thrombosis is an unusual complication of boils on the central face. Septicaemia may occur but is rare.

Differential diagnosis

The diagnosis is straightforward but hidradenitis suppurativa (p. 161) should be considered if only the groin and axillae are involved.

Investigations in chronic furunculosis

• General examination: look for underlying skin disease (e.g. scabies, pediculosis, eczema).
• Test the urine for sugar. Full blood count.
• Culture swabs from lesions, and carrier sites (nostrils, perineum) of the patient and immediate family.
• Immunological evaluation only if the patient has recurrent or unusual internal infections too.

Treatment

Acute episodes will respond to an appropriate antibiotic; incision speeds healing.

In chronic furunculosis (Fig. 14.3):
• Treat carrier sites such as the nose and groin twice daily for 6 weeks with an appropriate topical antiseptic or antibiotic (e.g. chlorhexidine solution, mupirocin cream or clindamycin solution). Treat family carriers in the same way.

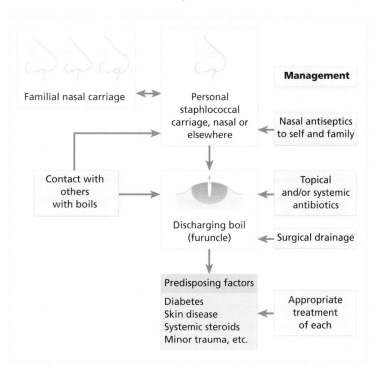

Fig. 14.3 Chronic furunculosis.

• Treat lesions with a topical antibiotic. In stubborn cases add 6 weeks of a systemic antibiotic chosen to cover organism's proven sensitivities.
• Daily bath using an antiseptic soap.
• Improve hygiene and nutritional state, if faulty.

Carbuncle

A group of adjacent hair follicles becomes deeply infected with *Staphylococcus aureus*, leading to a swollen painful suppurating area discharging pus from several points. The pain and systemic upset are greater than those of a boil. Diabetes must be excluded. Treatment needs both topical and systemic antibiotics. Incision and drainage has been shown to speed up healing, although it is not always easy when there are multiple deep pus-filled pockets. Consider the possibility of a fungal kerion (p. 216) in unresponsive carbuncles.

Scalded skin syndrome

In this condition the skin changes resemble a scald. Erythema and tenderness are followed by the loosening of large areas of overlying epidermis (Fig. 14.4). In

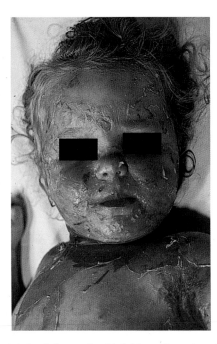

Fig. 14.4 Staphylococcal scalded skin syndrome in a child. The overlying epidermis is loosening in the red areas.

children the condition is usually caused by a staphylococcal infection elsewhere (e.g. impetigo or conjunctivitis). Organisms in what may be only a minor local infection release a toxin (exfoliatin) that causes a split to occur high in the epidermis. With systemic antibiotics the outlook is good.

This is in contrast to toxic epidermal necrolysis, which is usually drug-induced. The damage to the epidermis in toxic epidermal necrolysis is full thickness, and a skin biopsy will distinguish it from the scalded skin syndrome (p. 115).

Toxic shock syndrome

A staphylococcal toxin is also responsible for this condition, in which fever, a rash—usually a widespread erythema—and sometimes circulatory collapse are followed a week or two later by characteristic desquamation, most marked on the fingers and hands. Many cases have followed staphylococcal overgrowth in the vagina of women using tampons. Systemic antibiotics and irrigation of the infected site are needed.

Streptococcal infections

Erysipelas

The first warning of an attack is often malaise, shivering and a fever. After a few hours the affected area of skin becomes red, and the eruption spreads with a well-defined advancing edge. Blisters may develop on the red plaques (Fig. 14.5). Untreated, the condition can even be fatal, but it responds rapidly to systemic penicillin, sometimes given intravenously. The causative streptococci usually gain their entry through a split in the skin, e.g. between the toes or under an ear lobe.

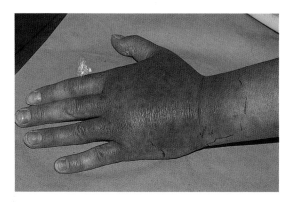

Fig. 14.5 Erysipelas—note sharp spreading edge, here demarcated with a ballpoint pen.

Episodes can affect the same area repeatedly and so lead to persistent lymphoedema. Low dosage long-term oral penicillin V will usually cut down the frequency of recurrences. The cause of the original skin split, perhaps a minor tinea pedis, should be treated too.

Cellulitis

This inflammation of the skin occurs at a deeper level than erysipelas. The subcutaneous tissues are involved; and the area is more raised and swollen, and the erythema less marginated than in erysipelas. Cellulitis often follows an injury and favours areas of hypostatic oedema. Streptococci, staphylococci or other organisms may be the cause. Treatment is elevation, rest—sometimes in hospital—and systemic antibiotics, sometimes given intravenously.

Necrotizing fasciitis

A mixture of pathogens, usually including streptococci and anaerobes, is responsible for this rare condition, which is a surgical emergency. At first the infection resembles a dusky, often painful, cellulitis, but it quickly turns into an extending necrosis of the skin and subcutaneous tissues. A deep 'stab' incision biopsy through the skin into the fascia may be necessary to obtain material for bacteriological culture. A magnetic resonance imaging (MRI) scan may help to establish how far the infection has spread. The prognosis is often poor despite early surgical debridement and prompt intravenous antibiotics, even when given before the bacteriological results are available.

Erysipeloid

It is convenient to mention this here, but the causative organism is *Erysipelothrix insidiosa* and not a streptococcus. It infects a wide range of animals, birds and fish. In humans, infections are most common in butchers, fishmongers and cooks, the organisms penetrating the skin after a prick from an infected bone. Such infections are usually mild, and localized to the area around the inoculation site. The swollen purple area spreads slowly with a clear-cut advancing edge. With penicillin the condition clears quickly; without it, resolution takes several weeks.

Cat-scratch disease

The infective agent is the bacillus *Rochalimaea henselae*. A few days after a cat bite or scratch, a reddish granulomatous papule appears at the site of inoculation. Tender regional lymphadenopathy follows some weeks later, and lasts for several weeks, often being accompanied by a mild fever. The glands may discharge before settling spontaneously. There is no specific treatment.

Spirochaetal infections

Syphilis

Cause

Infection with the causative organism, *Treponema pallidum*, may be congenital, acquired through transfusion with contaminated blood, or by accidental inoculation. The most important route, however, is through sexual contact with an infected partner.

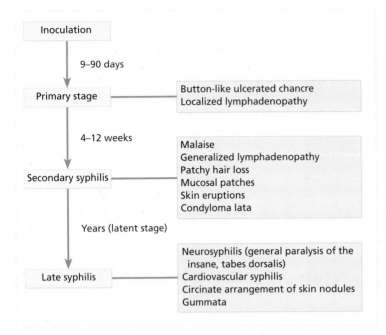

Fig. 14.6 The stages of syphilis.

Presentation

Congenital syphilis. If there is a high standard of antenatal care, syphilis in the mother will be detected and treated during pregnancy, and congenital syphilis will be rare. Otherwise, stillbirth is a common outcome, although some children with congenital syphilis may develop the stigmata of the disease only in late childhood.

Acquired syphilis. The features of the different stages are given in Fig. 14.6. After an incubation period (9–90 days), a primary chancre develops at the site of inoculation. Often this is genital, but oral and anal chancres are not uncommon. A typical chancre is an ulcerated, although not painful, button-like lesion of up to 1 cm in diameter accompanied by local lymphadenopathy. Untreated it lasts about 6 weeks and then clears leaving an inconspicuous scar.

The secondary stage may be reached while the chancre is still subsiding. Systemic symptoms and a generalized lymphadenopathy usher in eruptions that at first are macular and inconspicuous, and later papular and more obvious. Lesions are distributed symmetrically and are of a coppery ham colour. Sometimes they resemble pityriasis rosea. Classically, there are obvious lesions on the palms and soles. Annular lesions are also not uncommon. Condyloma lata are moist papules in the genital and anal areas. Other signs include a 'moth-eaten' alopecia and mucous patches in the mouth.

The skin lesions of late syphilis may be nodules that spread peripherally and clear centrally, leaving a serpiginous outline. Gummas are granulomatous areas; in the skin they quickly break down to leave punched-out ulcers that heal poorly, leaving papery white scars.

Clinical course

Even if left untreated, most of those who contract syphilis have no further problems after the secondary stage has passed. Others develop the cutaneous or systemic manifestations of late syphilis.

Differential diagnosis

The skin changes of syphilis can mimic many other skin diseases. Always consider the following.
1 Chancre: chancroid (multiple and painful), herpes simplex, anal fissure, cervical erosions.
2 Secondary syphilis:

- eruption—measles, rubella, drug eruptions, pityriasis rosea, lichen planus, psoriasis;
- condylomas—genital warts, haemorrhoids;
- oral lesions—aphthous ulcers, candidiasis.

3 Late syphilis: bromide and iodide reactions, other granulomas, erythema induratum.

Investigations

The diagnosis of syphilis in its infectious (primary and secondary) stages can be confirmed using dark field microscopy to show up spirochaetes in smears from chancres, oral lesions, or moist areas in a secondary eruption.

Serological tests for syphilis become positive only some 5–6 weeks after infection (usually a week or two after the appearance of the chancre). The traditional tests [Wasswemann reaction (WR) and Venereal Disease Research Laboratory (VDRL)] have now been replaced by more specific ones [e.g. the rapid plasma reagin (RPR) test and the fluorescent treponemal antibody/absorption (FTA/ABS) test]. These more sensitive tests do not become negative after treatment if an infection has been present for more than a few months.

Treatment

This should follow the current recommendations of the World Health Organization (WHO). Penicillin is still the treatment of choice (e.g. for early syphilis benzathine penicillin 1.2 million units given intramuscularly into each buttock at a single session, or procaine penicillin 600 000 units intramuscularly daily for 12 days), with long-term high-dose oral erythromycin and tetracycline being effective alternatives for those with penicillin allergy. The use of long-acting penicillin injections overcomes the ever-present danger of poor compliance with oral treatment. Every effort must be made to trace and treat infected contacts.

LEARNING POINTS

1 Syphilis is still around. Remember that today's general was yesterday's lieutenant.
2 It is still worth checking for syphilis in perplexing rashes.

Yaws

Yaws is distributed widely across the poorer parts of the tropics. The spirochaete, *Treponema pallidum* ssp. *pertenue*, gains its entry through skin abrasions. After an incubation period of up to 6 months, the primary lesion, a crusting and ulcerated papule known as the 'mother yaw', develops at the site of inoculation; later it may enlarge to an exuberant raspberry-like swelling which lasts for several months before healing to leave an atrophic pale scar. In the secondary stage, other lesions may develop in any area but do so especially around the orifices. They are not unlike the primary lesion but are smaller and more numerous ('daughter yaws'). Hyperkeratotic plaques may appear on the palms and soles. The tertiary stage is characterized by ulcerated gummatous skin lesions, hyperkeratosis of the palms and soles, and a painful periostitis that distorts the long bones. Serological tests for syphilis are positive. Treatment is with penicillin.

Lyme disease

The spirochaete *Borrelia burgdorferi* is responsible for this condition, named after the town in the USA where it was first recognized. It is transmitted to humans by ticks of the genus *Ixodes*, commonly harboured by deer. The site of the tick bite becomes the centre of a slowly expanding erythematous ring ('erythema migrans'; Fig. 14.7). Later, many annular non-scaly plaques may develop. In the USA, a few of those affected develop arthritis and heart disease, both of which are less common in European cases. Other internal complications include meningitis and cranial nerve palsies. Treated early, the condition clears well with a 21-day course of oral amoxycillin or doxycycline: patients affected systemically need longer courses of parenteral antibiotics. Infection can be confirmed by serology, although this is usually negative in the first few weeks after innoculation.

Other infections

Cutaneous anthrax

This condition is usually acquired through contact with infected livestock or animal products such as wool

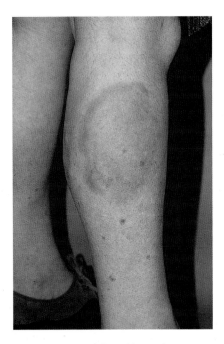

Fig. 14.7 A tick bite was followed by erythema migrans.

or bristles. Previously rare in industrialized countries, its importance has increased there since the recent wave of bio-terrorist attacks. The spores of *Bacillus anthracis*, the causative organism, are highly resistant to physical and chemical agents.

Anthrax has two main clinical variants: inhalational anthrax, which is outside the scope of this book; and cutaneous anthrax. The incubation period of the latter is usually between 2 and 5 days. A skin lesion then appears on an exposed part, often in association with a variable degree of cutaneous oedema, which can sometimes be massive, especially on the face. Within a day or two, the original small painless papule shows vesicles that quickly coalesce into a larger single blister. This ruptures to form an ulcer with a central dark eschar, which falls off after 1–2 weeks leaving a scar. The skin lesions are often accompanied by fever, headache, myalgia and regional lymphadenopathy. The mortality rate for untreated cutaneous anthrax is up to 20%; with appropriate antibiotic treatment, this falls to less than 1%.

Cultures of material taken from the vesicle may be positive in 12–48 h; a Gram stain will show Gram-positive bacilli, occurring singly or in short chains. Quicker results may be obtained by a direct fluorescent antibody test, or by an enzyme-linked immuno-absorbant assay (ELISA)—both of which are currently available only at reference laboratories. Before the results are available, it is wise to assume that the organism is penicillin- and tetracycline-resistant, and to start treatment with ciprofloxacin at 400 mg intravenously every 12 h or, for milder cases, ciprofloxacin 500 mg orally every 12 h. The latter dose is suitable for prophylactic use in those who are known to have been exposed to spores. A switch to an alternative regimen can be made once the antibiotic sensitivity of the organism has been established. At present, anthrax vaccine is in short supply; it requires six injections over 18 months, with subsequent boosters, to prevent anthrax.

Gonococcal septicaemia

Skin lesions are important clues to the diagnosis of this condition, in which the symptoms and signs of classical gonorrhoea are usually absent. The patient, usually a woman with recurring fever and joint pains, develops sparse crops of skin lesions, usually around the hands and feet. The grey, often haemorrhagic, vesicopustules are characteristic. Rather similar lesions are seen in chronic meningococcal septicaemia.

Mycobacterial infections

Tuberculosis

Most infections in the UK are caused by *Mycobacterium tuberculosis*. *Mycobacterium bovis* infection, endemic in cattle, can be spread to humans by milk, but human infection with this organism is now rare in countries where cattle have been vaccinated against tuberculosis and the milk is pasteurized. The steady decline of tuberculosis in developed countries has been reversed in some areas where AIDS is especially prevalent. Dormant tuberculosis of the skin can also be reactivated by systemic corticosteroids, immuno-suppressants and new anti TNF biological agents.

Inoculation tuberculosis

Lupus vulgaris (Fig. 14.8) can follow the inoculation of tubercle bacilli into the skin of a person with high immunity, the direct spread of the organism from an underlying infected lymph node, or blood-borne spread from a pulmonary lesion. Lesions occur most often around the head and neck. A reddish-brown scaly

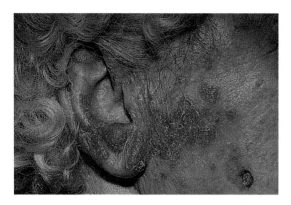

Fig. 14.8 A plaque with the brownish tinge characteristic of lupus vulgaris. Diascopy was positive.

plaque slowly enlarges, and can damage deeper tissues such as cartilage, leading to ugly mutilation. Scarring and contractures may follow.

Diascopy (p. 32) shows up the characteristic brownish 'apple jelly' nodules and the clinical diagnosis should be confirmed by a biopsy. A warty variant exists.

Scrofuloderma

The skin overlying a tuberculous lymph node or joint may become involved in the process. The subsequent mixture of lesions (irregular puckered scars, fistulae and abscesses) is most commonly seen in the neck.

Tuberculides

A number of skin eruptions have, in the past, been attributed to a reaction to internal foci of tuberculosis. Of these, the best authenticated—by finding mycobacterial DNA by polymerase chain reaction (PCR)—are the 'papulonecrotic tuberculides'—recurring crops of firm dusky papules, which may ulcerate, favouring the points of the knees and elbows.

Erythema induratum (Bazin's disease)

In erythema induratum, deep purplish ulcerating nodules occur on the backs of the lower legs, usually in women with a poor 'chilblain' type of circulation. Sometimes this is associated with a tuberculous focus elsewhere. Erythema nodosum (p. 101) may also be the result of tuberculosis elsewhere.

Investigations

Biopsy for:
• microscopy (tuberculoid granulomas);
• bacteriological culture; and
• detection of mycobacterial DNA by PCR.
Mantoux test.

Treatment

The treatment of all types of cutaneous tuberculosis should be with a full course of a standard multidrug antituberculosis regimen. There is no longer any excuse for the use of one drug alone.

Prevention

Outbreaks of pulmonary tuberculosis are reminders that this disease has not yet been conquered and that vigilance is important. Bacillus Calmette–Guérin (BCG) vaccination of schoolchildren, immunization of cattle and pasteurization of milk remain the most effective protective measures.

Leprosy

Cause

Mycobacterium leprae was discovered by Hansen in 1874, but has still not been cultured *in vitro*, although it can be made to grow in some animals (armadillos, mouse foot-pads, etc.). In humans the main route of infection is through nasal droplets from cases of lepromatous leprosy although, interestingly, some cases have occurred in Louisiana from eating infected armadillos.

Epidemiology

Some 15 million people suffer from leprosy. Most live in the tropics and subtropics, but the ease of modern travel means that some cases are seen in northern Europe and the USA.

Presentation

The range of clinical manifestations and complications depends upon the immune response of the patient (Fig. 14.9). Those with a high resistance develop a paucibacillary tuberculoid type (Fig. 14.10) and those

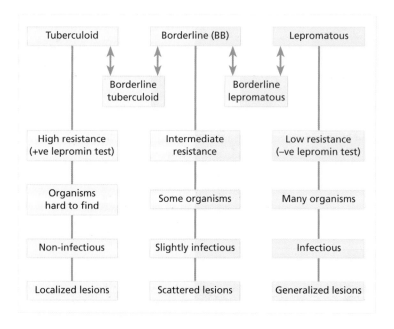

Fig. 14.9 The spectrum of leprosy: tuberculoid to lepromatous.

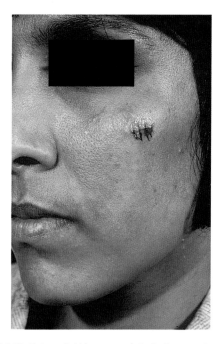

Fig. 14.10 Tuberculoid leprosy: subtle depigmentation with a palpable erythematous rim at the upper edge.

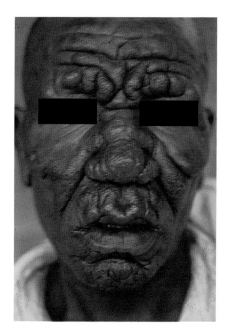

Fig. 14.11 The 'leonine' facies of lepromatous leprosy.

with low resistance a multibacillary lepromatous type. Nerve thickening is earlier and more marked in the tuberculoid than lepromatous type (Fig. 14.11). Between the extremes lies a spectrum of reactions clas-sified as 'borderline'. Those most like the tuberculoid type are known as borderline tuberculoid (BT) and those nearest to the lepromatous type as borderline lepromatous (BL). The clinical differences between the two polar types are given in Fig. 14.12.

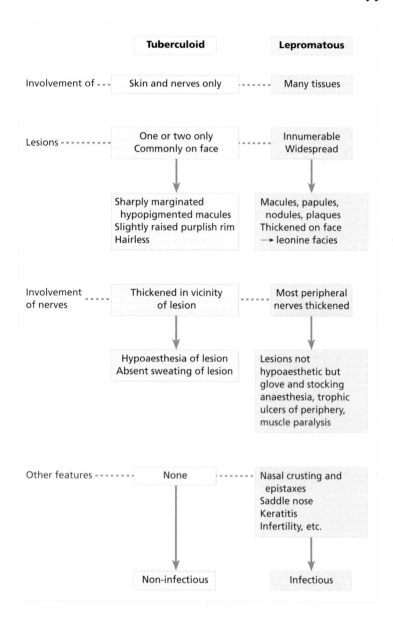

	Tuberculoid	Lepromatous
Involvement of	Skin and nerves only	Many tissues
Lesions	One or two only Commonly on face	Innumerable Widespread
	Sharply marginated hypopigmented macules Slightly raised purplish rim Hairless	Macules, papules, nodules, plaques Thickened on face → leonine facies
Involvement of nerves	Thickened in vicinity of lesion	Most peripheral nerves thickened
	Hypoaesthesia of lesion Absent sweating of lesion	Lesions not hypoaesthetic but glove and stocking anaesthesia, trophic ulcers of periphery, muscle paralysis
Other features	None	Nasal crusting and epistaxes Saddle nose Keratitis Infertility, etc.
	Non-infectious	Infectious

Fig. 14.12 Tuberculoid vs. lepromatous leprosy.

Differential diagnosis

Tuberculoid leprosy. Consider the following—in none of which is there any loss of sensation.
• Vitiligo (p. 246)—loss of pigment is usually complete.
• Pityriasis versicolor (p. 221)—scrapings show mycelia and spores.
• Pityriasis alba—a common cause of scaly hypopigmented areas on the cheeks of children.
• Postinflammatory depigmentation of any cause.

• Sarcoidosis, granuloma annulare, necrobiosis lipoidica.

Lepromatous leprosy. Widespread leishmaniasis can closely simulate lepromatous leprosy. The nodules seen in neurofibromatosis and mycosis fungoides, and multiple sebaceous cysts, can cause confusion, as can the acral deformities seen in yaws and systemic sclerosis. Leprosy is a great imitator.

Investigations

• Biopsy of skin or sensory nerve.
• Skin or nasal smears, with Ziehl–Nielsen or Fité stains, will show up the large number of organisms seen in the lepromatous type.
• Lepromin test. This is of no use in the diagnosis of leprosy but, once the diagnosis has been made, it will help to decide which type of disease is present (positive in tuberculoid type).

Treatment

The emergence of resistant strains of *M. leprae* means that it is no longer wise to treat leprosy with dapsone alone. It should now be used in combination, usually with rifampicin, and also with clofazimine for lepromatous leprosy. A brief period of isolation is needed only for patients with infectious lepromatous leprosy; with treatment they quickly become non-infectious and can return to the community. However, their management should remain in the hands of physicians with a special interest in the disease. Tuberculoid forms are usually treated for 6–12 months; multibacillary leprosy needs treatment for at least 2 years.

Special care is needed with the two types of lepra reaction that can occur during treatment:
• Type 1 (reversal) reactions are seen mainly in borderline tuberculoid disease (Fig. 14.13). Lesions become red and angry, and pain and paralysis follow neural inflammation. Treatment is with salicylates, chloroquine, non-steroidal and steroidal anti-inflammatory drugs.
• Type 2 reactions are common in lepromatous leprosy and include erythema nodosum, nerve palsies, lymphadenopathy, arthritis, iridocyclitis, epididymoorchitis and proteinuria. They are treated with the drugs used for type 1 reactions, and also with thalidomide.

The household contacts of lepromatous patients are at risk of developing leprosy and should be followed up. Child contacts may benefit from prophylactic therapy and BCG inoculation.

Other mycobacterial infections

Mycobacteria are widespread in nature, living as environmental saprophytes. Some can infect humans.

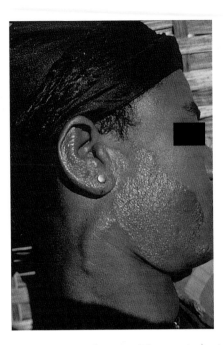

Fig. 14.13 Type 1 reversal reaction. The posterior auricular nerve is grossly swollen.

Mycobacterium marinum

Mycobacterium marinum lives in water. Human infections have occurred in epidemics centred on infected swimming pools. Another route of infection is through minor skin breaches in those who clean out tropical fish tanks (Fig. 14.14). After a 3-week incubation period, an indolent abscess or ulcerated nodule forms at the site of inoculation; later nodules may develop along the draining lymphatics (sporotrichoid spread; Fig. 14.15 and p. 222). The lesions heal spontaneously, but slowly. Resolution may be speeded by an 8-week course of trimethoprim/sulfamethoxazole or minocycline. Should these fail, rifampicin in combination with ethambutol is worth a trial.

Mycobacterium ulcerans

Infections are confined to certain humid tropical areas where the organism lives on the vegetation, and are most common in Uganda (Buruli ulcers). The necrotic spreading ulcers, with their undermined edges, are usually found on the legs. Drug therapy is often disappointing and the treatment of choice is probably the surgical removal of infected tissue.

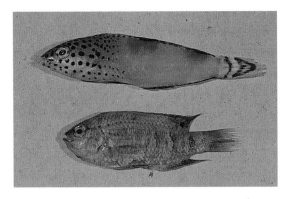

Fig. 14.14 Dead tropical fish picked out of the tank by the patient shown in Fig. 14.15.

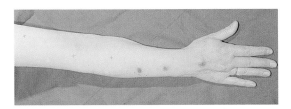

Fig. 14.15 The sporotrichoid spread of an atypical mycobacterial infection.

Leishmaniasis

Leishmania organisms are protozoa whose life cycle includes stages in phlebotomus flies, from which they are transmitted to humans. Different species, in different geographical areas, cause different clinical pictures.
• *Leishmania tropica* is found around the Mediterranean coast and in southern Asia; it causes chronically discharging skin nodules (oriental sores; Fig. 14.16).
• *Leishmania donovani* causes kala-azar, a disease characterized by fever, hepatosplenomegaly and anaemia. The skin may show an irregular darkening, particularly on the face and hands.
• *Leishmania mexicana* and *braziliensis* are found in South and Central America. They also cause deep sores, but up to 40% of those infected with *L. braziliensis* develop 'episodic', destructive metastatic lesions in the mucosa of the nose or month.

Diagnosis

This is confirmed by:
• histology—amastigote parasites, granulomatous reaction;
• touch smear—amastigote parasites;

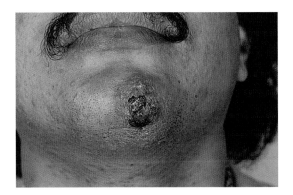

Fig. 14.16 Leishmaniasis acquired in the Middle East.

• culture; and
• polymerase chain reaction tests.

Treatment

Single nodules often resolve spontaneously and may not need treatment. Destructive measures, including cryotherapy, are sometimes used for localized skin lesions. Oral zinc sulphate (5 mg/kg/day for 4 weeks) showed promising results in a recent Indian trial.

Intralesional or intravenous antimony compounds are still the treatment of choice for most types of leishmaniasis, e.g. sodium stibogluconate (20 mg/kg/day for 20 days) with regular blood tests and electrocardiographic monitoring.

Viral infections

The viral infections dealt with here are those that are commonly seen in dermatology clinics. A textbook of infectious diseases should be consulted for details of systemic viral infections, many of which, like measles and German measles, have their own specific rashes.

Viral warts

Most people will have a wart at some time in their lives. Their prevalence is highest in childhood, and they affect an estimated 4–5% of schoolchildren in the UK.

Cause

Warts are caused by the human papilloma virus (HPV), which has still not been cultured *in vitro*. Nevertheless,

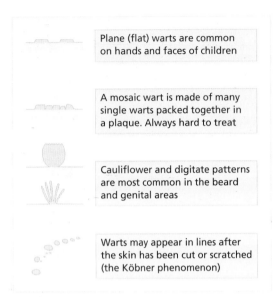

Plane (flat) warts are common on hands and faces of children

A mosaic wart is made of many single warts packed together in a plaque. Always hard to treat

Cauliflower and digitate patterns are most common in the beard and genital areas

Warts may appear in lines after the skin has been cut or scratched (the Köbner phenomenon)

Fig. 14.17 Viral warts—variations on the theme.

more than 70 'types' of the virus have been recognized by DNA sequencing; each has its own range of clinical manifestations. HPV-1, 2 and 4, for example, are found in common warts, whereas HPV-3 is found in plane warts, and HPV-6, 11, 16 and 18 are most common in genital warts. Infections occur when wart virus in skin scales comes into contact with breaches in the skin or mucous membranes.

Presentation

Warts adopt a variety of patterns (Fig. 14.17), some of which are described below.

Common warts (Figs 14.18 and 14.19). The first sign is a smooth skin-coloured papule, often more easily felt than seen. As the lesion enlarges, its irregular hyperkeratotic surface gives it the classic 'warty' appearance. Common warts usually occur on the hands but are also often on the face and genitals. They are more often multiple than single. Pain is rare.

Plantar warts. These have a rough surface, which protrudes only slightly from the skin and is surrounded by a horny collar (Fig. 14.20). On paring, the presence of bleeding capillary loops allows plantar warts to be distinguished from corns. Often multiple, plantar warts can be painful.

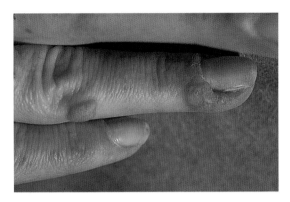

Fig. 14.18 Typical common warts on the fingers.

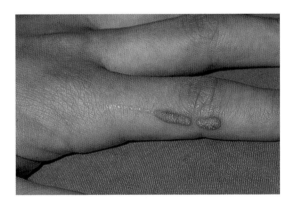

Fig. 14.19 Multiple hand warts in a fishmonger.

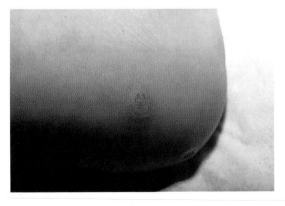

Fig. 14.20 Solitary plantar wart on the heel. (Courtesy of Dr E.C. Benton, The Royal Infirmary of Edinburgh, Edinburgh, UK.)

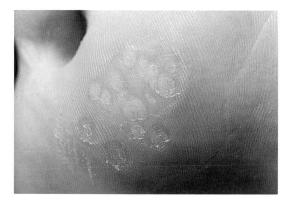

Fig. 14.21 Group of warts under the forefoot pared to show mosaic pattern.

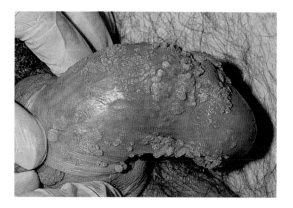

Fig. 14.23 Massive penile warts in an immunosuppressed patient.

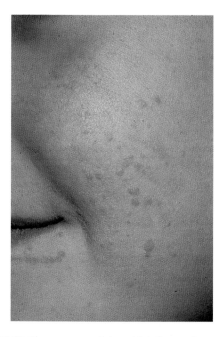

Fig. 14.22 Plane warts resolving with inflammation.

Mosaic warts (Fig. 14.21). These rough marginated plaques are made up of many small tightly packed but discrete individual warts. They are most common on the soles but are also seen on palms and around fingernails. Usually they are not painful.

Plane warts (Fig. 14.22). These smooth flat-topped papules are most common on the face and brow, and on the backs of the hands. Usually skin-coloured or light brown, they become inflamed as a result of an immunological reaction, just before they resolve spontaneously. Lesions are multiple, painless and, like common warts, are sometimes arranged along a scratch line.

Facial warts. These are most common in the beard area of adult males and are spread by shaving. A digitate appearance is common. Lesions are often ugly but are painless.

Anogenital warts (condyloma acuminata) (Fig. 14.23). Papillomatous cauliflower-like lesions, with a moist macerated vascular surface, can appear anywhere in this area. They may coalesce to form huge lesions causing discomfort and irritation. The vaginal and anorectal mucosae may be affected. The presence of anogenital warts in children raises the spectre of sexual abuse, but is usually caused by autoinoculation from common warts elsewhere.

Course

Warts resolve spontaneously in the healthy as the immune response overcomes the infection. This happens within 6 months in some 30% of patients, and within 2 years in 65%. Such spontaneous resolution, sometimes heralded by a punctate blackening caused by capillary thrombosis (Fig. 14.24), leaves no trace. Mosaic warts are notoriously slow to resolve and often resist all treatments. Warts persist and spread in immunocompromised patients (e.g. those on immunosuppressive therapy or with lymphoreticular disease).

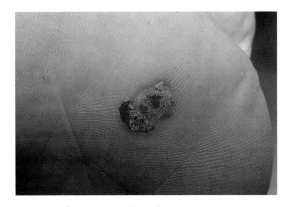

Fig. 14.24 Spontaneous resolution of a group of plantar warts. The blackness is caused by capillary thrombosis.

Seventy per cent of renal allograft recipients will have warts 5 years after transplantation.

Complications

1 Some plantar warts are very painful.
2 Epidermodysplasia verruciformis is a rare inherited disorder in which there is a universal wart infection, usually with HPV of unusual types. An impairment of cell-mediated immunity (p. 26) is commonly found and ensuing carcinomatous change frequently occurs.
3 Malignant change is otherwise rare, although infections with HPV of certain genital strains predispose to cervical and penile carcinoma. HPV infections in immunocompromised patients (e.g. renal allograft recipients) have also been linked with skin cancer, especially on light-exposed areas.

Differential diagnosis

Most warts are easily recognized. The following must be ruled out.
• *Molluscum contagiosum* (p. 209) are smooth, dome-shaped and pearly, with central umbilication.
• *Plantar corns* are found on pressure areas; there is no capillary bleeding on paring. They have a central keratotic core and are painful.
• *Granuloma annulare* lesions (p. 284) have a smooth surface, as the lesions are dermal; and their outline is often annular.
• *Condyloma lata* are seen in syphilis. They are rare but should not be confused with condyloma acuminata (warts). The lesions are flatter, greyer and less well

defined. If in doubt, look for other signs of secondary syphilis (p. 193) and carry out serological tests.
• *Amelanotic melanomas and other epithelial malignancies* can present as verrucose nodules—those in patients over the age of 40 years should be examined with special care. Mistakes have been made in the past.

Treatment

Many warts give no trouble, need no treatment and will go away by themselves. Otherwise treatment will depend on the type of wart. In general terms, destruction by cryotherapy is less likely to cause scars than excision or electrosurgery.

Palmoplantar warts

Home treatment is best, with one of the many wart paints now available (Formulary 1, p. 335). Most contain salicylic acid (12–20%). The success rate is good if the patient is prepared to persist with regular treatment. Paints should be applied once daily, after moistening the warts in hot water for at least 5 min. After drying, dead tissue and old paint are removed with an emery board or pumice stone. Enough paint to cover the surface of the wart, but not the surrounding skin, is applied and allowed to dry. Warts on the plantar surface should be covered with plasters although this is not necessary elsewhere. Side-effects are rare if these instructions are followed. Wart paints should not be applied to facial or anogenital skin, or to patients with adjacent eczema.

If no progress is being made after the regular and correct use of a salicylic acid wart paint for 12 weeks, then a paint containing formaldehyde or glutaraldehyde is worth trying. A useful way of dealing with multiple small plantar warts is for the area to be soaked for 10 min each night in a 4% formalin solution, although a few patients become allergic to this.

Cryotherapy with liquid nitrogen (at –196°C) is more effective than the less cold, dry ice or dimethyl ether/propane techniques. However, it is painful. A cotton-tipped applicator dipped into liquid nitrogen is applied to the wart until a small frozen halo appears in the surrounding normal skin (Fig. 14.25). The human papilloma virus, and also other viruses such as HIV, can survive in stored liquid nitrogen and so, once used, a bud should not be dipped back into the flask. Treatment with a liquid nitrogen spray gun does not

Fig. 14.25 A wart treated with cryotherapy: area includes a small frozen halo of normal surrounding skin.

carry the risk of cross-infecting patients, and is quicker and just as effective. The use of two freeze–thaw cycles increases the clearance rate of plantar warts but not of hand warts. If further treatments are necessary, the optimal interval is 3 weeks. The cure rate is higher if plantar warts are pared before they are frozen, but this makes no difference to warts elsewhere. If there has been no improvement after four or five treatments there is little to be gained from further freezings.

A few minutes tuition from a dermatologist will help practitioners wishing to start cryotherapy. Blisters should not be provoked intentionally, but occur from time to time, and will not alarm patients who have been forewarned.

Anogenital warts

Women with anogenital warts, or who are the partners of men with anogenital warts, should have their cervical cytology checked regularly as the wart virus can cause cervical cancer.

The focus has shifted towards self-treatment using podophyllotoxin (0.5% solution or 0.15% cream) or imiquimod (5% cream). Both are irritants and should be used carefully according to the manufacturer's instructions. Imiquimod is an immune response modifier that induces keratinocytes to produce cytokines, leading to wart regression, and may help to build cell-mediated immunity for longlasting protection. It is applied as a thin layer three times weekly and washed off with a mild soap 6–10 h after application. Podophyllin paint (15%) is used much less often now. It should be applied carefully to the warts and allowed to dry

before powdering with talcum. On the first occasion it should be washed off with soap and water after 2 h but, if there has been little discomfort, this can be increased stepwise to 6 h. Treatment is best carried out weekly by a doctor or nurse, but not by the patient. Podophyllin must not be used in pregnancy. Cryotherapy, electrosurgery and laser treatment are all effective treatments in the clinic.

Facial common warts

These are best treated with electrocautery or a hyfrecator, but also surrender to careful cryotherapy. Scarring is an unwanted complication. Shaving, if essential, should be with a brushless foam and a disposable razor.

Plane warts

On the face these are best left untreated and the patient or parent can be reasonably assured that spontaneous resolution will occur. When treatment is demanded, the use of a wart paint or imiquimod cream is reasonable. Gentle cryotherapy of just a few warts may help to induce immunity.

Solitary, stubborn or painful warts

These can be removed under local anaesthetic with a curette, although cure is not assured with this or any other method, and a scar often follows. Surgical excision is never justifiable (Fig. 14.26). Bleomycin can also be injected into such warts with success but this treatment should only be undertaken by a specialist.

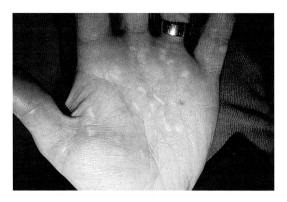

Fig. 14.26 Multiple scars following the injudicious surgical treatment of warts.

Varicella (chickenpox)

Cause

The herpes virus varicella-zoster is spread by the respiratory route; its incubation period is about 14 days.

Presentation and course

Slight malaise is followed by the development of papules, which turn rapidly into clear vesicles, the contents of which soon become pustular. Over the next few days the lesions crust and then clear, sometimes leaving white depressed scars. Lesions appear in crops, are often itchy, and are most profuse on the trunk and least profuse on the periphery of the limbs (centripetal). Second attacks are rare. Varicella can be fatal in those who are immunologically compromised.

Complications

• Pneumonitis, with pulmonary opacities on X-ray.
• Secondary infection of skin lesions.
• Haemorrhagic or lethal chickenpox in the immunocompromised.
• Scarring.

Differential diagnosis

Smallpox, mainly centrifugal anyway, has been universally eradicated, and the diagnosis of chickenpox is seldom in doubt.

Investigations

None are usually needed.

Treatment

Aciclovir, famciclovir and valaciclovir (Formulary 2, p. 344) should be reserved for severe attacks and for immunocompromised patients; for the latter, prophylactic aciclovir can also be used to prevent disease if given within a day or two of exposure. In mild attacks, calamine lotion topically is all that is required. A live attenuated vaccine is now available, and being more widely used. It is not universally effective and should not be given to patients with immunodeficiencies or blood dyscrasias who might not be able to resist even the attenuated organism.

Herpes zoster

Cause

Shingles too is caused by the herpes virus varicella-zoster. An attack is a result of the reactivation, usually for no obvious reason, of virus that has remained dormant in a sensory root ganglion since an earlier episode of chickenpox (varicella). The incidence of shingles is highest in old age, and in conditions such as Hodgkin's disease, AIDS and leukaemia, which weaken normal defence mechanisms. Shingles does not occur in epidemics; its clinical manifestations are caused by virus acquired in the past. However, patients with zoster can transmit the virus to others in whom it will cause chickenpox (Fig. 14.27).

Presentation and course

Attacks usually start with a burning pain, soon followed by erythema and grouped, sometimes blood-filled, vesicles scattered over a dermatome. The clear vesicles quickly become purulent, and over the space of a few days burst and crust. Scabs usually separate in 2–3 weeks, sometimes leaving depressed depigmented scars.

Zoster is characteristically unilateral (Fig. 14.28). It may affect more than one adjacent dermatome. The thoracic segments and the ophthalmic division of the trigeminal nerve are involved disproportionately often.

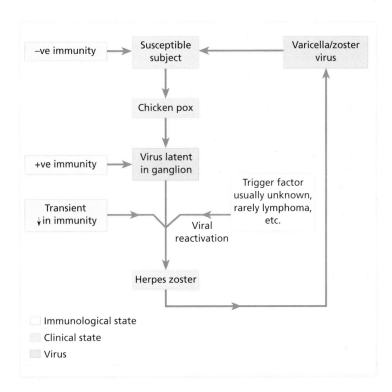

Fig. 14.27 Zoster–varicella relationships.

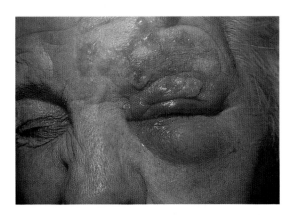

Fig. 14.28 Herpes zoster of the left ophthalmic division of the trigeminal nerve. No nasociliary involvement (see text); this is reassuring.

It is not uncommon for a few pock-like lesions to be found outside the main segment of involvement, but a generalized chickenpox-like eruption accompanying segmental zoster should raise suspicions of an underlying immunocompromised state or malignancy, par-ticularly if the lesions are unusually haemorrhagic or necrotic.

Complications

- Secondary bacterial infection is common.
- Motor nerve involvement is uncommon, but has led to paralysis of ocular muscles, the facial muscles, the diaphragm and the bladder.
- Zoster of the ophthalmic division of the trige-minal nerve can lead to corneal ulcers and scarring. A good clinical clue here is involvement of the naso-ciliary branch (vesicles grouped on the side of the nose).
- Persistent neuralgic pain, after the acute episode is over, is most common in the elderly.

Differential diagnosis

Occasionally, before the rash has appeared, the initial pain is taken for an emergency such as acute appendicitis or myocardial infarction. Otherwise, the dermatomal distribution, and the pain, allow zoster to be distinguished easily from herpes simplex, eczema and impetigo.

Investigations

Cultures are of little help as they take 5–7 days, and are only positive in 70% of cases. Biopsy or Tzanck smears show multinucleated giant cells and a ballooning degeneration of keratinocytes, indicative of a herpes infection. Any clinical suspicions about underlying conditions, such as Hodgkin's disease, chronic lymphatic leukaemia or AIDS, require further investigation.

Treatment

Systemic treatment should be given to all patients if diagnosed in the early stages of the disease. It is essential that this treatment should start within the first 5 days of an attack. Famciclovir and valaciclovir are as effective as aciclovir (Formulary 2, p. 344); they depend on virus-specific thymidine kinase for their antiviral activity. All three drugs are safe, and using them may cut down the chance of getting postherpetic neuralgia, particularly in the elderly.

If diagnosed late in the course of the disease, systemic treatment is not likely to be effective and treatment should be supportive with rest, analgesics and bland applications such as calamine. Secondary bacterial infection should be treated appropriately.

A trial of systemic carbamazepine, gabapentin or amitriptyline, or 4 weeks of topical capsaicin cream (Formulary 1, p. 339), despite the burning sensation it sometimes causes, may be worthwhile for established post-herpetic neuralgia.

LEARNING POINTS

1 Post-herpetic neuralgia affects the elderly rather than the young.
2 Systemic aciclovir works best if given early in the course of the disease.
3 Look for an underlying cause when there is dissemination outside the main affected dermatomes.

Herpes simplex

Cause

Herpesvirus hominis is the cause of herpes simplex. The virus is ubiquitous and carriers continue to shed virus particles in their saliva or tears. It has been separated into two types. The lesions caused by type II virus occur mainly on the genitals, while those of type I are usually extragenital; however, this distinction is not absolute.

The route of infection is through mucous membranes or abraded skin. After the episode associated with the primary infection, the virus may become latent, possibly within nerve ganglia, but still capable of giving rise to recurrent bouts of vesication (recrudescences).

Presentation

Primary infection

The most common recognizable manifestation of a primary type I infection in children is an acute gingivostomatitis accompanied by malaise, headache, fever and enlarged cervical nodes. Vesicles, soon turning into ulcers, can be seen scattered over the lips and mucous membranes. The illness lasts about 2 weeks.

Primary type II virus infections, usually transmitted sexually, cause multiple and painful genital or perianal blisters which rapidly ulcerate.

The virus can also be inoculated directly into the skin (e.g. during wrestling). A herpetic whitlow is one example of this direct inoculation. The uncomfortable pus-filled blisters on a fingertip are seen most often in medical personnel attending patients with unsuspected herpes simplex infections.

Recurrent (recrudescent) infections

These strike in roughly the same place each time. They may be precipitated by respiratory tract infections (cold sores), ultraviolet radiation, menstruation or even stress. Common sites include the face (Fig. 14.29) and lips (type I), and the genitals (type II), but lesions can occur anywhere. Tingling, burning or even pain is followed within a few hours by the development of erythema and clusters of tense vesicles. Crusting occurs within 24–48 h and the whole episode lasts about 12 days.

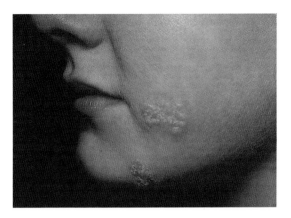

Fig. 14.29 The grouped vesicles of herpes simplex, here provoked by sunlight. Those in the lower group are beginning to crust.

Complications

• Herpes encephalitis or meningitis can occur without any cutaneous clues.
• Disseminated herpes simplex: widespread vesicles may be part of a severe illness in newborns, debilitated children or immunosuppressed adults.
• Eczema herpeticum: patients with atopic eczema are particularly susceptible to widespread cutaneous herpes simplex infections. Those looking after patients with atopic eczema should stay away if they have cold sores.
• Herpes simplex can cause recurrent dendritic ulcers leading to corneal scarring.
• In some patients, recurrent herpes simplex infections are regularly followed by erythema multiforme (p. 99).

Investigations

None are usually needed. Doubts over the diagnosis can be dispelled by culturing the virus from vesicle fluid. Antibody titres rise with primary, but not with recurrent infections.

Treatment

'Old-fashioned' remedies suffice for occasional mild recurrent attacks; sun block may cut down their frequency. Dabbing with surgical spirit is helpful, and secondary bacterial infection can be reduced by topical bacitracin, mupirocin, framycetin or fusidic acid. For more severe and frequent attacks, aciclovir cream, if used at the first sign of the recrudescence, and applied five or six times a day for the first 4 days

of the episode, cuts down the length of attacks and perhaps increases the intervals between them.

Aciclovir tablets (Formulary 2, p. 344), 200 mg five times daily for 5 days, is more effective and can be given to those with widespread or systemic involvement. Recurrences in the immunocompromised can usually be prevented by long-term treatment at a lower dosage. Famciclovir and valaciclovir are metabolized by the body into aciclovir and are as effective as aciclovir, having the additional advantage of needing fewer doses per day.

Molluscum contagiosum

Cause

This common pox virus infection can be spread by direct contact; e.g. sexually or by sharing a towel at the swimming bath.

Presentation and course

The incubation period ranges from 2 to 6 weeks. Often several members of one family are affected. Individual lesions are shiny, white or pink, and hemispherical; they grow slowly up to 0.5 cm in diameter. A central punctum, which may contain a cheesy core, gives the lesions their characteristic umbilicated look.

On close inspection a mosaic appearance may be seen. Multiple lesions are common (Fig. 14.30) and their distribution depends on the mode of infection. Atopic individuals and the immunocompromised are prone to especially extensive infections, spread by scratching and the use of topical steroids.

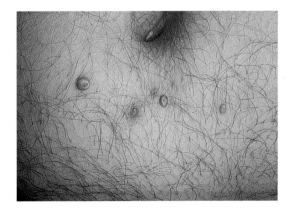

Fig. 14.30 An umbilicus surrounded by umbilicated papules of molluscum contagiosum.

Untreated lesions usually clear in 6–9 months, often after a brief local inflammation. Large solitary lesions may take longer. Some leave depressed scars.

Complications

Eczematous patches often appear around mollusca. Traumatized or overtreated lesions may become secondarily infected.

Differential diagnosis

Inflamed lesions can simulate a boil. Large solitary lesions in adults can be confused with a keratocanthoma (p. 262), an intradermal naevus (p. 259), or even a cystic basal cell carcinoma (p. 266). Confusion with warts should not arise as these have a rough surface and no central pore.

Investigations

None are usually needed, but the diagnosis can be confirmed by looking under the microscope for large swollen epidermal cells, easily seen in unstained preparations of debris expressed from a lesion.

Treatment

Many simple destructive measures cause inflammation and then resolution. They include squeezing out the lesions with forceps, piercing them with an orange stick (preferably without phenol), and curettage. Liquid nitrogen may also be helpful.

These measures are fine for adults, but young children dislike them and it is reasonable to play for time using imiquimod or chlortetracycline cream, or instructing the mother carefully how to apply a wart paint once a week to lesions well away from the eyes.

LEARNING POINTS

1 If you cannot tell mollusca from warts, buy a lens.
2 Do not hurt young children with mollusca. You will not be able to get near them next time something more serious goes wrong.

Sometimes a local anaesthetic cream (EMLA; see Formulary 1, p. 339), under polythene occlusion for an hour, will help children to tolerate more attacking treatment. Sparse eyelid lesions can be left alone but patients with numerous lesions may need to be referred to an ophthalmologist for curettage. Common sense measures help to limit spread within the family.

Orf

Cause

Contagious pustular dermatitis is common in lambs. Its cause is a parapox virus that can be transmitted to those handling infected animals. The condition is therefore most commonly seen on the hands of shepherds, of their wives who bottle-feed lambs, and of butchers, vets and meat porters.

Presentation and course

The incubation period is 5–6 days. Lesions, which may be single or multiple, start as small firm papules that change into flat-topped apparently pustular nodules with a violaceous and erythematous surround (Fig. 14.31). The condition clears up spontaneously in about a month.

Complications

- Lymphadenitis and malaise are common.
- Erythema multiforme.
- 'Giant' lesions can appear in the immunosuppressed.

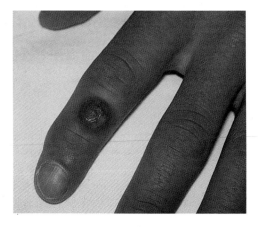

Fig. 14.31 The pseudopustular nodule of orf.

Differential diagnosis

Diagnosis is usually simple if contact with sheep is recognized. Milker's nodules, a pox virus infection acquired from cow's udders, can look like orf, as can staphylococcal furuncles.

Investigations

None are usually needed. If there is any doubt, the diagnosis can be confirmed by the distinctive electron microscopic appearance of the virus obtained from crusts.

Treatment

A topical antibiotic helps to prevent secondary infection; otherwise no active therapy is needed.

Acquired immunodeficiency syndrome (AIDS)

The AIDS epidemic was first recognized in the USA in 1981. The early cases were male homosexuals with pneumocystis pneumonia or Kaposi's sarcoma and immunosuppression. Later it became clear that the human immunodeficiency virus (HIV) could be acquired from contaminated body fluids, particularly semen and blood, in many ways, the importance of which varies from country to country. In the UK and the USA, for example, most cases have been homosexual or bisexual men; in parts of Africa, on the other hand, the disease is most often spread heterosexually.

Other groups at high risk are intravenous drug abusers who share contaminated needles and syringes, and haemophiliacs who were given infected blood products. Up to a half of babies born to infected mothers will be infected transplacentally.

The global epidemic is not slackening off though the pattern of transmission in industrialized nations is changing. Heterosexual transmission now accounts for 25–30% of new cases in Europe and the USA. In 1999, about 5.4 million people were newly infected with HIV.

Pathogenesis

The human immunodeficiency viruses, HIV-1 and HIV-2 (mainly in West Africa), are RNA retroviruses containing reverse transcriptase enzymes, which allow the viral DNA copy to be incorporated into the chromosomes of the host cell. Their main target is a subset of T lymphocytes (helper/inducer cells) that express glycoprotein CD4 molecules on their surface (p. 19). These bind to the surface envelope of the HIV. Viral replication within the helper/inducer cells kills them, and their depletion leads to the loss of cell-mediated immunity so characteristic of HIV infection. A variety of opportunistic infections may then follow.

Course

The original infection may be asymptomatic, or followed by a glandular fever-like illness at the time of seroconversion. After a variable latent phase, which may last several years, a persistent generalized lymphadenopathy develops. The term 'AIDS-related complex' refers to the next stage, in which many of the symptoms of AIDS (e.g. fever, weight-loss, fatigue or diarrhoea) may be present without the opportunistic infections or tumours characteristic of full-blown AIDS. Not all of those infected with HIV will develop AIDS but, for those who do, the average time from infection to the onset of AIDS is about 10 years. Once AIDS develops, if untreated, about half will die within 1 year and three-quarters within 4 years.

Skin changes in AIDS

Skin conditions are often the first clue to the presence of AIDS. The following are important:
1 *Kaposi's sarcoma* (Figs 14.32–14.34) is the initial presentation in a decreasing percentage of AIDS patients, particularly homosexual men. The lesions of classical Kaposi's sarcoma are multiple purplish patches or nodules (see Fig. 19.49). In AIDS the lesions may be atypical, sometimes looking like bruises or pyogenic granulomata (p. 277). The diagnosis can easily be missed and the mouth must always be examined.
2 *Seborrhoeic eczema and folliculitis* (Fig. 14.35) are seen in at least 50% of patients, often starting at an early stage of immunosuppression. The underlying cause may be an overgrowth of *Pityrosporum* yeasts. An itchy folliculitis of the head, neck and trunk, and an eosinophilic folliculitis, possibly as a result of the multiplication of *Demodex folliculorum*, have also been described.
3 *Skin infections*—florid, unusually extensive or atypical examples of common infections may be seen with

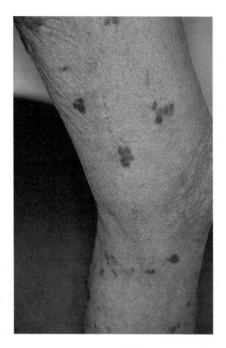

Fig. 14.32 Disseminated Kaposi's sarcoma in AIDS.

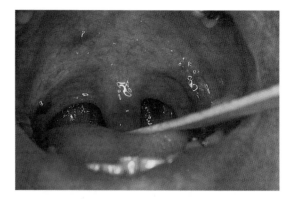

Fig. 14.34 Kaposi's sarcoma of hard palate, anterior fauces and uvula in AIDS.

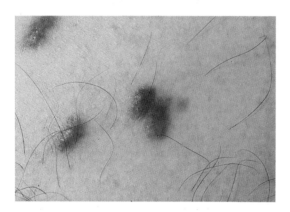

Fig. 14.33 Kaposi's sarcoma in AIDS.

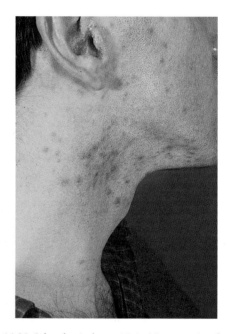

Fig. 14.35 Seborrhoeic dermatitis (otitis externa) and seborrhoeic folliculitis in HIV disease.

one or more of the following: herpes simplex, herpes zoster, molluscum contagiosum, oral and cutaneous candida, tinea, pityriasis versicolor, scabies and staphylococci. Facial and perianal warts are common. Hairy leukoplakia (Fig. 14.36), often on the sides of the tongue, may be caused by proliferation of the Epstein–Barr virus. Bacillary angiomatosis may look like Kaposi's sarcoma and is caused by the bacillus that causes cat-scratch fever. Syphilis can coexist with AIDS, as can mycobacterial infections.

4 *Other manifestations*—dry skin is common in AIDS; so is pruritus. Psoriasis may start or worsen with AIDS. Diffuse alopecia is not uncommon. Drug eruptions are often seen in AIDS patients.

Management

The clinical diagnosis of HIV infection is confirmed by a positive blood test for antibodies to the virus. Patients should be counselled before and after testing

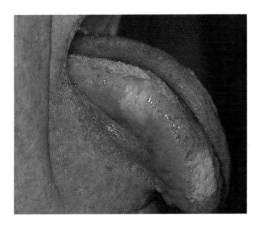

Fig. 14.36 Hairy leukoplakia on the side of the tongue.

for HIV antibody. Sexual contacts of infected individuals should be traced.

Modern drugs for HIV infections increase life expectancy, but are not 'cures' in the usual sense. They reduce the viral load but are expensive and sometimes toxic. Guidelines on how to use them change constantly, and so the drug treatment of HIV infections should be directed by specialists in the field, who will monitor the plasma viral load and CD4 count regularly (Table 14.1). Difficult decisions to be made include the timing of treatment—the benefits of starting early have to be balanced against the risk of toxicity—and choosing the right drug combination of highly active antiretroviral treatment (HAART)—usually triple therapy with two nucleoside reverse transcriptase inhibitors plus either a non-nucleoside reverse transcriptase inhibitor or a protease inhibitor. The regimen will be changed if there is clinical or

Table 14.1 Recommendations for starting highly active antiretroviral treatment (HAART) in the adult.

Disease stage	Decision
Symptomatic	Treat
Asymptomatic	
CD4 < 200×10^6/L	Treat
CD4 200–350×10^6/L	Treatment generally offered
CD4 > 350×10^6/L	Defer treatment unless high viral load

virological deterioration, or if the patient becomes pregnant, although the teratogenic potential of most of these drugs is still not known.

Treatment otherwise is symptomatic and varies according to the type of opportunistic infection detected. Prophylactic treatment against a number of life-threatening infections is also worthwhile, and prolongs life expectancy. Educating the public to avoid risky behaviour, such as unprotected sexual intercourse, is still hugely important.

Mucocutaneous lymph node syndrome (Kawasaki's disease)

The cause may be a recent parvovirus infection. The disease affects young children whose erythema, although often generalized, becomes most marked in a glove and stocking distribution; it may be associated with indurated oedema of the palms and soles. Peeling around the fingers and toes is one obvious feature but is not seen at the start. Bilateral conjunctival injection and erythema of the lips, buccal mucosa and tongue ('strawberry tongue') are common.

The episode is accompanied by fever and usually resolves within 2 weeks. Despite its name, not all patients have lymphadenopathy. The danger of this condition lies in the risk of developing myocarditis and coronary artery disease. The pathology is close to that of polyarteritis nodosa. Aspirin and intravenous gammaglobulin are the mainstay of treatment; both should be given early in the disease and reduce the risk of coronary artery involvement.

Gianotti–Crosti syndrome

This is a rather uncommon reaction to an infection with hepatitis B virus in childhood. Small reddish papules erupt bilaterally over the limbs and face, and fade over the course of a few weeks. Jaundice is uncommon, although tests of liver function give abnormal results.

Herpangina

This is an acute infectious illness, caused by group A Coxsackie viruses. The patient is usually a child with a fever, and a severe sore throat covered in many small vesicles, which rapidly become superficial ulcers. Episodes resolve in about a week.

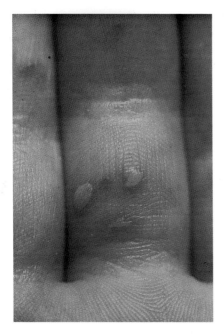

Fig. 14.37 The typical vesicles of hand, foot and mouth disease.

Hand, foot and mouth disease

This is usually caused by Coxsackie A16. Minor epidemics occur in institutions. The oral vesicles are larger and fewer than those of herpangina. The hand and foot lesions are small greyish vesicles with a narrow rim of redness around (Fig. 14.37). The condition settles within a few days.

Measles

An incubation period of 10 days is followed by fever, conjunctival injection, photophobia and upper respiratory tract catarrh. Koplik's spots (pinhead sized white spots with a bright red margin) are seen at this stage on the buccal mucosa. The characteristic 'net-like' rash starts after a few days, on the brow and behind the ears, and soon becomes extensive before fading with much desquamation. Prevention is by immunization with the combined MMR (measles/mumps/rubella) vaccine.

Rubella

After an incubation period of about 18 days, lymphadenopathy occurs a few days before the evanescent pink macular rash, which fades, first on the trunk, over the course of a few days. Rubella during the first trimester of pregnancy carries a risk of damage to the unborn child. Prevention is by immunization with the combined MMR vaccine.

Erythema infectiosum (fifth disease)

This is caused by the human parvovirus B19 and occurs in outbreaks, often in the spring. A slapped cheek erythema is quickly followed by a reticulate erythema of the shoulders. The affected child feels well, and the rash clears over the course of a few days. Other features, sometimes not accompanied by a rash, include transient anaemia and arthritis.

Fungal infections

Dermatophyte infections (ringworm)

Cause

Three genera of dermatophyte fungi cause tinea infections (ringworm).
• *Trichophyton*—skin, hair and nail infections.
• *Microsporum*—skin and hair.
• *Epidermophyton*—skin and nails.
Dermatophytes invade keratin only, and the inflammation they cause is due to metabolic products of the fungus or to delayed hypersensitivity. In general, zoophilic fungi (those transmitted to humans by animals) cause a more severe inflammation than anthropophilic ones (spread from person to person).

Presentation and course

This depends upon the site and on the strain of fungus involved.

Tinea pedis (athlete's foot)

This is the most common type of fungal infection in humans. The sharing of wash places (e.g. in showers) and of swimming pools, predisposes to infection; occlusive footwear encourages relapses.

Most cases are caused by one of three organisms: *Trichophyton rubrum* (the most common and the

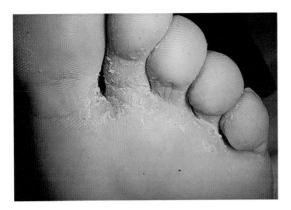

Fig. 14.38 Tinea pedis. Scaly area spreading to the sole from the toe webs.

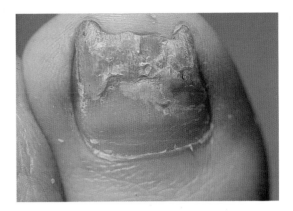

Fig. 14.40 Chronic tinea of the big toe nail. Starting distally, the thickness and discoloration are spreading proximally.

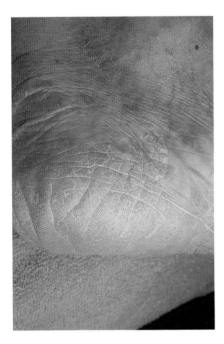

Fig. 14.39 Powdery scaling, most obvious in the skin creases, caused by a *Trychophyton rubrum* infection.

most stubborn), *Trichophyton mentagrophytes* var. *interdigitale* and *Epidermophyton floccosum*.

There are three common clinical patterns.
1 Soggy interdigital scaling, particularly in the fourth and fifth interspace (all three organisms; Fig. 14.38).
2 A diffuse dry scaling of the soles (usually *T. rubrum*; Fig. 14.39).
3 Recurrent episodes of vesication (usually *T. mentagrophytes* var. *interdigitale* or *E. floccosum*).

Tinea of the nails

Toenail infection is usually associated with tinea pedis. The initial changes occur at the free edge of the nail, which becomes yellow and crumbly (Fig. 14.40). Subungual hyperkeratosis, separation of the nail from its bed, and thickening may then follow. Usually only a few nails are infected but rarely all are. Fingernail lesions are similar, but less common, and are seldom seen without a chronic *T. rubrum* infection of the skin of the hands.

Tinea of the hands

This is usually asymmetrical and associated with tinea pedis. *T. rubrum* may cause a barely perceptible erythema of one palm with a characteristic powdery scale in the creases.

Tinea of the groin

This is common and affects men more often than women. The eruption is sometimes unilateral or asymmetrical. The upper inner thigh is involved and lesions expand slowly to form sharply demarcated plaques with peripheral scaling (Fig. 14.41). In contrast to candidiasis of the groin area, the scrotum is usually spared. A few vesicles or pustules may be seen within the lesions. The organisms are the same as those causing tinea pedis.

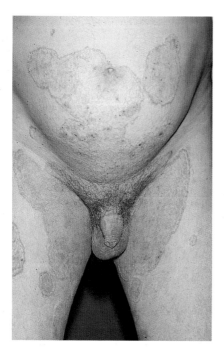

Fig. 14.41 A very gross example of tinea of the groin. The *T. rubrum* infection has spread on to the abdomen and thighs, aided by the use of topical steroids.

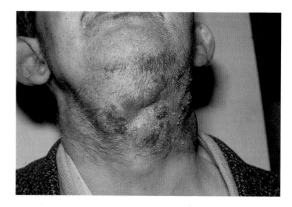

Fig. 14.42 Animal ringworm of the beard area showing boggy inflamed swellings (kerion).

Tinea of the trunk and limbs

Tinea corporis is characterized by plaques with scaling and erythema most pronounced at the periphery. A few small vesicles and pustules may be seen within them. The lesions expand slowly and healing in the centre leaves a typical ring-like pattern.

Tinea of the scalp (tinea capitis)

This is usually a disease of children. The causative organism varies from country to country.

Fungi coming from animal sources (zoophilic fungi) induce a more intense inflammation than those spread from person to person (anthropophilic fungi). In ringworm acquired from cattle, for example, the boggy swelling, with inflammation, pustulation and lymphadenopathy, is often so fierce that a bacterial infection is suspected; such a lesion is called a kerion and the hair loss associated with it may be permanent. Tinea of the beard area is usually caused by zoophilic species and shows the same features (Fig. 14.42). Anthropophilic organisms cause bald rather scaly areas, with minimal

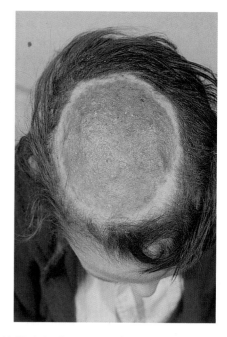

Fig. 14.43 Animal ringworm of a child's scalp: not truly a kerion as flat and non-pustular.

inflammation and hairs broken off 3–4 mm from the scalp. In favus, caused by *Trichophyton schoenleini*, the picture is dominated by foul-smelling yellowish crusts surrounding many scalp hairs, and sometimes leading to scarring alopecia.

Complications

1 Fierce animal ringworm of the scalp (Fig. 14.43) can lead to a permanent scarring alopecia.

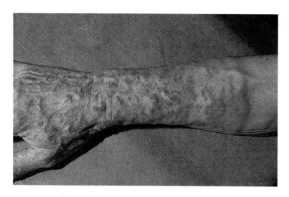

Fig. 14.44 'Tinea incognito'. Topical steroid applications have thinned the skin and altered much of the morphology. A recognizable active spreading edge is still visible.

2 A florid fungal infection anywhere can induce vesication on the sides of the fingers and palms (a trichophytide).
3 Epidemics of ringworm occur in schools.
4 The usual appearance of a fungal infection can be masked by mistreatment with topical steroids (tinea incognito; Fig. 14.44).

Differential diagnosis

This varies with the site. Some of the more common problems are listed in Table 14.2.

Investigations

The microscopic examination of a skin scraping, nail clipping or plucked hair is a simple procedure. The

Table 14.2 Common problems in the differential diagnosis of dermatophyte infections.

Area	Differential diagnosis
Scalp	Alopecia areata, psoriasis, seborrhoeic eczema, carbuncle, abscess, trichotillomania
Feet	Erythrasma, interdigital intertrigo, eczema
Trunk	Discoid eczema, psoriasis, candidiasis, pityriasis rosea
Nails	Psoriasis, paronychia, trauma, ageing changes
Hand	Chronic eczema, granuloma annulare, xerosis, dyshidrotic eczema

scraping should be taken from the scaly margin of a lesion, with a small curette or a scalpel blade, and clippings/scrapings from the most crumbly part of a nail. Broken hairs should be plucked with tweezers. Specimens are cleared in potassium hydroxide (p. 35). Branching hyphae can easily be seen (see Fig. 3.7) using a scanning ($\times$ 10) or low-power ($\times$ 25) objective lens, with the iris diaphragm almost closed, and the condenser racked down. Hyphae may also be seen within a cleared hair shaft, or spores may be noted around it.

Cultures should be carried out in a mycology or bacteriology laboratory. Transport medium is not necessary, and specimens should be sent in folded black paper. The report may take as long as a month; microscopy is much quicker.

Wood's light (ultraviolet light) examination of the scalp usually reveals a green fluorescence of the hairs in *Microsporum audouini* and *M. canis* infections. The technique is useful for screening children in institutions where outbreaks of tinea capitis still sometimes occur, but some fungi (e.g. *Trichophyton tonsurans*) do not fluoresce.

Treatment

Local

This is all that is needed for minor skin infections. The more recent imidazole preparations (e.g. miconazole and clotrimazole) and the allylamines such as terbinafine (Formulary 1, p. 335), have largely superseded time-honoured remedies such as benzoic acid ointment (Whitfield's ointment) and tolnaftate. They should be applied twice daily. Magenta paint (Castellani's paint), although highly coloured, is helpful for exudative or macerated areas in body folds or toe webs. Occasional dusting with an antifungal powder is useful to prevent relapses.

Topical nail preparations. Many patients now prefer to avoid systemic treatment. For them a nail lacquer containing amorolfine is worth a trial. It should be applied once or twice a week for 6 months; it is effective against stubborn moulds such as *Hendersonula* and *Scopulariopsis*. Both amorolfine and tioconazole nail solutions (Formulary 1, p. 335) can be used as adjuncts to systemic therapy (see below).

Systemic

This is needed for tinea of the scalp or of the nails, and for widespread or chronic infections of the skin that have not responded to local measures.

Terbinafine (Formulary 2, p. 342) has now largely superceded griseofulvin. It acts by inhibiting fungal squalene epoxidase and does not interact with the cytochrome P-450 system. It is fungicidal and so cures chronic dermatophyte infections more quickly and more reliably than griseofulvin. For tinea capitis in children, for example, a 4-week course of terbinafine is as effective as an 8-week course of griseofulvin. Cure rates of 70–90% can be expected for infected fingernails after a 6-week course of terbinafine, and for infected toenails after a 3-month course. It is not effective in pityriasis versicolor or *Candida* infections.

Griseofulvin (Formulary 2, p. 343) was for many years the drug of choice for chronic dermatophyte infections. It has proved to be a safe drug, but treatment may have to be stopped because of persistent headache, nausea, vomiting or skin eruptions. The drug should not be given in pregnancy or to patients with liver failure or porphyria. It interacts with coumarin anticoagulants, the dosage of which may have to be increased. Its effectiveness falls if barbiturates are being taken at the same time.

Griseofulvin is fungistatic and treatment for infected nails has to be prolonged (an average of 12 months for fingernails, and at least 18 months for toenails). The disappointing results for toenail infections seen in some 30–40% of cases can be improved by the concomitant use of topical nail preparations (see above).

LEARNING POINTS

1 Do not prescribe griseofulvin, terbinafine or itraconazole for psoriasis of the nails or chronic paronychia. Get mycological proof first.
2 Your patient's asymmetrical 'eczema' is spreading despite local steroids—think of a dermatophyte infection.
3 Consider tinea in acute inflammatory and purulent reactions of the scalp and beard.

Itraconazole (Formulary 2, p. 343) is now preferred to ketoconazole, which occasionally damages the liver, and is a reasonable alternative to terbinafine and griseofulvin if these are contraindicated. It is effective in tinea corporis, cruris and pedis; and also in nail infections, although without a licence for this use in many countries. Fungistatic rather than fungicidal, it interferes with the cytochrome P-450 system, so a review of any other medication being taken is needed before a prescription is issued. Its wide spectrum makes it useful also in pityriasis versicolor and candidiasis.

Candidiasis

Cause

Candida albicans is a classic opportunistic pathogen. Even in transient and trivial local infections in the apparently fit, one or more predisposing factors such as obesity, moisture and maceration, diabetes, pregnancy, the use of broad-spectrum antibiotics, or perhaps the use of the contraceptive pill, will often be found to be playing some part. Opportunism is even more obvious in the overwhelming systemic infections of the immunocompromised (Fig. 14.45).

Presentation

This varies with the site (Fig. 14.46).

Oral candidiasis (see also Chapter 13)

One or more whitish adherent plaques (like bread sauce) appear on the mucous membranes. If wiped off they leave an erythematous base. Under dentures, candidiasis will produce sore red areas. Angular stomatitis, usually in denture wearers (Fig. 14.47), may be candidal.

Candida intertrigo

A moist glazed area of erythema and maceration appears in a body fold; the edge shows soggy scaling, and outlying satellite papulopustules. These changes are most common under the breasts, and in the armpits and groin, but can also occur between the fingers of those whose hands are often in water.

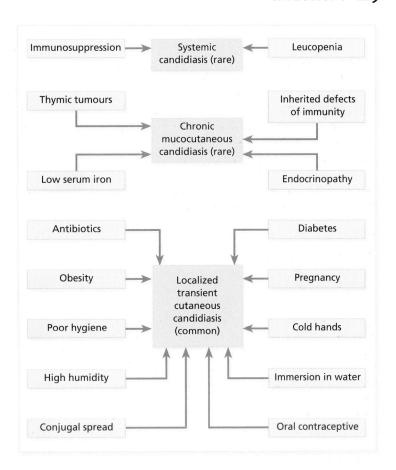

Fig. 14.45 Factors predisposing to the different types of candidiasis.

Genital candidiasis

Most commonly presents as a sore itchy vulvovaginitis, with white curdy plaques adherent to the inflamed mucous membranes, and a whitish discharge. The eruption may extend to the groin folds. Conjugal spread is common; in males similar changes occur under the foreskin (Fig. 14.48) and in the groin.

Diabetes, pregnancy and antibiotic therapy are common predisposing factors.

Paronychia

Acute paronychia is usually bacterial, but in chronic paronychia *Candida* may be the sole pathogen, or be found with other opportunists such as *Proteus* or *Pseudomonas*. The proximal and sometimes the lateral nail folds of one or more fingers become bolstered and red (see Fig. 13.28). The cuticles are lost and small amounts of pus can be expressed. The adjacent nail plate becomes ridged and discoloured. Predisposing factors include wet work, poor peripheral circulation and vulval candidiasis.

Chronic mucocutaneous candidiasis

Persistent candidiasis, affecting most or all of the areas described above, can start in infancy. Sometimes the nail plates as well as the nail folds are involved. *Candida* granulomas may appear on the scalp. Several different forms have been described including those with autosomal recessive and dominant inheritance patterns. In the *Candida* endocrinopathy syndrome, chronic candidiasis occurs with one or more endocrine defects, the most common of which are hypoparathyroidism, and Addison's disease. A few late-onset cases have underlying thymic tumours.

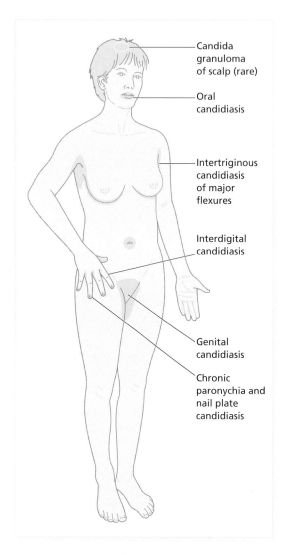

Candida
granuloma
of scalp (rare)

Oral
candidiasis

Intertriginous
candidiasis
of major
flexures

Interdigital
candidiasis

Genital
candidiasis

Chronic
paronychia and
nail plate
candidiasis

Fig. 14.46 Sites susceptible to *Candida* infection.

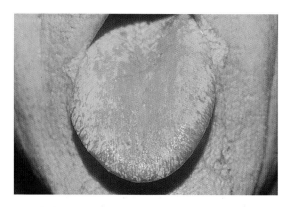

Fig. 14.47 Candidal angular stomatitis associated with severe candidiasis of the tongue.

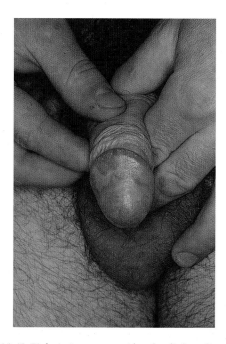

Fig. 14.48 Pink circinate areas with only a little scaling. Consider Reiter's syndrome or candidiasis.

Systemic candidiasis

This is seen against a background of severe illness, leucopenia and immunosuppression. The skin lesions are firm red nodules, which can be shown by biopsy to contain yeasts and pseudohyphae.

Investigations

Swabs from suspected areas should be sent for culture. The urine should always be tested for sugar. In chronic mucocutaneous candidiasis, a detailed immunological work-up will be needed, focusing on cell-mediated immunity.

Treatment

Predisposing factors should be sought and eliminated; e.g. denture hygiene may be important. Infected skin folds should be separated and kept dry. Those with chronic paronychia should keep their hands warm and dry.

Amphotericin, nystatin and the imidazole group of compounds are all effective topically. For the mouth, these are available as oral suspensions, lozenges and oral gels (Formulary 1, p. 334). False teeth should be removed at night, washed and steeped in a nystatin solution. For other areas of candidiasis, creams, ointment and pessaries are available (Formulary 1, p. 335). Magenta paint is also a useful but messy remedy for the skin flexures. In chronic paronychia, the nail folds can be packed with an imidazole cream or drenched in an imidazole solution several times a day. Genital candidiasis responds well to a single day's treatment with either itraconazole and fluconazole (Formulary 2, p. 343). Both are also valuable for recurrent oral candidiasis of the immunocompromised, and for the various types of chronic mucocutaneous candidiasis.

Pityriasis versicolor

Cause

The old name, tinea versicolor, should be dropped as the disorder is caused by commensal yeasts (*Pityrosporum orbiculare*) and not by dermatophyte fungi. Overgrowth of these yeasts, particularly in hot humid conditions, is responsible for the clinical lesions.

Carboxylic acids released by the organisms inhibit the increase in pigment production by melanocytes that occurs normally after exposure to sunlight. The term 'versicolor' refers to the way in which the superficial scaly patches, fawn or pink on non-tanned skin (Fig. 14.49), become paler than the surrounding skin after exposure to sunlight (Fig. 14.50). The condition should be regarded as non-infectious.

Presentation and course

The fawn or depigmented areas, with their slightly branny scaling and fine wrinkling, look ugly. Other-

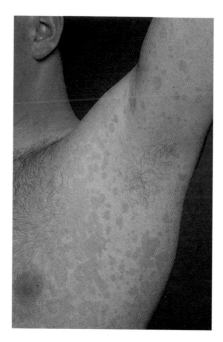

Fig. 14.49 Pityriasis versicolor: fawn areas stand out against the untanned background.

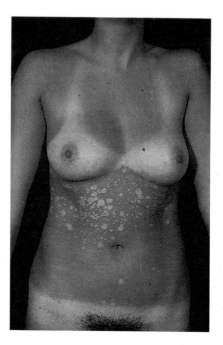

Fig. 14.50 This patient's holiday was spoilt by versicolor ruining her expensive tan.

wise they are symptom-free or only slightly itchy. Lesions are most common on the upper trunk but can become widespread. Untreated lesions persist, and depigmented areas, even after adequate treatment, are slow to regain their former colour. Recurrences are common.

Differential diagnosis

In vitiligo (p. 246), the border is clearly defined, scaling is absent, lesions are larger, the limbs and face are often affected, and depigmentation is more complete; however, it may sometimes be hard to distinguish vitiligo from the pale non-scaly areas of treated versicolor. Seborrhoeic eczema of the trunk tends to be more erythematous, and is often confined to the presternal or interscapular areas. Pityriasis alba often affects the cheeks. Pityriasis rosea, tinea corporis, secondary syphilis and erythrasma seldom cause real confusion.

Investigations

Scrapings, prepared and examined as for a dermatophyte infection (p. 35), show a mixture of short branched hyphae and spores (a 'spaghetti and meatballs' appearance). Culture is not helpful.

Treatment

A topical preparation of one of the imidazole group of antifungal drugs (Formulary 1, p. 335) can be applied at night to all affected areas for 2–4 weeks. Equally effective, but messier and more irritant, is a 2.5% selenium sulphide mixture in a detergent base (Selsun shampoo). This should be lathered on to the patches after an evening bath, and allowed to dry. Next morning it should be washed off. Three applications at weekly intervals are adequate. A shampoo containing ketoconazole is now available (Formulary 1, p. 329) and is less messy, but just as effective as the selenium ones. Alternatively, selenium sulphide lotion (USA) can be applied for 10 min, rinsed off and re-applied daily for 1 week. For widespread or stubborn infections systemic itraconazole (200 mg daily for 7 days) has been shown to be curative, but interactions with other drugs must be avoided (Formulary 2, p. 343). Recurrence is common after any treatment.

LEARNING POINTS

1 This is not a dermatophyte infection, so do not try griseofulvin or terbinafine.
2 Patients think the treatment has not worked if their pale patches do not disappear straight away—warn them about this in advance.

Deep fungal infections

Histoplasmosis

Histoplasma capsulatum is found in soil and in the droppings of some animals (e.g. bats). Airborne spores are inhaled and cause lung lesions, which are in many ways like those of tuberculosis. Later, granulomatous skin lesions may appear, particularly in the immunocompromised. Amphotericin B or itraconazole, given systemically, is often helpful.

Coccidioidomycosis

The causative organism, *Coccidioides immitis*, is present in the soil in arid areas in the USA. Its spores are inhaled, and the pulmonary infection may be accompanied by a fever. At this stage erythema nodosum (p. 101) may be seen. In a few patients the infection becomes disseminated, with ulcers or deep abscesses in the skin. Treatment is with amphotericin B or itraconazole.

Blastomycosis

Infections with *Blastomyces dermatitidis* are virtually confined to rural areas of the USA. Rarely, the organism is inoculated into the skin; more often it is inhaled and then spreads systemically from the pulmonary focus to other organs including the skin. There the lesions are wart-like, hyperkeratotic nodules, which spread peripherally with a verrucose edge, while tending to clear and scar centrally. Treatment is with systemic amphotericin B or itraconazole.

Sporotrichosis

The causative fungus, *Sporotrichum schencki*, lives saprophytically in soil or on wood in warm humid countries.

Infection is through a wound, where later a lesion like an indolent boil arises. Later still, nodules appear in succession along the draining lymphatics (Fig. 14.15). Potassium iodide or itraconazole are both effective.

Actinomycosis

The causative organism, *Actinomyces israeli*, is bacterial but traditionally considered with the fungi. It has long branching hyphae and is part of the normal flora of the mouth and bowel. In actinomycosis, a lumpy induration and scarring coexist with multiple sinuses discharging pus containing 'sulphur granules', made up of tangled filaments. Favourite sites are the jaw, and the chest and abdominal walls. Long-term penicillin is the treatment of choice.

Mycetoma (Madura foot)

Various species of fungus or actinomycetes may be involved. They gain access to the subcutaneous tissues, usually of the feet or legs, via a penetrating wound. The area becomes lumpy and distorted, later enlarging and developing multiple sinuses. Pus exuding from these shows tiny diagnostic granules. Surgery may be a valuable alternative to the often poor results of medical treatment, which is with systemic antibiotics or antifungal drugs, depending on the organism isolated.

Further reading

Diven, D.G. (2001) An overview of poxviruses. *Journal of the American Academy of Dermatology* **44**, 1–14.

Gupta, A.K., Bluhm, R. and Summerbell, R. (2002) Pityriasis versicolor. *Journal of the European Academy of Dermatology and Venereology* **16**, 19–33.

Higgins, E.M., Fuller, L.C. & Smith, C.H. (2000) Guidelines for the management of tinea capitis. *British Journal of Dermatology* **143**, 53–58.

Lesher, J.L. Jr. (2000) *An Atlas of Microbiology of the Skin.* Parthenon, London.

Manders, M. (1998) Toxin-mediated streptococcal and staphylococcal disease. *Journal of the American Academy of Dermatology* **39**, 383–398.

Roberts, D.T. (1999) Onychomycosis: current treatment and future challenges. *British Journal of Dermatology* **141** (Suppl. 56), 1–4.

Sterling, J.C., Handfield-Jones, S., & Hudson. P. (2001) Guidelines for the treatment of cutaneous warts. *British Journal of Dermatology* **144**, 4–11.

Tyring, S.K., McCrary, M.L. & Severson, J. (1999) Varicella zoster virus. *Journal of the American Academy of Dermatology* **41**, 1–14.

Infestations

Infestation, the presence of animal parasites on or in the body, is common in tropical countries and less so in temperate ones. Infestations fall into two main groups:

1 those caused by arthropods; and
2 those caused by worms.

Arthropods

Table 15.1 lists some of the ways in which arthropods affect the skin. Only a few can be discussed here.

Insect bites

The skin changes are partly a result of the injection of pharmacologically active substances, and partly of sensitization to injected antigens. A wheal may appear within a few minutes, to be followed by a firm itchy persistent papule, often with a central haemorrhagic punctum. Bullous reactions are common on the legs of children. The diagnosis is usually obvious; when it is not, the term papular urticaria is sometimes used.

Papular urticaria

Cause

This term, with its hint that the condition is a variant of ordinary urticaria, is a misnomer. Papular urticaria is nothing more than an excessive, possibly allergic, reaction to insect bites. The source of the bites may be simple garden pests but more often is a parasite on

Table 15.1 Arthropods and their effects on the skin.

Type of arthropod	Manifestations
Insects	
Hymenoptera	Bee and wasp stings
	Ant bites
Lepidoptera	Caterpillar dermatitis
Coleoptera	Blisters from cantharidin
Diptera	Mosquito and midge bites
	Myiasis
Aphaniptera	Human and animal fleas
Hemiptera	Bed bugs
Anoplura	Lice infestations
Mites	
Demodex folliculorum	Normal inhabitant of facial hair follicles
Sarcoptes scabei	Human and animal scabies
Food mites	Grain itch, grocer's itch, etc.
Harvest mites	Harvest itch
House dust mite	Possible role in atopic eczema
Cheyletiella	Papular urticaria
Ticks	Tick bites. Vector of rickettsial infections and erythema chronicum migrans (p. 195)

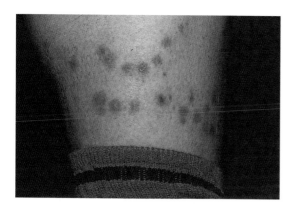

Fig. 15.1 Florid insect bites on the leg. Note the tendency of the lesions to lie in lines and groups.

a domestic pet. Human fleas are now rather uncommon. Often the source cannot be traced.

Presentation

Lesions are usually most common on the arms or legs. They consist of groups or lines of small itchy excoriated smooth urticarial papules (Fig. 15.1) of a uniform size that may become bullous and infected. Some clear to leave small scars or pigmented areas.

Course

Lesions tend to start after infancy, and an affected child will usually 'grow out' of the problem in a few years, even if the source of the bites is not dealt with. Individual lesions last for 1 or 2 weeks and recur in distinct crops, especially in the summer—hence the lay term 'heat bumps'. The lesions will disappear with any change of environment, for example by going on holiday. Surprisingly often only one member of a family is affected, perhaps because the others have developed immunological tolerance after repeated bites.

Complications

Itching leads to much discomfort and loss of sleep. Impetiginization is common.

Differential diagnosis

The grouped excoriated papules of papular urticaria are quite different from the skin changes of scabies, in which burrows are the diagnostic feature. Atopic prurigo may be more difficult to distinguish but here there is usually a family history of atopy and frankly eczematous plaques are found in a typical distribution.

Investigations

The parents should be encouraged to act as detectives in their own environment, but some resist the idea that the lesions are caused by bites, asking why the other family members are not affected. This attitude is often supported by veterinarians who, after a superficial look at infested animals, pronounce them clear. In such cases the animal should be brushed vigorously while standing on a polythene sheet. Enough dandruff-like material can then be obtained to send to a reliable veterinary laboratory. Often the cause is a *Cheyletiella* mite infestation.

Treatment

Local treatment with Eurax HC ointment or calamine lotion, and the regular use of insect repellents, may be of some help but the ultimate solution is to trace the source of the bites.

Infested animals should be treated by a veterinarian, and insecticidal powders should be used for soft furnishings in the home. Sometimes professional exterminators are needed; but even measures such as these can meet with little success.

Bed bugs (Hemiptera)

During the day, bed bugs hide in crevices in walls and furniture; at night they can travel considerable distances to reach a sleeping person. Burning wheals, turning into firm papules, occur in groups wherever the crawling bugs have easy access to the skin, the face, neck and hands being the most common sites. Treatment should be based on the application of insecticides to walls and furniture likely to be harbouring the bugs.

Myiasis

The larvae of several species of fly develop only if deposited in living flesh; humans are one of several possible hosts. The skin lesions look like boils, but movement may be detected within them. The diagnosis is proved by incising the nodule and extracting the larva.

Lice infestations (pediculosis)

Lice are flattened wingless insects that suck blood. Their eggs, attached to hairs or clothing, are known as nits. The main feature of all lice infestations is severe itching, followed by scratching and secondary infection.

Two species are obligate parasites in humans: *Pediculus humanus* (with its two varieties *P. humanus capitis*, the head louse, and *P. humanus corporis*, the body louse) and *Phthirus pubis* (the pubic louse).

Head lice

Cause

Head lice are still common, affecting up to 10% of children even in the smartest schools. The head louse itself measures some 3–4 mm in length and is greyish, and often rather hard to find. However, its egg cases (nits) can be seen easily enough, firmly stuck to the hair shafts. Spread from person to person is achieved by head-to-head contact, and perhaps by shared combs or hats.

Presentation and course

The main symptom is itching, at first around the sides and back of the scalp and then more generally over it. Scratching and secondary infection soon follow and, in heavy infestations, the hair becomes matted and smelly. Draining lymph nodes often enlarge.

Complications

Secondary bacterial infection may be severe enough to make the child listless and feverish.

Differential diagnosis

All patients with recurrent impetigo or crusted eczema on their scalps should be carefully examined for the presence of nits.

Investigations

None are usually required.

Treatment

Malathion, carbaryl and permethrin preparations (Formulary 1, p. 336) are probably the treatments of choice now. They kill lice and eggs effectively; malathion has the extra value of sticking to the hair and so protecting against reinfection for 6 weeks. The policy whereby public health authorities rotate their use, with the aim of lessening the risk of resistant strains emerging, has fallen out of favour now.

Lotions should remain on the scalp for at least 12 h, and are more effective than shampoos. The application should be repeated after 1 week so that any lice that survive the first application and hatch out in that interval can be killed. Other members of the family and school mates should be checked. A toothcomb helps to remove nits but occasionally matting is so severe that the hair has to be clipped short. A systemic antibiotic may be needed to deal with severe secondary infection. Some recommend, as an alternative to the treatments mentioned above, that the hair should be combed repeatedly and meticulously with a special 'detection comb'—but the efficacy of this method has still to be established. However, a head louse repellent, containing 2% piperonal, is available over the counter and may be worth a trial for those who are repeatedly reinfested. Systemic ivermectin therapy is reserved for infestations resisting the treatments listed above.

Body lice

Cause

Body louse infestations are now uncommon except in the unhygienic and socially deprived. Morphologically the body louse looks just like the head louse, but lays its eggs in the seams of clothing in contact with the skin. Transmission is via infested bedding or clothing.

Presentation and course

Self-neglect is usually obvious; against this background there is severe and widespread itching, especially on the trunk. The bites themselves are soon obscured by excoriations and crusts of dried blood or serum. In chronic untreated cases ('vagabond's disease') the skin becomes generally thickened, eczematized and pigmented; lymphadenopathy is common.

Differential diagnosis

In scabies, characteristic burrows are seen (p. 227). Other causes of chronic itchy erythroderma include eczema and lymphomas, but these are ruled out by the finding of lice and nits.

Investigations

Clothing should be examined for the presence of eggs in the inner seams.

Treatment

First and foremost treat the infested clothing and bedding. Lice and their eggs can be killed by high temperature laundering, by dry cleaning and by tumble-drying. Less competent patients will need help here. Once this has been achieved, 5% permethrin cream rinse or 1% lindane lotion (USA only) (Formulary 1, p. 335) may be used on the patient's skin.

Pubic lice

Cause

Pubic lice (crabs) are broader than scalp and body lice, and their second and third pairs of legs are well adapted to cling on to hair. They are usually spread by sexual contact, and most commonly infest young adults.

Presentation

Severe itching in the pubic area is followed by eczematization and secondary infection. Among the excoriations will be seen small blue-grey macules of altered blood at the site of bites. The shiny translucent nits are less obvious than those of head lice (Fig. 15.2). Pubic lice spread most extensively in hairy males and may even affect the eyelashes.

Differential diagnosis

Eczema of the pubic area gives similar symptoms but lice and nits are not seen.

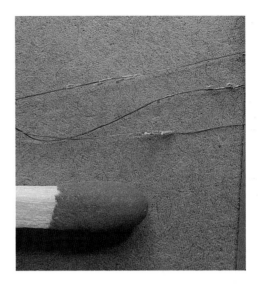

Fig. 15.2 Pediculosis pubis. Numerous eggs (nits) can be seen on the plucked pubic hairs.

Investigations

The possibility of coexisting sexually transmitted diseases should be kept in mind.

Treatment

Carbaryl, permethrin and malathion are all effective treatments. Aqueous solutions are less irritant than alcoholic ones. They should be applied for 12 h or overnight to all parts of the trunk, including the perianal area and to the limbs, and not just to the pubic area. Treatment should be repeated after 1 week, and infected sexual partners should also be treated. Shaving the area is not necessary.

Infestation of the eyelashes is particularly hard to treat, as this area is so sensitive that the mechanical removal of lice and eggs can be painful. Applying a thick layer of petrolatum twice a day for 2 weeks has been recommended. Aqueous malathion is effective for eyelash infestations but does not have a product licence for this purpose.

Scabies

Cause

Scabies is caused by the mite *Sarcoptes scabiei* var. *hominis* (Fig. 15.3). Adult mites are 0.3–0.4 mm long

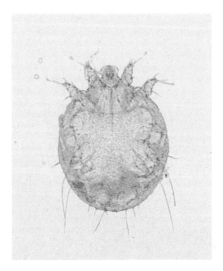

Fig. 15.3 The adult female acarus (scabies mite).

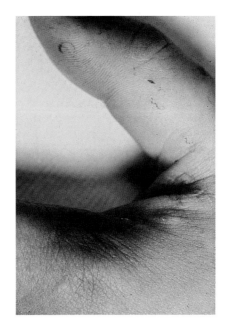

Fig. 15.4 Typical burrows seen on the side of the thumb.

and therefore just visible, although hard to see except through a lens. It is now well established that the mites are transferred from person to person by close bodily contact and not via inanimate objects.

Once on the skin, fertilized female mites burrow through the stratum corneum at the rate of about 2 mm per day, and produce two or three oval eggs each day. These turn into sexually mature mites in 2–3 weeks. The number of mites varies from case to case, from less than 10 in a clean adult to many more in an unwashed child. The generalized eruption of scabies, and its itchiness, are thought to be caused by a sensitization to the mites or their products.

Epidemiology

The prevalence of scabies in many populations rises and falls cyclically, peaking every 15–20 years. The idea of 'herd immunity' has been put forward to explain this, spread being most easy when a new generation of susceptible individuals has arisen.

Presentation

For the first 4–6 weeks after infestation there may be no itching, but thereafter pruritus dominates the picture, often affecting several people and being particularly severe at night.

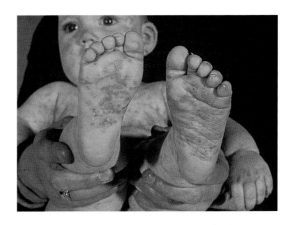

Fig. 15.5 The characteristic plantar lesions of scabies in infancy.

The most dramatic part of the eruption—excoriated, eczematized or urticarial papules—is usually on the trunk, but these changes are non-specific and a burrow has to be identified to confirm the diagnosis (Fig. 15.4).

Most burrows lie on the sides of the fingers, finger webs, sides of the hand and on the flexural aspects of the wrists. Other favourite sites include the elbows, ankles and feet (especially in infants; Fig. 15.5), nipples and genitals (Fig. 15.6). Only in infancy does scabies affect the face. Burrows are easily missed grey-white

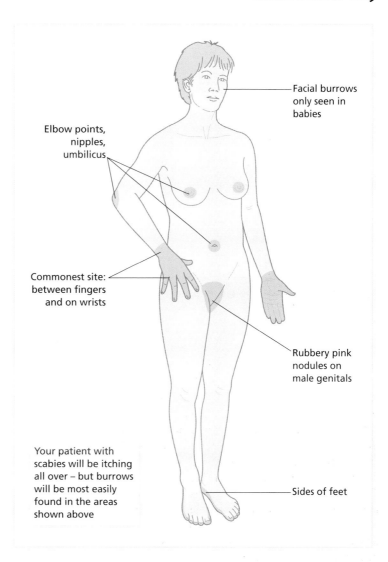

Facial burrows
only seen in
babies

Elbow points,
nipples,
umbilicus

Commonest site:
between fingers
and on wrists

Rubbery pink
nodules on
male genitals

Your patient with
scabies will be itching
all over – but burrows
will be most easily
found in the areas
shown above

Sides of feet

Fig. 15.6 Common sites of burrows
in scabies.

slightly scaly tortuous lines of up to 1 cm in length. The acarus may be seen through a lens as a small dark dot at the most recent least scaly end of the burrow. With experience it can be removed for microscopic confirmation (p. 35). On the genitals, burrows are associated with erythematous rubbery nodules (Fig. 15.7).

Course

Scabies persists indefinitely unless treated. In the chronic stage, the number of mites may be small and diagnosis is correspondingly difficult. Relapses after apparently adequate treatment are common and can be put down to reinfestation from undetected and untreated contacts.

Complications

• Secondary infection, with pustulation, is common (Fig. 15.8). Rarely, glomerulonephritis follows this.
• Repeated applications of scabicides can cause skin irritation and eczema.
• Persistent itchy red nodules may remain on the genitals or armpits of children for some months after adequate treatment.

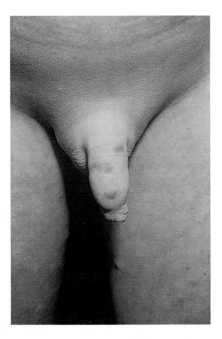

Fig. 15.7 Unmistakable rubbery nodules on the penis, diagnostic of scabies.

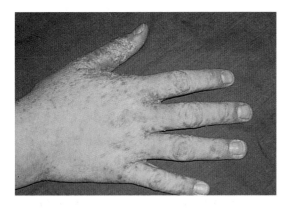

Fig. 15.8 Scabies with bacterial super infection.

• Venereal disease may be acquired at the same time as scabies.

• Crusted (Norwegian) scabies, which may not be itchy, is a widespread crusted eruption in which vast numbers of mites are found. It affects people with learning difficulties or the immunosuppressed, and can be the unsuspected source of epidemics of ordinary scabies.

Differential diagnosis

Only scabies shows characteristic burrows. Animal scabies from pets induces an itchy rash in humans but this lacks burrows. The lesions of papular urticaria (p. 224) are excoriated papules, in groups, mainly on the legs. Late-onset atopic eczema (p. 81), cholinergic urticaria (p. 95), lichen planus (p. 64), neurotic excoriations (p. 297) and dermatitis herpetiformis (p. 113) have their own distinctive features. Fibreglass can also cause epidemics of itching.

Investigations

With practice an acarus can be picked neatly with a needle from the end of its burrow and identified microscopically; failing this, eggs and mites can be seen microscopically in burrow scrapings mounted in potassium hydroxide (p. 35) or mineral oil. Some find dermatoscopy (p. 33) a quick and reliable way to identify the mite.

Treatment

• Use an effective scabicide; there are many on the market now (Formulary 1, p. 335). In the UK, the preferred treatment is with malathion or permethrin; lindane is no longer available. Topical treatment plus ivermectin (on a named patient basis in the UK), in a single dose of 200 µg/kg by mouth, is effective for Norwegian scabies and scabies that does not respond to topical measures alone.

• For babies over 2 months, toddlers and young children we advise permethrin cream, 25% benzyl benzoate emulsion diluted with three parts of water, or 6% precipitated sulphur in white soft paraffin (petrolatum).

• It is still not clear which scabicides can be safely used to treat pregnant women or those who are breast-feeding. Despite the absence of convincing evidence that unborn children can be damaged by topical scabicides, we prefer to use the same measures that we use to treat babies (above).

• Do not just treat the patient: treat all members of the family and sexual contacts, whether they are itching or not (Fig. 15.9).

• Have a printed sheet to give to the patient and go through it with them—scabies victims are notoriously confused.

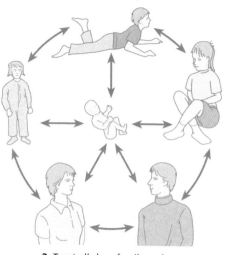

1 Scabicide must be applied to all areas below the neck. Special care to burrow-bearing areas

2 Treat all close family and sex partners – whether itchy or not

Fig. 15.9 The treatment of scabies.

- One convenient way to apply scabicides to the skin is with a 5 cm (2 inch) paintbrush. The number of applications recommended varies from dermatologist to dermatologist. There is no doubt that some preparations, such as malathion, disappear quickly from the skin, leaving it vulnerable to any mites which hatch out from eggs that have survived. A second application, a week after the first, is then essential. With permethrin, this may be less important. The main reason for recommending a second application is that it will cover areas left out during an inefficient first application.
- Make sure that patients grasp the fact that scabicides have to be applied to all areas of skin below the jaw line, including the genitals, soles of the feet, and skin under the free edge of the nails. If the hands are washed, the scabicide should be reapplied. A hot bath before treatment is no longer recommended.
- Ordinary laundering deals satisfactorily with clothing and sheets. Mites die in clothing unworn for 1 week.
- Residual itching may last for several days, or even a few weeks, but this does not need further applications of the scabicide. Rely instead on calamine lotion or crotamiton.

Parasitic worms

A textbook of tropical medicine should be consulted for more details on this subject.

Onchocerciasis

This is endemic in much of Central America and Africa where it is an important cause of blindness. The buffalo gnat (*Simulium* species) carries the filarial worm to humans. Infested humans become itchy with an excoriated papular eruption. Later the skin may thicken and become hyper- or hypopigmented. Dermal nodules are found, mainly near bony prominences, and contain both mature worms and microfilariae. It is the latter that invade the eye, leading to blindness. The diagnosis is confirmed by detecting active microfilariae in skin snips teased out in saline and examined microscopically. Ivermectin is now the treatment of choice. A single dose produces a prolonged reduction of microfilarial levels, and should be repeated every year until the adult worms die out. Diethylcarbamazine and suramin are now obsolete.

Filariasis

This is endemic throughout much of the tropics. The adult filarial worms, usually *Wuchereria bancrofti*, inhabit the lymphatics where they excite an inflammatory reaction with episodes of lymphangitis and fever, gradually leading to lymphatic obstruction and lymphoedema, usually of the legs or scrotum. Such swellings can be massive (elephantiasis). There is an eosinophilia and microfilariae are found in the peripheral blood, mainly at night; their vector from human to human is the mosquito, in which the larvae mature. Diethylcarbamazine or ivermectin is the treatment of choice.

Larva migrans

The larvae of hookworms that go through their full life cycle only in cats or dogs can penetrate human skin when it is in contact with soil or sand contaminated by the faeces of these animals. The larvae move under the skin creating tortuous red itchy lines (Fig. 15.10) that advance at the rate of a few millimetres a day. The larvae do eventually die, but this can be speeded up by a single oral dose of ivermectin.

Other worm infestations

• Threadworm (pinworm) infestation in children can cause severe anal and vulval pruritus. The small worms are seen best at night-time when the itch is worst. Treatment is with piperazine.
• Swimmer's itch, in tropical and lake waters, may be caused by the penetration through the skin of the cercariae of schistosomes of human and non-human origin. The skin should be towelled off immediately

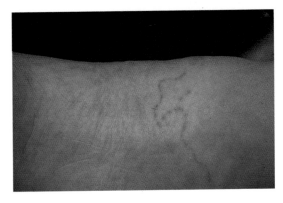

Fig. 15.10 Larva migrans—a red serpiginous line on the instep.

after swimming to prevent the schistosomes penetrating the skin as it dries.
• The larval stages of the pork tapeworm (cysticercosis) can present as multiple firm nodules in the skin.
• Larger fluctuant cysts may be caused by hydatid disease.

Further reading

Mehlhorn, H. (2001) *Encyclopedic Reference of Parasitology*. Springer, Berlin.

Skin reactions to light

Ultraviolet radiation (UVR) can be helpful when used to treat diseases such as psoriasis, but it can also be harmful (Fig. 16.1). It is the leading cause of skin cancers, and causes or worsens several skin disorders. UVR is non-ionizing, but changes the skin chemically by reacting with endogenous light-absorbing chemicals (chromophores), which include DNA, RNA, urocanic acid and melanin. Different types of skin (now conventionally divided into six types; Table 16.1) react differently to UVR, and require different degrees of protection against the sun.

The UVR spectrum is divided into three parts (Fig. 16.2), each having different effects on the skin, although UVC does not penetrate the ozone layer of the atmosphere and is therefore currently irrelevant to skin disease. Virtually all of the UVB is absorbed in the epidermis, whereas some 30% of UVA reaches the dermis. The B wavelengths (UVB: 290–320 nm) cause sunburn and are effectively screened out by window glass. The A spectrum (UVA) is long-wave ultraviolet light, from 320 nm to the most violet colour perceptible to the eye (about 400 nm). It ages and tans the skin. The differences between the wavelengths can be recorded conveniently in the form of action spectra, which show how effective each is at producing different biological effects, such as clearing psoriasis or causing erythema.

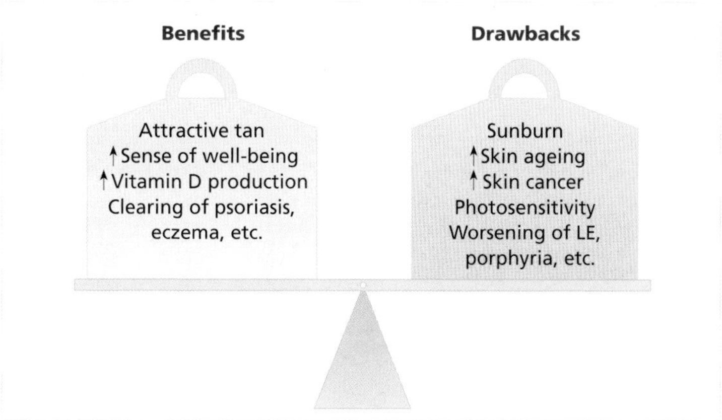

Benefits

Attractive tan
↑Sense of well-being
↑Vitamin D production
Clearing of psoriasis,
eczema, etc.

Drawbacks

Sunburn
↑Skin ageing
↑ Skin cancer
Photosensitivity
Worsening of LE,
porphyria, etc.

Fig. 16.1 The balance between the benefits and drawbacks of sun exposure.

Table 16.1 Skin types classified by their reactions to UVR.

Type	Definition	Description
I	Always burns but never tans	Pale skin, red hair, freckles
II	Usually burns, sometimes tans	Fair skin
III	May burn, usually tans	Darker skin
IV	Rarely burns, always tans	Mediterranean
V	Moderate constitutional pigmentation	Latin American, Middle Eastern
VI	Marked constitutional pigmentation	Black

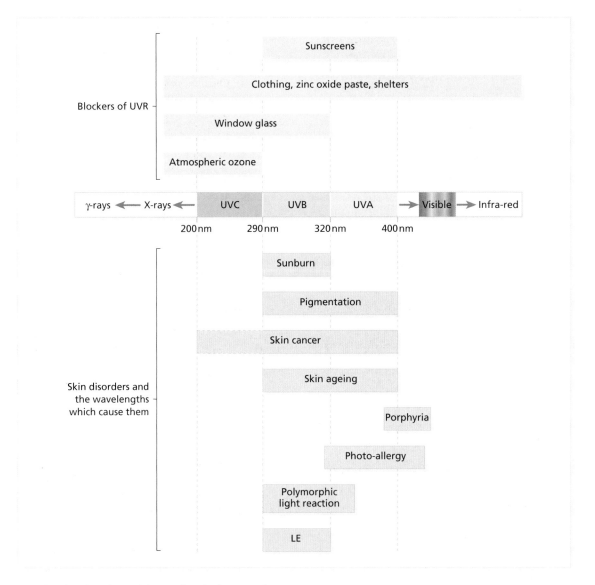

Fig. 16.2 Skin disorders and the wavelengths that cause them.

Sunburn

Cause

UVB penetrates the epidermis and superficial dermis, stimulating the production and release of prostaglandins, leukotrienes, histamine, interleukin 1 (IL-1) and tumour necrosis factor α (TNF-α), which cause pain and redness.

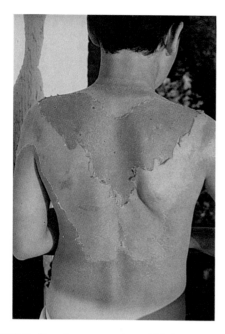

Fig. 16.3 Peeling after acute sunburn. This doctor's son should have known better.

Presentation and course

Skin exposed to too much UVB smarts and becomes red several hours later. Severe sunburn is painful and may blister. The redness is maximal after 1 day and then settles over the next 2 or 3 days, leaving sheet-like desquamation (Fig. 16.3), diffuse pigmentation (a 'tan') and, sometimes, discrete lentigines.

Differential diagnosis

Phototoxic reactions caused by drugs are like an exaggerated sunburn.

Investigations

None are required.

Treatment

The treatment is symptomatic. Baths may be cooling and oily shake lotions (e.g. oily calamine lotion), oil-in-water lotions or creams comforting. Potent topical corticosteroids (Formulary 1, p. 331) help if used early and briefly. Oral aspirin (a prostaglandin synthesis

Table 16.2 Drugs commonly causing photosensitivity.

Amiodarone
Chlorpropamide
Nalidixic acid
Oral contraceptives
Phenothiazines
Psoralens
Quinidine
Sulphonamides
Tetracyclines
Thiazides

inhibitor) relieves the pain. Sprays containing benzocaine also relieve pain, but occasionally sensitize.

Phototoxicity

Basic photochemical laws require a drug to absorb UVR to cause such a reaction. Most drugs listed in Table 16.2 absorb UVA as well as UVB, and so window glass, protective against sunburn, does not protect against most phototoxic drug reactions.

Presentation and course

Tenderness and redness occur only in areas exposed both to sufficient drug and to sufficient UVR (Fig. 16.4). The signs and symptoms are those of sunburn. The skin may later develop a deep tan.

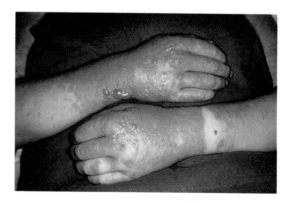

Fig. 16.4 Extreme photosensitivity of a patient taking griseofulvin. Note sparing of the area covered by the watch strap and ring.

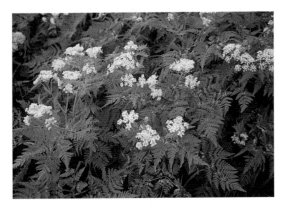

Fig. 16.5 Cow parsley contains psoralens and is a common cause of photodermatitis.

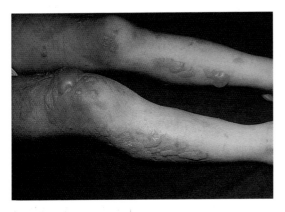

Fig. 16.6 Severe bullous eruption in areas in contact with giant hogweed (contains psoralens) and then exposed to sunlight (phytophotodermatitis).

Cause

These reactions are not immunological. Everyone exposed to enough of the drug, and to enough UVR, will develop the reaction. Some drugs that can cause phototoxic reactions are listed in Table 16.2. In addition, contact with psoralens in plants (Fig. 16.5) can cause a localized phototoxic dermatitis (phyto-photodermatitis; Fig. 16.6). These areas burn and may blister, leaving pigmentation in linear streaks and bizarre patterns.

Differential diagnosis

Photoallergic reactions are difficult to distinguish; the more so as the same drugs can often cause both photoallergic and phototoxic reactions. The main differ-ences between phototoxicity and photoallergy are shown in Table 16.3.

Investigations

None are usually required. In difficult cases, photo-testing can be carried out in special centres. The action spectrum (the wavelengths that cause the reaction) may incriminate a particular drug.

Treatment

This is the same as for sunburn. Drugs should be stopped if further exposure to ultraviolet light is likely.

Photoallergy

Drugs, topical or systemic, and chemicals on the skin, can interact with UVR and cause immunological reactions.

Cause

UVR converts an immunologically inactive form of a drug into an antigenic molecule. An immunological reaction, analogous to allergic contact dermatitis (p. 26), is induced if the antigen remains in the skin or is formed there on subsequent exposure to the drug and UVR. Many of the same drugs that cause photo-toxic reactions can also cause photoallergic ones.

Presentation

Photoallergy is often similar to phototoxicity. The areas exposed to UVR become inflamed, but the reaction is more likely to be eczematous. The eruption will be on exposed areas such as the hands, the V of the neck, the nose, the chin and the forehead. There is also a tendency to spare the upper lip under the nose, the eyelids and the submental region (Fig. 16.7). Often the eruption does not occur on the first expos-ure to ultraviolet, but only after a second or further exposures. A lag phase of one or more weeks is needed to induce an immune response.

Course

The original lesions are red patches, plaques, vesicles or bullae, which usually become eczematous. They tend

Table 16.3 Features distinguishing phototoxicity from photoallergy.

Phototoxicity	Photoallergy
Erythematous and smooth (may blister)	Eczematous and rough (may weep)
Immediate onset	Delayed onset (when immunity develops; may not occur on first exposure)
Hurts	Itches
Photopatch testing negative	Photopatch testing positive

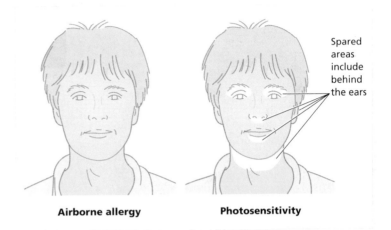

Airborne allergy　　　　**Photosensitivity**

Spared areas include behind the ears

Fig. 16.7 Features distinguishing airborne allergy from photosensitivity.

to resolve when either the drug or the exposure to UVR is stopped, but this may take several weeks.

Complications

Some drugs, such as the sulphonamides, can cause a persistent light reaction (see below).

Investigations

Photopatch testing by an expert can confirm the diagnosis. The chemical is applied for 24 h and the skin is then irradiated with UVA. An acute photoallergic contact dermatitis is then elicited. A control patch, not irradiated, rules out ordinary allergic contact dermatitis.

Treatment

The drug should be stopped and the patient protected from further ultraviolet exposure (avoidance,

clothing and sunscreens). Potent topical corticosteroids or a short course of a systemic corticosteroid will hasten resolution and provide symptomatic relief.

Chronic actinic dermatitis (actinic reticuloid)

Some patients with a photoallergic reaction never get over it and go on developing sun-induced eczematous areas long after the drug has been stopped.

Cause

This is not clear but some believe minute amounts of the drug persist in the skin indefinitely.

Presentation

This is the same as a photoallergic reaction to a drug. The patient goes on to develop a chronic dermatitis, with thick plaques on sun-exposed areas.

Course

These patients may be exquisitely sensitive to UVR. They are usually middle-aged or elderly men who react after the slightest exposure, even through window glass or from fluorescent lights. Affected individuals also become allergic to a range of contact allergens, especially oleoresins in some plants (e.g. chrysanthemums).

Complications

None, but the persistent severe pruritic eruption can lead to depression and even suicide.

Differential diagnosis

Airborne allergic contact dermatitis may be confused, but does not require sunlight. Sometimes the diagnosis is difficult as exposure both to sunlight and to the airborne allergen occurs only out of doors. Airborne allergic contact dermatitis also affects sites which sunlight is less likely to reach, such as under the chin (Fig. 16.7). A continuing drug photoallergy, a polymorphic light eruption (see below) or eczema as a result of some other cause must also be considered.

Histology shows a dense lymphocytic infiltrate and sometimes atypical lymphocytes suggestive of a lymphoma, but the disorder seldom becomes malignant.

Investigations

Persistent light reaction can be confirmed experimentally by exposing uninvolved skin to UVA or UVB. Patch tests and photopatch tests help to distinguish between photoallergy and airborne allergic contact dermatitis, and the action spectrum may point to a certain drug. This sort of testing is difficult, and should be carried out only in specialist centres.

Treatment

Usually cared for by specialists, these patients need extreme measures to protect their skin from UVR. These include protective clothing and frequent applications of combined UVA and UVB blocking agents (Formulary 1, p. 330). Patients must protect themselves from UVR coming through windows or from fluorescent lights. Some can only go out at night. As even the most potent topical steroids are often

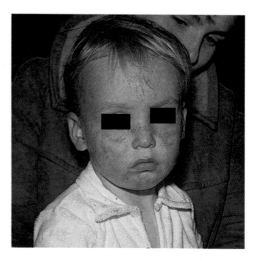

Fig. 16.8 Polymorphic light eruption: eczematous plaques on the face of a sad freckly boy. Persists throughout the summer but fades in the winter.

ineffective, systemic steroids or immunosuppressants (e.g. azathioprine) may be needed for long periods.

Polymorphic light eruption

This is the most frequent cause of a so-called 'sun allergy'.

Cause

It is speculated that UVR causes a natural body chemical to change into an allergen. Mechanisms are similar to those in drug photoallergy.

Presentation

Small itchy red papulovesicles or eczematous plaques arise from 2 h to 5 days, most commonly at 24 h, after exposure to UVR. The eruption is itchy and usually confined to sun-exposed areas (Fig. 16.8), remembering that some UVR passes through thin clothing.

Course

The disorder tends to recur each spring after UVR exposure. Tanning protects some patients so that if the initial exposures are limited, few or no symptoms occur later. Such patients can still enjoy sun exposure and outdoor activities. Others are so sensitive, or their skin pigments so poorly, that fresh exposures continue to induce reactions throughout the summer. These patients require photoprotection, and must limit their sun exposure and outdoor activities. The rash disappears during the winter.

Differential diagnosis

Phototoxic reactions, photoallergic reactions, miliaria rubra, chronic actinic dermatitis, ordinary eczemas, allergic reactions to sunscreens and airborne allergic contact dermatitis should be considered.

Investigations

It may be possible to reproduce the dermatitis by testing non-sun-exposed skin with UVB and UVA.

Treatment

If normal tanning does not confer protection, sunscreens (Formulary 1, p. 330) should be used. Protective clothing, such as wide-brimmed hats, long-sleeved shirts and long trousers, is helpful. In some patients, a 4-week PUVA course (p. 59) in the late spring can create enough tan to confer protection for the rest of the season. Moderately potent topical steroids (Formulary 1, p. 331) usually improve the eruption. Hydroxychloroquine (Formulary 2, p. 351) may be effective when used over the sunny season.

Actinic prurigo

This is clinically distinct from a polymorphic light eruption although its unknown cause may be the same. Papules, crusts and excoriations arise on sun-exposed areas and sometimes also on other sites. Lesions may persist through the winter. It is common among North American Indians and may resemble excoriated acne, bites, eczema, erythropoetic protoporphyria or neurotic excoriations. It may be associated with atopy.

Solar urticaria

This is discussed in Chapter 8. Wheals occur in the sun-exposed areas, within minutes. Some patients have erythropoietic protoporphyria (p. 119) and this should be considered particularly if solar urticaria starts in infancy.

Actinic keratoses

These are discussed in Chapter 18.

Actinic cheilitis

This is discussed in Chapter 13 and see Fig. 24.14.

Lupus erythematosus

Many patients with lupus erythematosus (p. 119) become worse after exposure to UVR, especially to UVB. They should be warned about this, and protect themselves from the sun (avoidance, clothing and sunscreens).

Carcinomas

The sun can cause basal cell carcinomas, squamous cell carcinomas and malignant melanomas. These are discussed in Chapter 18.

Exacerbated diseases

UVR is useful in the treatment of many skin diseases, but it can also make some worse (Table 16.4).

Porphyria cutanea tarda

This is described in Chapter 19.

LEARNING POINTS

If the skin reacts badly to light through glass then:
1 Sunscreens are usually ineffective.
2 Think of drugs or porphyria.

Cutaneous ageing

The trouble with old skin is the way it looks rather than the way it behaves. Skin chronically damaged by UVR during childhood thereafter looks old. This 'photoageing' effect causes the skin to become thin on the extremities, so that it bruises and tears easily (Fig. 16.9). The elastic fibres become clumped and

Helps	Worsens
Atopic eczema	Darier's disease
Cutaneous T-cell lymphoma	Herpes simplex
Parapsoriasis	Lupus erythematosus
Pityriasis lichenoides	Pellagra
Pityriasis rosea	Photoallergy/toxicity
Pruritus of renal failure, liver disease	Porphyrias (excluding acute intermittent)
AIDS	Xeroderma pigmentosum
Psoriasis	

Table 16.4 The effect of sunlight on some skin diseases.

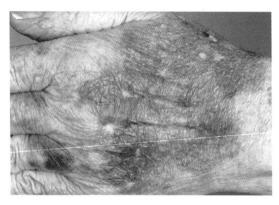

Fig. 16.9 Thin skin on the back of the hand. The whitish areas are stellate pseudoscars, the skin having never been broken. The pseudoscars follow the dispersion of senile purpura.

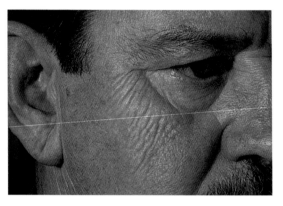

Fig. 16.10 Prolonged sun exposure has caused this furrowed yellowish thickened area on the cheek (solar elastosis).

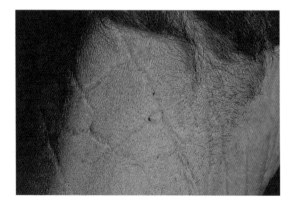

Fig. 16.11 'Sailor's skin' (cutis rhomboidalis nuchae): the deep creases on the back of the neck contain many comedones.

amorphous, leading clinically to a yellow pebbly look called actinic elastosis (Figs 16.10 and 16.11). Chronic exposure to sunlight, or to UVR in tanning parlours, also causes lentigines, freckles, xerosis and, of course, skin cancers. The bronzed young skins of today will become the wrinkled spotted rough prune-like ones of tomorrow.

Wrinkles occur when the dermis loses its elastic recoil, failing to snap back properly into shape. UVR damages elastic tissue and hastens this process. Although face-lifts can smooth wrinkles out, there is no way to reverse the damage fully; however, tretinoin cream (Formulary 1, p. 336) seems to help some patients. Prevention (reducing exposure to UVR) is better than any cure, and is especially important in sunny climates (Table 16.5).

Skin ages even in sun protected areas, but much more slowly. The dermis thins, skin collagen falls

by about 1% per year throughout adult life, and becomes more stable (less elastic). Fibroblasts become sparser in the dermis, accounting for reduced collagen synthesis and slower wound healing.

Table 16.5 Tips to avoid skin damage for those living in a sunny climate.

1 Apply sunscreen daily to all exposed parts—rain or shine, reapply after 20 min
2 Reapply sunscreen often when outdoors
3 Use a sunscreen with a protective factor (SPF) of at least 15
4 Wear protective clothing, including wide-brimmed hats
5 Target outdoor activities for early morning or late afternoon
6 Seek the shade
7 Avoid tanning salons
8 Do not sunbathe
9 Wear cosmetics, including lipstick
10 Help your children to protect themselves

Further reading

Berneburg, M., Plettenberg, H. & Krutmann, J. (2000) Photoaging of human skin. *Photodermatology, Photoimmunology and Photomedicine* **16**, 239–244.

Epstein, J.H. (1999) Phototoxicity and photoallergy. *Seminars in Cutaneous Medicine and Surgery* **18**, 274–284.

Gonzalez, E. & Gonzalez, S. (1996) Drug photosensitivity, idiopathic photodermatitis, and sunscreens. *Journal of the American Academy of Dermatology* **35**, 871–875.

Johnson, B.E. & Ferguson, J. (1990) Drug and chemical photosensitivity. *Seminars in Dermatology* **9**, 39–46.

Krutman, J., Hönigsmann, H., Elmets, C.A. & Bergstresser, P.R. (2001) *Dermatological Phototherapy and Photodiagnostic Methods*. Springer, Berlin.

Disorders of pigmentation

Normal skin colour

The colour of normal skin comes from a mixture of pigments. Untanned Caucasoid skin is pink, from oxyhaemoglobin in the blood within the papillary loops and superficial horizontal plexus (see Fig. 2.10). Melanin (see below) blends with this colour, e.g. after a suntan. Melanin is, of course, also responsible for the shades of brown seen in Negroid skin. Other hues are caused by the addition to these pigments of yellow from carotene, found mainly in subcutaneous fat and in the horny layer of the epidermis. There is no natural blue pigment: when blue is seen it is either because of an optical effect from normal pigment (usually melanin) in the dermis, or the presence of an abnormal pigment.

Melanogenesis

Tyrosine, formed in the liver by hydroxylation of the essential amino acid phenylalanine under the influence of phenylalanine hydroxylase, is the substrate for the reactions that occur in melanocytes (Fig. 17.1). These are the only cells in the epidermis to contain tyrosinase (dopa oxidase), the rate-limiting enzyme in melanogenesis. This copper-dependent enzyme converts tyrosine to melanin. Dopa is formed by the oxidation of tyrosine, and further enzymic action leads to the formation of dopaquinone. Eumelanins, brown or black pigments, are then formed by polymerization. Phaeomelanins and trichochromes, the pigments in red hair, are synthesized in a similar way, except that cysteine reacts with dopaquinone and is incorporated

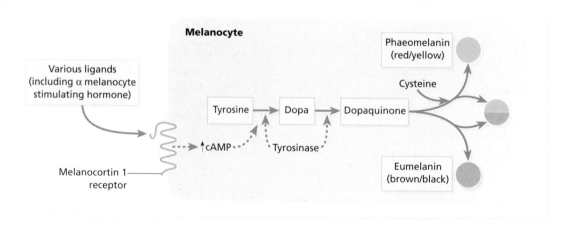

Fig. 17.1 The control of melanogenesis. Melanocortin 1 receptor (MC1R) activity is both constitutive and rate limiting when promoting melanogenesis, via cyclic adenosine monophosphate (cAMP) production and tyrosinase stimulation. The MC1R is activated by ligands such as α-melanocyte-stimulating hormone (α-MSH) and other pituitary peptides. In the absence of such ligands or the MC1R itself (knockout animals), and with loss-of-function mutations of the MC1R, phaeomelanin is produced. The precise mechanism by which ultraviolet radiation stimulates melanogenesis remains uncertain.

into the subsequent polymers. Phaeomelanins and eumelanins may intermesh to form mixed melanin polymers.

Eumelanins and phaeomelanins differ from neuro-melanins, the pigments found in the substantia nigra and in cells of the chromaffin system (adrenal medulla, sympathetic ganglia, etc.). The latter are derived from tyrosine using a different enzyme, tyrosine hydroxy-lase, which is not found in melanocytes.

Melanin is made within melanosomes, tiny part-icles measuring about 0.1×0.7 µm, shaped either like American footballs (eumelanosomes, containing eume-lanin) or British soccer balls (phaeomelanosomes, containing phaeomelanin). Eventually, fully melanized melanosomes pass into the dendritic processes of the melanocyte to be injected into neighbouring keratin-ocytes. Once there, the melanosomes are engulfed in lysosomal packages (melanosome complexes) and distributed throughout the cytoplasm.

Negroids are not black because they have more melanocytes than Caucasoids, but because their melanocytes produce more and larger melanosomes, which are broken down less rapidly in the melano-some complexes. Melanins protect against ultraviolet radiation (UVR) damage by absorbing and scattering the rays, and by scavenging free radicals.

The control of melanogenesis

Melanogenesis can be increased by several stimuli, the most important of which is UVR. Tanning involves two distinct reactions.

1 An immediate reaction occurs within 5 min of exposure to long-wave ultraviolet (UVA: 320–400 nm) and may be because of the photo-oxidation of preformed melanin. This pigment-darkening reac-tion, which lasts about 15 min, is responsible for the well-known phenomenon of a 'false tan'.

2 The production of *new* pigment is delayed for some 24 h after exposure to medium wave ultraviolet (UVB: 290–320 nm) and UVA. It depends on the pro-liferation of melanocytes, an increase in tyrosinase activity and melanosome production, and an increased transfer of new melanosomes to their surrounding keratinocytes.

A neat control mechanism involving glutathione has been postulated. Reduced glutathione in the epi-dermis, produced by the action of glutathione reduc-tase on glutathione, inhibits tyrosinase. UVR and

some inflammatory skin conditions may induce pig-mentation by oxidizing glutathione and so blocking its inhibition of melanogenesis.

Melanocytes are also influenced by melanocyte-stimulating hormone (MSH; peptides from the pitu-itary and other areas of the brain) (Fig. 17.1). Their melanocyte-stimulating activity is caused by a com-mon heptapeptide sequence, cleaved from the pre-cursor protein, pro-opiomelanocortin, as a result of two proconvertase enzymes. However, MSH peptides may play little part in the physiological control of pig-mentation. Hypophysectomy will not cause a black skin to lighten and only large doses of adrenocorti-cotrophic hormone (ACTH), in pathological states (see below), will increase skin pigmentation. It is now known that pro-opiomelanocortin and MSH peptides are also produced by both keratinocytes and melanocytes in the skin; so MSH may have a paracrine or autocrine function. In the skin, α-MSH also acts as an anti-inflammatory agent by antagonizing the effects of interleukin 1 (IL-1) in inducing IL-2 receptors on lym-phocytes (p. 12) and in inducing pyrexia.

Animal experiments indicate that oestrogens, progestogens and, possibly, testosterone may, in some circumstances, stimulate melanogenesis, either directly or by increasing the release of MSH peptides from the pituitary.

Genetics and skin pigmentation

Genetic differences determine the pigmentation of the different races. The black person living in Britain, and the white person living in Africa remain black and white, respectively. None the less, there is some phe-notypic variation in skin colour, e.g. tanning after sun exposure. Recently, red hair has been shown to be a result of genetic variations in the amino acid sequence of the melanocortin 1 receptor (MC1R) (Fig. 17.1). Some genodermatoses with abnormal pigmentation are described in Chapter 21.

Abnormal skin colours

These may be caused by an imbalance of the normal pigments mentioned above (e.g. in cyanosis, chloasma and carotenaemia) or by the presence of abnormal pigments (Table 17.1). Sometimes it is difficult to dis-tinguish between the colours of these pigments; e.g.

Table 17.1 Some abnormal pigments.

Endogenous

Haemoglobin-derived

Methaemoglobin	blue colour in vessels,
Sulphaemoglobin	cyanosis
Carboxyhaemoglobin	pink
Bilirubin	
Biliverdin	yellow-green
Haemosiderin	brown

Drugs

Gold	blue-grey (chrysiasis)
Silver	blue-grey (argyria)
Bismuth	grey
Mepacrine	yellow
Clofazamine	red
Phenothiazines	slate-grey
Amiodarone	blue-grey

Diet

Carotene	orange

Exogenous

Tattoo pigments

Carbon	blue-black
Coal dust	blue-black
Cobalt	blue
Chrome	green
Cadmium	yellow
Mercury	red
Iron	brown

Local medications

Silver nitrate	black
Magenta paint	magenta
Gentian violet	violet
Eosin	pink
Potassium permanganate	brown
Dithranol (anthralin)	purple
Tar	brown
Iodine	yellow

Table 17.2 Some causes of hypopigmentation.

Genetic	Albinism
	Piebaldism
	Phenylketonuria
	Waardenburg's syndrome
	Chediak–Higashi syndrome: autosomal recessive lysosomal defect, pale skin with sparse silvery-grey or blond hair, susceptible to infections
	Tuberous sclerosis (p. 302)
Endocrine	Hypopituitarism
Chemical	Contact with substituted phenols (in rubber industry) Chloroquine and hydroxychloroquine
Postinflammatory	Eczema
	Pityriasis alba
	Psoriasis
	Sarcoidosis
	Lupus erythematosus
	Lichen sclerosus et atrophicus
	Cryotherapy
Infections	Leprosy
	Pityriasis versicolor
	Syphilis, yaws and pinta
Tumours	Halo naevus
	Malignant melanoma
Miscellaneous	Vitiligo
	Idiopathic guttate hypomelanosis

the gingery brown colour of haemosiderin is readily confused with melanin. Histological stains may be needed to settle the issue. In practice, apart from tattoos, most pigmentary problems are caused by too much, or too little melanin.

Decreased melanin pigmentation

Some conditions in which there is a lack of melanin are listed in Table 17.2. A few of the more important,

and the mechanisms involved, are summarized in Fig. 17.2.

Oculocutaneous albinism

In this condition, little or no melanin is made either in the skin and eyes (oculocutaneous albinism) or in the eyes alone (ocular albinism—not discussed further here). The prevalence of albinism of all types ranges from 1 in 20 000 in the USA and UK to 5% in some communities.

Cause

The hair bulb test (see Investigations) separates oculocutaneous albinism into two main types: tyrosinase-negative and tyrosinase-positive. Roughly

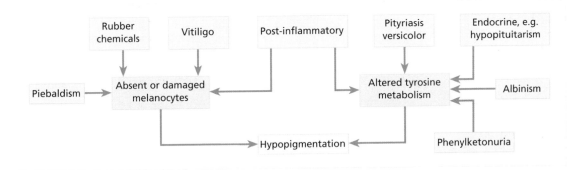

Fig. 17.2 The mechanisms involved in some types of hypopigmentation.

equal numbers of the two types are found in most communities, both being inherited as autosomal recessive traits. This explains how children with two albino parents can sometimes themselves be normally pigmented, the genes being complementary in the double heterozygote (Fig. 17.3).

The tyrosinase gene lies on chromosome 11q14-q21. More than 20 allelic variations have been found there in patients with tyrosinase-negative albinism. The gene for tyrosinase-positive human albinism has been mapped to chromosome 15q11-q13. It probably encodes for an ion channel protein in the melanosome involved in the transport of tyrosine.

Presentation and course

The whole skin is white and pigment is also lacking in the hair, iris and retina (Fig. 17.3). Albinos have poor sight, photophobia and a rotatory nystagmus. As they grow older tyrosinase-positive albinos gain a little pigment in their skin, iris and hair. Negroid skin becomes yellow-brown and the hair becomes yellow. Albinos may also develop freckles. Sunburn is common on unprotected skin. As melanocytes are present, albinos have non-pigmented melanocytic naevi and may develop amelanotic malignant melanomas.

Complications

In the tropics these unfortunate individuals develop numerous sun-induced skin tumours even when they are young, confirming the protective role of melanin.

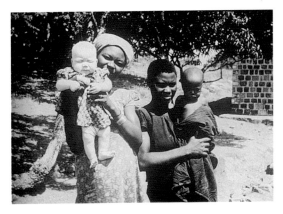

Fig. 17.3 Oculocutaneous albinism. An albino baby born to a normally pigmented African family (autosomal recessive inheritance).

Differential diagnosis

Piebaldism and vitiligo are described below.

Investigations

Prenatal diagnosis of albinism is now possible but may not be justifiable in view of the good prognosis. A biopsy from fetal skin, taken at 20 weeks, is examined by electron microscopy for arrested melanosome development.

The hair bulb test, in which plucked hairs are incubated in dihydroxyphenylalanine, distinguishes tyrosinase-positive from tyrosinase-negative types. Those whose hair bulbs turn black (tyrosine-positive) are less severely affected.

Treatment

Avoidance of sun exposure, and protection with opaque clothing, wide-brimmed hats and sunscreen creams (Formulary 1, p. 330), are essential and allow albinos in temperate climates to live a relatively normal life. Early diagnosis and treatment of skin tumours is critical. In the tropics the outlook is less good and the termination of affected pregnancies may be considered.

Piebaldism

These patients often have a white forelock of hair and patches of depigmentation lying symmetrically on the limbs, trunk and central part of the face, especially the chin. The condition is present at birth and is inherited as an autosomal dominant trait. A genetic abnormality in mice (dominant white spotting) provided the clue that allowed the human piebaldism gene to be mapped to chromosome 4q12, where the *KIT* protooncogene lies. This encodes the tyrosine kinase transmembrane cellular receptor on certain stem cells; without this they cannot respond to normal signals for development and migration. Melanocytes are absent from the hypopigmented areas. The depigmentation, often mistaken for vitiligo, may improve with age. There is no effective treatment. Waardenburg's syndrome includes piebaldism (with a white forelock in 20% of cases), hypertelorism, a prominent inner third of the eyebrows, irides of different colour and deafness.

Phenylketonuria

This rare metabolic cause of hypopigmentation has a prevalence of about 1 : 25 000. It is described in Chapter 20.

Hypopituitarism

The skin changes here may alert an astute physician to the diagnosis. The complexion has a pale, yellow tinge; there is thinning or loss of the sexual hair; the skin itself is atrophic. The hypopigmentation is caused by a decreased production of pituitary melanotrophic hormones (see above).

Vitiligo

The word vitiligo comes from the Latin word *vitellus*, which means 'veal' (pale, pink flesh). It is an acquired circumscribed depigmentation, found in all races; its prevalence may be as high as 0.5–1%; its inheritance is polygenic.

Cause and types

There is a complete loss of melanocytes from affected areas. There are two main patterns: a common generalized one and a rare segmental type. *Generalized vitiligo*, including the acrofacial variant, usually starts after the second decade. There is a family history in 30% of patients and this type is most frequent in those with autoimmune diseases such as diabetes, thyroid disorders and pernicious anaemia. It is postulated that in this type melanocytes are the target of a cell-mediated autoimmune attack. *Segmental vitiligo* is restricted to one part of the body, but not necessarily to a dermatome. It occurs earlier than generalized vitiligo, and is not associated with autoimmune diseases. Trauma and sunburn can precipitate both types.

Clinical course

Generalized type. The sharply defined, usually symmetrical (Fig. 17.4), white patches are especially common on the backs of the hands, wrists, fronts of knees, neck and around body orifices. The hair of the scalp and beard may depigment too. In Caucasoids, the surrounding skin is sometimes hyperpigmented.

The course is unpredictable: lesions may remain static or spread; occasionally they repigment spontaneously from the hair follicles.

Segmental type. The individual areas look like the generalized type but their segmental distribution is striking. Spontaneous repigmentation occurs more often in this type than in generalized vitiligo (Fig. 17.5).

Differential diagnosis

Contact with depigmenting chemicals, such as hydroquinones and substituted phenols in the rubber industry, should be excluded. Pityriasis versicolor (p. 221) must be considered; its fine scaling and less

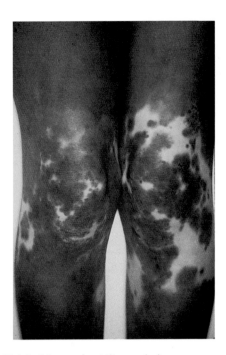

Fig. 17.4 Striking patchy vitiligo on the knees.

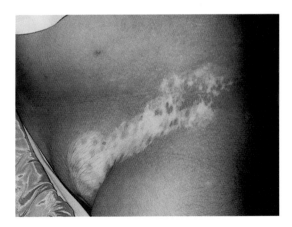

Fig. 17.5 Vitiligo: patchy repigmentation is caused by the migration of melanocytes from the depths of the hair follicles.

complete pigment loss separate it from vitiligo. Postinflammatory depigmentation (see below) may look very like vitiligo but is less white and improves spontaneously. The patches of piebaldism are present at birth. Sometimes leprosy must be excluded—by sensory testing and a general examination. Other tropical

diseases that cause patchy hypopigmentation are leishmaniasis (p. 201), yaws (p. 195) and pinta.

Treatment

Treatment is unsatisfactory. Recent patches may respond to a potent or very potent topical steroid, applied for 1–2 months. After this, the strength should be gradually tapered to a mildly potent steroid for maintenance treatment. Some patients improve with psoralens (trimethylpsoralen or 8-methoxypsoralen, in a dosage of 0.4–0.6 mg/kg body weight), taken 1–2 h before graduated exposure to natural sunshine or to artificial UVA (PUVA; p. 59). Narrow band (311 nm) UVB may also be effective. Therapy is given 2–3 times weekly for at least 6 months; new lesions seem to respond best. Autologous skin grafts are becoming popular in some centres although they remain experimental. The two most common procedures are minigrafting (implants of 1 mm grafts from unaffected skin) and suction blister grafting (using the epidermal roofs of suction blisters from unaffected skin for grafting). Melanocyte and stem cell transplants, in which single cell suspensions are made from unaffected skin and applied to dermabraded vitiliginous skin, are also being investigated. The use of these techniques may be limited by cost, and by the development of vitiligo (Köbner phenomenon) at donor sites.

As a general rule, established vitiligo is best left untreated in most white people, although advice about suitable camouflage preparations (Formulary 1, p. 330) to cover unsightly patches should be given. Sun avoidance and screening preparations (Formulary 1, p. 330) are needed to avoid sunburn of the affected areas and a heightened contrast between the pale and dark areas. Black patients with extensive vitiligo can be completely and irreversibly depigmented by creams containing the monobenzyl ether of hydroquinone.

LEARNING POINTS

1 Vitiligo looks ugly and sunburns easily. Treat with cosmetic cover and sunscreens or sun avoidance.
2 Do not promise a cure.

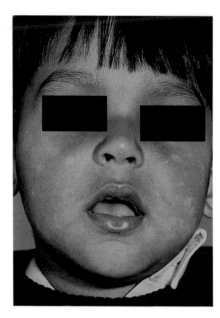

Fig. 17.6 Pityriasis alba.

The social implications of this must be discussed and carefully considered, and written consent given before such treatment is undertaken.

Postinflammatory depigmentation

This may follow eczema, psoriasis, sarcoidosis, lupus erythematosus and, rarely, lichen planus. It may also result from cryotherapy or a burn. In general, the more severe the inflammation, the more likely pigment is to decrease rather than increase in its wake. These problems are most significant in Negroids or Asians. With time, the skin usually repigments. Pityriasis alba is common on the faces of children. The initial lesion is probably a variant of eczema (pinkish with fine scaling), which fades leaving one or more pale, slightly scaly, areas (Fig. 17.6). Exposure to the sun makes the patches more obvious.

White hair

Melanocytes in hair bulbs become less active with age and white hair (canities) is a universal sign of ageing. Early greying of the hair is seen in the rare premature ageing syndromes, such as Werner's syndrome, and in autoimmune conditions such as pernicious anaemia, thyroid disorders and Addison's disease.

Disorders with increased pigmentation (hypermelanosis)

Some of these disorders are listed in Table 17.3. The most common will be described below and the mechanisms involved are summarized in Fig. 17.7.

Table 17.3 Some causes of hyperpigmentation.

Genetic	Freckles
	Lentigines
	Café au lait macules
	Peutz–Jeghers syndrome
	Xeroderma pigmentosum (Chapter 21)
	Albright's syndrome: segmental hyperpigmentation, fibrous dysplasia of bones, precocious puberty
Endocrine	Addison's disease
	Cushing's syndrome
	Pregnancy
	Renal failure
Metabolic	Biliary cirrhosis
	Haemochromatosis
	Porphyria
Nutritional	Malabsorption
	Carcinomatosis
	Kwashiorkor
	Pellagra
Drugs	Photosensitizing drugs
	ACTH and synthetic analogues
	Oestrogens and progestogens
	Psoralens
	Arsenic
	Busulfan
	Minocycline
Postinflammatory	Lichen planus
	Eczema
	Secondary syphilis
	Systemic sclerosis
	Lichen and macular amyloidosis
	Cryotherapy
Poikiloderma	
Tumours	Acanthosis nigricans (p. 283)
	Pigmented naevi (p. 257)
	Malignant melanoma (p. 268)
	Mastocytosis (p. 279)

ACTH, adenocorticotrophic hormone.

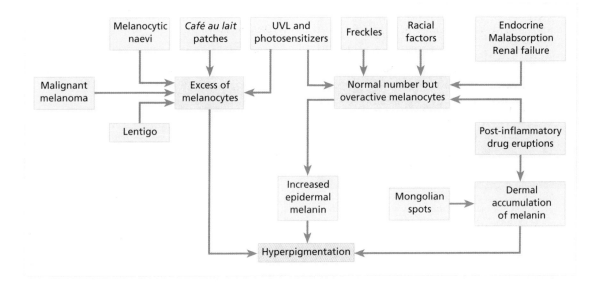

Fig. 17.7 The mechanisms of some types of hyperpigmentation.

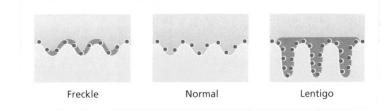

Freckle   Normal   Lentigo

Fig. 17.8 Histology of a freckle and a lentigo.

Freckles (ephelides)

Freckles are so common that to describe them seems unnecessary. They are seen most often in the red-haired or blond person as sharply demarcated light brown-ginger macules, usually less than 5 mm in diameter. They multiply and become darker with sun exposure.

Increased melanin is seen in the basal layer of the epidermis without any increase in the number of melanocytes, and without elongation of the rete ridges (Fig. 17.8). No treatment is necessary.

Melanotic macule of the lip

This common lesion (Fig. 17.9) worries doctors but is benign. Its histology is similar to that of a freckle (Fig. 17.8).

Lentigo

Simple and senile lentigines look alike. They are light or dark brown macules, ranging from 1 mm to 1 cm across. Although usually discrete, they may have an irregular outline. Simple lentigines arise most often in childhood as a few scattered lesions, often on areas not exposed to sun, including the mucous membranes. Senile or solar lentigines are common after middle age on the backs of the hands ('liver spots'; Fig. 17.10) and on the face (Fig. 17.11) In contrast to freckles, lentigines have increased numbers of melanocytes. They should be distinguished from freckles, from junctional melanocytic naevi (p. 258) and from a lentigo maligna (p. 271). Treatment is usually unnecessary but melanin-specific high energy lasers (e.g. pigmented lesion dye laser, 510 nm; Q-switched ruby laser, 694 nm; Q-switched alexandrite laser, 755 nm) are extremely

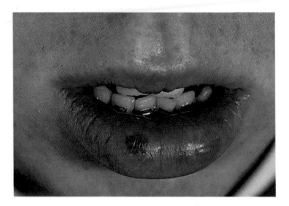

Fig. 17.9 Melanotic macule of the lip: slow to evolve and benign, as suggested by its even colour and sharp margin.

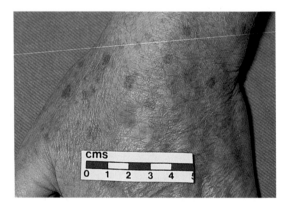

Fig. 17.10 Senile lentigines on the back of an elderly hand ('liver spots'). Note accompanying atrophy.

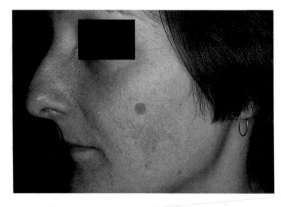

Fig. 17.11 A simple lentigo showing a sharp edge and an even distribution of pigment.

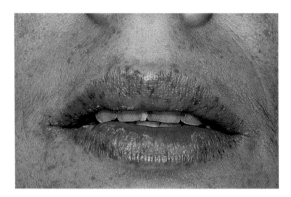

Fig. 17.12 Profuse lentigines on and around the lips in the Peutz–Jeghers syndrome.

effective for treating ugly lesions. Liver spots associated with actinic damage lighten or clear with the daily application of 0.1% tretinoin cream (Formulary 1, p. 336) or 3% hydroquinone (Formulary 1, p. 330).

Conditions associated with multiple lentigines

Three rare but striking syndromes feature multiple lentigines.

Peutz–Jeghers syndrome

Profuse lentigines are seen on and around the lips in this autosomal dominant condition (Fig. 17.12). Scattered lentigines also occur on the buccal mucosa, gums, hard palate, hands and feet. The syndrome is important because of its association with polyposis of the small intestine, which may lead to recurrent intussusception and, rarely, to malignant transformation of the polyps. Ten per cent of affected women have ovarian tumours.

Cronkhite–Canada syndrome

This consists of multiple lentigines on the backs of the hands and a more diffuse pigmentation of the palms and volar aspects of the fingers. It may also associate with gastrointestinal polyposis. Alopecia and nail abnormalities complete the rare but characteristic clinical picture.

LEOPARD syndrome

This is an acronym for generalized Lentiginosis associated with cardiac abnormalities demonstrated by ECG,

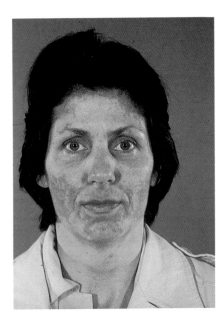

Fig. 17.13 Chloasma worsened by sun exposure.

Ocular hypertelorism, Pulmonary Stenosis, Abnormal genitalia, Retardation of growth and Deafness.

Chloasma

Chloasma is a patterned pigmentation of the face occurring in women during pregnancy or when taking oral contraceptives. The areas of increased pigmentation are well defined, symmetrical and their edges are often scalloped (the mask of pregnancy; Fig. 17.13). Most of the extra melanin lies in the epidermis, but there is some in the dermis too, making treatment more difficult. If the area is viewed under Wood's light, an increase in contrast or in pigmentation suggests mainly epidermal pigmentation, whereas loss of contrast suggests dermal pigment. The light brown colour becomes darker after exposure to the sun. The placenta may secrete hormones that stimulate melanocytes. Chloasma should be differentiated from a phototoxic reaction to a scented cosmetic or to a drug. Treatment is unsatisfactory, although some find bleaching agents that contain hydroquinone helpful. The optimal effect is achieved with preparations containing 2–5% hydroquinone, applied for 6–10 weeks. After this, maintenance treatment should be with preparations containing no more than 2% hydroquinone. A sunscreen will make the pigmentation less obvious during the summer and will minimize the chance of spread.

Endocrine hyperpigmentation

Addison's disease

Hyperpigmentation caused by the overproduction of ACTH is often striking. It may be generalized or limited to the skin folds, creases of the palms, scars and the buccal mucosa.

Cushing's syndrome

Increased ACTH production may cause a picture like that of Addison's disease. The hyperpigmentation may become even more marked after adrenalectomy (Nelson's syndrome).

Pregnancy

There is a generalized increase in pigmentation during pregnancy, especially of the nipples and areolae, and of the linea alba. Chloasma (see above) may also occur. The nipples and areolae remain pigmented after parturition.

Chronic renal failure

The hyperpigmentation of chronic renal failure and of patients on haemodialysis is caused by an increase in levels of pituitary melanotrophic peptides, normally cleared by the kidney.

Porphyria

Formed porphyrins, especially uroporphyrins, are produced in excess in cutaneous hepatic porphyria and congenital erythropoietic porphyria (p. 287). These endogenous photosensitizers induce hyperpigmentation on exposed areas; skin fragility, blistering, milia and hypertrichosis are equally important clues to the diagnosis.

Nutritional hyperpigmentation

Any severe wasting disease, such as malabsorption, AIDS, tuberculosis or cancer, may be accompanied by diffuse hyperpigmentation. Kwashiorkor presents a

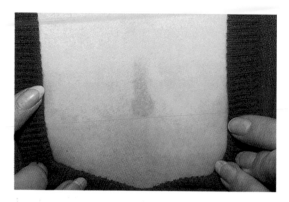

Fig. 17.14 A drop of psoralen-containing perfume photosensitized this pendant-shaped area, which became pigmented after exposure to the sun.

mixed picture of generalized hypopigmentation and patchy postinflammatory hyperpigmentation, and in this condition the hair is red-brown or grey.

Chemicals causing hyperpigmentation

Table 16.2 lists drugs that commonly photosensitize. All can cause hyperpigmentation of the exposed skin. Psoralens are used in the photochemotherapy of psoriasis (Chapter 5) and, more rarely, of vitiligo.

The term 'berloque dermatitis' (Fig. 17.14) refers to a 'pendant' of hyperpigmentation, often on the side of the neck, where cosmetics have been applied which contain the photosensitizing 5-methoxypsoralen. Cosmetics for men (pre- and aftershaves, etc.) are a thriving source of these.

Arsenic is not used medically nowadays. Once it caused 'raindrop' depigmentation within a diffuse bronzed hyperpigmentation.

Busulfan and bleomycin, used to treat some forms of leukaemia, frequently cause diffuse hyperpigmentation but may also cause brown streaks (flagellate hyperpigmentation). Minocycline can leave blue-black drug deposits in inflamed acne spots on the shins or on the mucosae. They can be removed successfully with Q-switched ruby laser (694 nm) treatment.

Postinflammatory hyperpigmentation

This is common after lichen planus (p. 64). It is also a feature of systemic sclerosis (p. 126) and some types of cutaneous amyloidosis, and is often an unwelcome sequel of cryotherapy.

Poikiloderma

Poikiloderma is the name given to a triad of signs: reticulate pigmentation, atrophy and telangiectasia. It is not a disease but a reaction pattern with many causes including X-irradiation, photocontact reactions, and connective tissue and lymphoreticular disorders. Congenital variants (Rothmund–Thomson syndrome, Bloom's syndrome and Cockayne's syndrome) associated with photosensitivity, dwarfism and mental retardation also occur.

Further reading

Hann, S-K. and Nordlund, J.J. (2000) *Vitiligo.* Blackwell Science, Oxford.

Nordlund, J.J., Boissy, R.E., Hearing, V.J., King, R. & Ortonne, J-P. (1998) *The Pigmentary System.* Oxford University Press, New York.

Taylor, S.C. (2002) Understanding skin of color. *Journal of the American Academy of Dermatology.* Suppl. 46/2.

18 Skin tumours

This chapter deals both with skin tumours arising from the epidermis and its appendages, and from the dermis (Table 18.1).

Prevention

Many skin tumours (e.g. actinic keratoses, lentigines, keratoacanthomas, basal cell carcinomas, squamous cell carcinomas, malignant melanomas and, arguably, acquired melanocytic naevi) would all become less common if Caucasoids, especially those with a fair skin, protected themselves adequately against sunlight. The education of those living in sunny climates or holidaying in the sun has already reaped great rewards here (Fig. 18.1). Successful campaigns have focused on regular self-examination and on reducing sun exposure by avoidance, clothing and sunscreen preparations (Figs 18.2 and 18.3). Public compliance has been encouraged by imaginative slogans like the Australian 'sun smart' and 'slip, slap and slop' (slip on the shirt, slap on the hat and slop on the sunscreen) advice, the

Table 18.1 Skin tumours.

Derived from	Benign	Premalignant/carcinoma in situ	Malignant
Epidermis and appendages	Viral wart Squamous cell papilloma Seborrhoeic keratosis Skin tag Linear epidermal naevus Milium Melanocytic naevus Epidermoid/pilar cyst Chondrodermatitis nodularis helicis (although, strictly, an inflammation)	Keratoacanthoma Intraepidermal carcinoma Actinic keratosis Sebaceous naevus	Basal cell carcinoma Squamous cell carcinoma Malignant melanoma Paget's disease of the nipple (although, strictly, a breast tumour)
Dermis	Haemangioma Lymphangioma Glomus tumour Pyogenic granuloma Dermatofibroma Neurofibroma Neuroma Keloid Lipoma Lymphocytoma cutis Mastocytosis		Kaposi's sarcoma Lymphoma Dermatofibrosarcoma protuberans Metastases

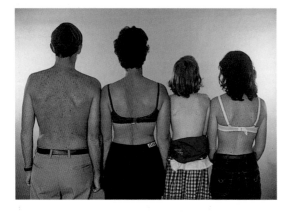

Fig. 18.1 This family lived in the tropics. No prizes for guessing which of them avoided the sun.

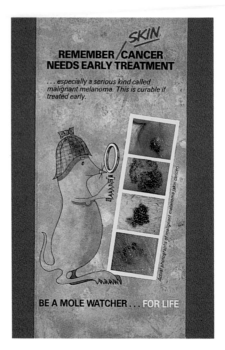

Fig. 18.2 An eye-catching and effective way of teaching the public how to look at their moles. A pamphlet produced by the Cancer Research Campaign in the UK.

American Academy of Dermatology 'ABCs' (away, block, cover up, shade) leaflet and that lovable American creature Joel Mole.

Tumours of the epidermis and its appendages

Benign

Viral warts

These are discussed in Chapter 13, but are mentioned here for two reasons: first, solitary warts are sometimes misdiagnosed on the face or hands of the elderly; and, secondly, a wart is one of the few tumours in humans that is, without doubt, caused by a virus. Seventy per cent of transplant patients who have been immunosuppressed for over 5 years have multiple viral warts and there is growing evidence that immunosuppression, viral warts and ultraviolet radiation interact in this setting to cause squamous cell carcinoma (p. 267).

Squamous cell papilloma

This common tumour, arising from keratinocytes, may resemble a viral wart clinically. Sometimes an excessive hyperkeratosis produces a horn-shaped excrescence (a 'cutaneous horn'). Excision, or curet-

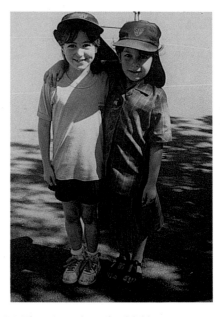

Fig. 18.3 These Australian schoolchildren are wearing legionnaire's caps with large peaks and flaps. These are becoming fashionable after several clever campaigns, and the 'no hat, no play' rule has become an accepted way of life.

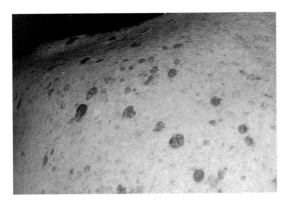

Fig. 18.4 Typical multiple seborrhoeic warts on the shoulder. Each individual lesion might look worryingly like a malignant melanoma but, in the numbers seen here, the lesions must be benign.

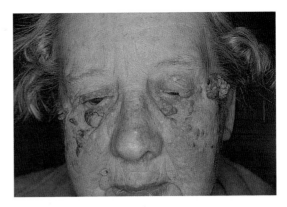

Fig. 18.5 Numerous unsightly seborrhoeic warts of the face.

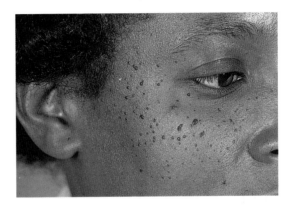

Fig. 18.6 Dermatosis papulosa nigra.

tage with cautery to the base, is the treatment of choice. The histology should be checked.

Seborrhoeic keratosis (basal cell papilloma, seborrhoeic wart)

This is a common benign epidermal tumour, unrelated to sebaceous glands. The term 'senile wart' should be avoided as it offends many patients.

Cause

Usually unexplained but:
• multiple lesions may be inherited (autosomal dominant);
• occasionally follow an inflammatory dermatosis; or
• very rarely, the sudden eruption of hundreds of itchy lesions is associated with an internal neoplasm (Leser–Trélat sign).

Presentation

Seborrhoeic keratoses usually arise after the age of 50 years, but flat inconspicuous lesions are often visible earlier. They are often multiple (Figs 18.4 and 18.5) but may be single. Lesions are most common on the face and trunk. The sexes are equally affected.
   Physical signs:
• a distinctive 'stuck-on' appearance;
• may be flat, raised or pedunculated;

• colour varies from yellow to dark brown; and
• surface may have greasy scaling and scattered keratin plugs ('currant bun' appearance).

Clinical course

Lesions may multiply with age but remain benign.

Differential diagnosis

Seborrhoeic keratoses are easily recognized. Occasionally they can be confused with a pigmented cellular naevus, a pigmented basal cell carcinoma and, most importantly, with a malignant melanoma. Some Afro-Caribbeans have many dark warty papules on their faces (dermatosis papulosa nigra; Fig. 18.6). Histologically these are like seborrhoeic warts.

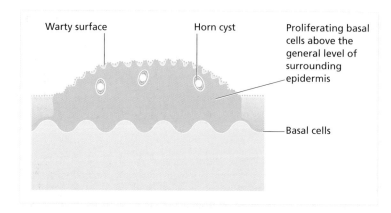

Fig. 18.7 Histology of a seborrhoeic keratosis.

Investigations

Biopsy is needed only in rare dubious cases. The histology is diagnostic (Fig. 18.7): the lesion lies above the general level of the surrounding epidermis and consists of proliferating basal cells and horn cysts.

Treatment

Seborrhoeic keratoses can safely be left alone, but ugly or easily traumatized ones can be removed with a curette under local anaesthetic (this has the advantage of providing histology), or by cryotherapy.

LEARNING POINT

If you cannot tell most seborrhoeic warts from a melanoma you will send too many elderly people unnecessarily to the pigmented lesion clinic.

Skin tags (acrochordon)

These common benign outgrowths of skin affect mainly the middle-aged and elderly.

Cause

This is unknown but the trait is sometimes familial. Skin tags are most common in obese women, and rarely are associated with tuberous sclerosis (p. 302), acanthosis nigricans (p. 383) or acromegaly, and diabetes.

Presentation and clinical course

Skin tags occur around the neck and within the major flexures. They look unsightly and may catch on clothing and jewellery. They are soft skin-coloured or pigmented pedunculated papules (Fig. 18.8).

Differential diagnosis

The appearance is unmistakable. Tags are rarely confused with small melanocytic naevi.

Treatment

Small lesions can be snipped off with fine scissors, frozen with liquid nitrogen, or destroyed with a hyfrecator without local anaesthesia. There is no way of preventing new ones from developing.

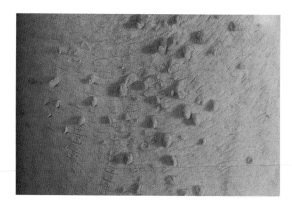

Fig. 18.8 Numerous axillary skin tags.

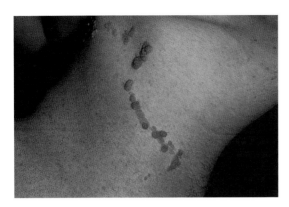

Fig. 18.9 Linear warty epidermal naevus.

Linear epidermal naevus

These lesions are an example of cutaneous mosaicism (p. 300) and so tend to follow Blaschko's lines (Fig. 18.9).

Melanocytic naevi

The term 'naevus' refers to a lesion, often present at birth, which has a local excess of one or more normal constituents of the skin. Melanocytic naevi (moles) are localized benign proliferations of melanocytes. Their classification (Table 18.2) is based on the site of the aggregations of naevus cells (Fig. 18.10).

Cause and evolution

The cause is unknown. A genetic factor is likely in many families, working together with excessive sun exposure during childhood.

Table 18.2 Classification of melanocytic naevi.

Congenital melanocytic naevi
Acquired melanocytic naevi
    Junctional naevus
    Compound naevus
    Intradermal naevus
    Spitz naevus
    Blue naevus
    Atypical melanocytic naevus

With the exception of congenital melanocytic naevi (see below), most appear in early childhood, often with a sharp increase in numbers during adolescence. Further crops may appear during pregnancy, oestrogen therapy or, rarely, after cytotoxic chemotherapy and immunosuppression, but new lesions come up less often after the age of 20 years.

Melanocytic naevi in childhood are usually of the 'junctional' type, with proliferating melanocytes in clumps at the dermo-epidermal junction. Later, the melanocytes round off and 'drop' into the dermis. A 'compound' naevus has both dermal and junctional components. With maturation the junctional component disappears so that the melanocytes in an 'intradermal' naevus are all in the dermis (Fig. 18.10).

Presentation

Congenital melanocytic naevi (Figs 18.11 and 18.12). These are present at birth or appear in the neonatal period and are seldom less than 1 cm in diameter. Their colour varies from brown to black or blue-black. With maturity some become protuberant

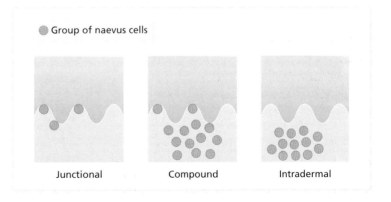

Group of naevus cells

Junctional   Compound   Intradermal

Fig. 18.10 Types of acquired melanocytic naevi.

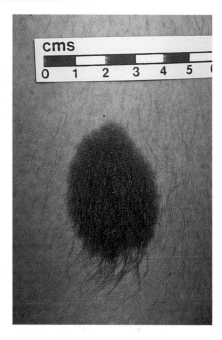

Fig. 18.11 Congenital melanocytic naevus.

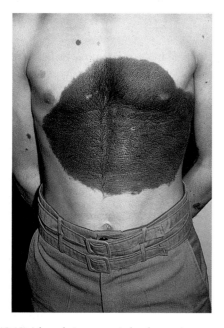

Fig. 18.12 A large hairy congenital melanocytic naevus. (Courtesy of Dr Auf Qaba, St John's Hospital, Livingstone.)

and hairy, with a cerebriform surface. Such lesions can be disfiguring, e.g. a 'bathing trunk' naevus, and carry an increased risk of malignant transformation.

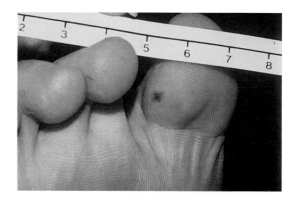

Fig. 18.13 Junctional melanocytic naevus.

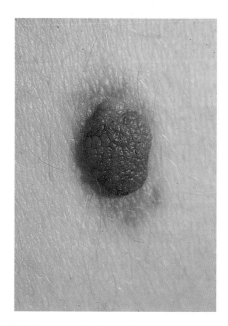

Fig. 18.14 Compound melanocytic naevus. No recent change.

Junctional melanocytic naevi (Fig. 18.13). These are roughly circular macules. Their colour ranges from mid to dark brown and may vary even within a single lesion. Most naevi of the palms, soles and genitals are of this type.

Compound melanocytic naevi (Fig. 18.14). These are domed pigmented nodules of up to 1 cm in diameter. They may be light or dark brown but their colour is more even than that of junctional naevi. Most are smooth, but larger ones may be cerebriform, or even hyperkeratotic and papillomatous; many bear hairs.

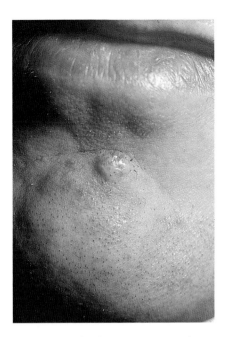

Fig. 18.15 Intradermal melanocytic naevus with numerous shaved hairs.

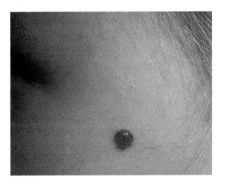

Fig. 18.16 Spitz naevus.

Intradermal melanocytic naevi (Fig. 18.15). These look like compound naevi but are less pigmented and often skin-coloured.

Spitz naevi (juvenile melanomas; Fig. 18.16). These are usually found in children. They develop over a month or two as solitary pink or red nodules of up to 1 cm in diameter and are most common on the face and legs. Although benign, they are often excised because of their rapid growth.

Blue naevi (Fig. 18.17). So-called because of their striking slate grey-blue colour, blue naevi usually

appear in childhood and adolescence, on the limbs, buttocks and lower back. They are usually solitary.

Mongolian spots. Pigment in dermal melanocytes is responsible for these bruise-like greyish areas seen on the lumbosacral area of most Down's syndrome and many Asian and black babies. They usually fade during childhood.

Atypical mole syndrome (dysplastic naevus syndrome; Fig. 18.18). Clinically atypical melanocytic naevi can

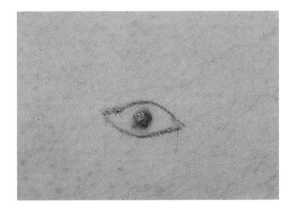

Fig. 18.17 The blue ink matches the blue naevus.

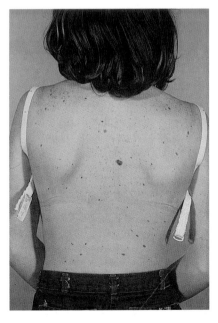

Fig. 18.18 Atypical moles in a 12-year-old girl. Note the malignant melanoma lying between the scapulae.

occur sporadically or run in families as an autosomal dominant trait, with incomplete penetrance, affecting several generations. Some families with atypical naevi are melanoma-prone. Genes for susceptibility to melanoma have been mapped to chromosomes 1p36 and 9p13 in a few of these families. The many large irregularly pigmented naevi are most obvious on the trunk but some may be present on the scalp. Their edges are irregular and they vary greatly in size—many being over 1 cm in diameter. Some are pinkish and an inflamed halo may surround them. Some have a mamillated surface. Patients with multiple atypical melanocytic or dysplastic naevi with a positive family history of malignant melanoma should be followed up 6-monthly for life.

Differential diagnosis of melanocytic naevi

• *Malignant melanomas.* This is the most important part of the differential diagnosis. Melanomas are very rare before puberty, single and more variably pigmented and irregularly shaped (other features are listed below under Complications).
• *Seborrhoeic keratoses.* These can cause confusion in adults but have a stuck-on appearance and are warty. Tell-tale keratin plugs and horny cysts may be seen with the help of a lens.
• *Lentigines.* These may be found on any part of the skin and mucous membranes. More profuse than junctional naevi, they are usually grey-brown rather than black, and develop more often after adolescence.
• *Ephelides* (freckles). These are tan macules less than 5 mm in diameter. They are confined to sun-exposed areas, being most common in blond or red-haired people.
• *Haemangiomas.* Benign proliferations of blood vessels, including haemangiomas and pyogenic granulomas, may be confused with a vascular Spitz naevus or an amelanotic melanoma.

Histology

Most acquired lesions fit into the scheme given in Fig. 18.10: orderly nests of benign naevus cells are seen in the junctional region, in the dermis, or in both. However, some types of melanocytic naevi have their own distinguishing features. In congenital naevi the naevus cells may extend to the subcutaneous fat, and hyperplasia of other skin components (e.g. hair follicles)

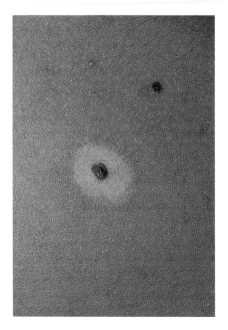

Fig. 18.19 Halo naevus.

may be seen. A Spitz naevus has a histology worryingly similar to that of a melanoma. It shows dermal oedema and dilatated capillaries, and is composed of large epithelioid and spindle-shaped naevus cells, some of which may be in mitosis.

In a blue naevus, naevus cells are seen in the mid and deep dermis.

The main features of clinically atypical ('dysplastic') naevi are lengthening and bridging of rete ridges, and the presence of junctional nests showing melanocytic dysplasia (nuclear pleomorphism and hyperchromatism). Fibrosis of the papillary dermis and a lymphocytic inflammatory response are also seen.

Complications

• *Inflammation.* Pain and swelling are common but are not features of malignant transformation. They are caused by trauma, bacterial folliculitis or a foreign body reaction to hair after shaving or plucking.
• *Depigmented halo* (Fig. 18.19). So-called 'halo naevi' are uncommon but benign. There may be vitiligo elsewhere. The naevus in the centre often involutes spontaneously before the halo repigments.
• *Malignant change.* This is extremely rare except in congenital melanocytic naevi, where the risk has

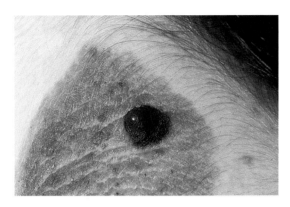

Fig. 18.20 Malignant melanoma developing within a congenital melanocytic naevus.

been estimated at between 3 and 6% depending on their size (Fig. 18.20), and in the atypical naevi of melanoma-prone families. It should be considered if the following changes occur in a melanocytic naevus:

- itch;
- enlargement;
- increased or decreased pigmentation;
- altered shape;
- altered contour;
- inflammation;
- ulceration; or
- bleeding.

If changing lesions are examined carefully, remembering the 'ABCDE' features of malignant melanoma (Table 18.3), few malignant melanomas should be missed.

Treatment

Excision is needed when:
1 a naevus is unsightly;
2 malignancy is suspected or is a known risk, e.g. in a large congenital melanocytic naevus; or
3 a naevus is repeatedly inflamed or traumatized.

Table 18.3 The ABCDE of malignant melanoma.

Asymmetry
Border irregularity
Colour variability
Diameter greater than 0.5 cm
Elevation irregularity

LEARNING POINT

Even if you think it is harmless, do not be afraid to refer a mole that has changed to a dermatologist.

Epidermoid and pilar cysts

Often incorrectly called 'sebaceous cysts', these are common and can occur on the scalp, face, behind the ears and on the trunk. They often have a central punctum; when they rupture, or are squeezed, foul-smelling cheesy material comes out. Histologically, the lining of a cyst resembles normal epidermis (an epidermoid cyst) or the outer root sheath of the hair follicle (a pilar cyst). Occasionally an adjacent foreign body reaction is noted. Treatment is by excision, or by incision followed by expression of the contents and removal of the cyst wall.

Milia

Milia are small subepidermal keratin cysts (Fig. 18.21). They are common on the face in all age groups and appear as tiny white millet seed-like papules of from 0.5 to 2 mm in diameter. They are occasionally seen at the site of a previous subepidermal blister (e.g. in epidermolysis bullosa and porphyria cutanea tarda). The contents of milia can be picked out with a sterile needle without local anaesthesia.

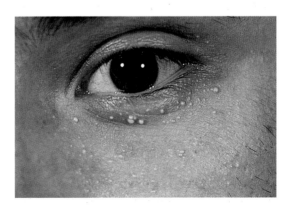

Fig. 18.21 Milia.

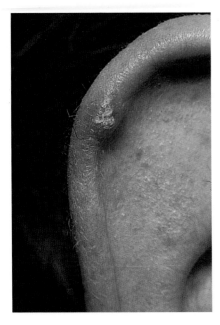

Fig. 18.22 Chondrodermatitis nodularis helicis. The inflammation of the underlying cartilage is painful enough to wake up patients repeatedly at night.

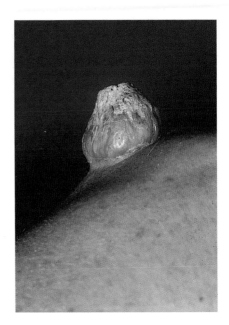

Fig. 18.23 Keratoacanthoma with its epidermal shoulders and central plug of keratin.

Chondrodermatitis nodularis helicis (painful nodule of the ear, ear corn; Fig. 18.22)

This terminological mouthful is, strictly, not a neoplasm, but a chronic inflammation. A painful nodule develops on the helix or antehelix of the ear, most often in men. It looks like a small corn, is tender and prevents sleep if that side of the head touches the pillow. Histologically, a thickened epidermis overlies inflamed cartilage. Wedge resection under local anaesthetic is effective if cryotherapy or intralesional triamcinolone injection fails.

Premalignant tumours

Keratoacanthoma

Some argue that this rapidly growing tumour should be classed as benign, but a very few transform into a squamous cell carcinoma.

Cause

Photosensitizing chemicals such as tar and mineral oils can act as cocarcinogens with ultraviolet radiation. They may also follow therapeutic immunosuppression.

Clinical features

They occur mainly on the exposed skin of fair individuals. More than two-thirds are on the face and most of the rest are on the arms. The lesion starts as a pink papule that rapidly enlarges; it may reach a diameter of 1 cm in a month or two. After 5 or 6 weeks the centre of the nodule forms either a keratinous plug or a crater (Fig. 18.23). If left, the lesion often resolves spontaneously over 6–12 months but leaves an ugly depressed scar.

Differential diagnosis

Squamous cell carcinoma is the main tumour to be distinguished from a keratoacanthoma. However, carcinomas grow more slowly and usually lack symmetry.

Histology

It is not possible to tell a keratoacanthoma from a squamous cell carcinoma histologically unless the architecture of the whole lesion can be assessed, including its base (Fig. 18.24). A typical lesion is symmetrical and composed of proliferating fronds

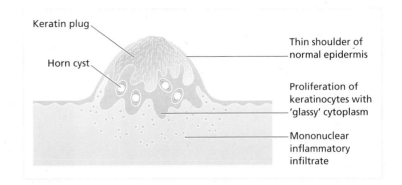

Keratin plug

Horn cyst

Thin shoulder of
normal epidermis

Proliferation of
keratinocytes with
'glassy' cytoplasm

Mononuclear
inflammatory
infiltrate

Fig. 18.24 Histology of
keratoacanthoma.

of epidermis that show mitotic activity but retain a well-differentiated squamous appearance with the production of much 'glassy' keratin. The centre of the cup-shaped mass is filled with keratin.

Treatment

Excision or curettage and cautery are both effective. Occasionally, a further curetting may be needed but this should be performed only once; if this is still ineffective, the lesion must be excised.

Intraepidermal carcinoma (Bowen's disease)

Usually single, these slowly expanding pink scaly plaques (Fig. 18.25) take years to reach a diameter of a few centimetres. Their border is sharply defined, with reniform projections and notches. About 3%

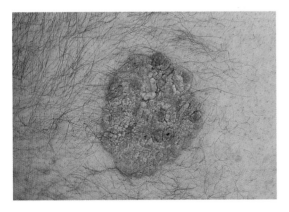

Fig. 18.25 Intraepidermal carcinoma: a slowly expanding warty plaque. Note the reniform projections and notches so suggestive of an *in situ* malignancy.

progress into an invasive squamous cell carcinoma. The presence of several may be a clue to previous exposure to carcinogens (e.g. excessive sun exposure, arsenic in a tonic when young).

Differential diagnosis

An intraepidermal carcinoma is often mistaken for psoriasis (Chapter 5), discoid eczema (p. 89), superficial basal cell carcinoma (see below) or for Paget's disease in the peri-anal region.

Treatment

These lesions are unaffected by local steroids. Small lesions may occasionally be left under observation in the frail and elderly. Cryotherapy or curettage are the treatments of choice for small lesions on a site where healing should be good (e.g. face or trunk); excision is an alternative. Photodynamic therapy (p. 325) is useful for large lesions on a poor healing site (e.g. the lower legs of the elderly). Topical 5-fluorouracil or imiquimod is helpful for multiple lesions (see Guidelines in Further reading).

Actinic keratoses

These discrete rough-surfaced lesions crop up on sun-damaged skin. They are premalignant, although only a few turn into a squamous cell carcinoma.

Cause

The effects of sun exposure are cumulative. Those with fair complexions living near the equator are most at risk and invariably develop these 'sun warts'.

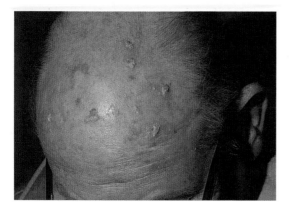

Fig. 18.26 Typical rough-surfaced actinic keratoses on the scalp.

A recent UK survey showed that one-third of men over 70 years had actinic keratoses. Melanin protects, and actinic keratoses are not seen in black skin. Conversely, albinos are especially prone to develop them.

Presentation

They affect the middle-aged and elderly in temperate climates, but younger people in the tropics. The pink or grey rough scaling macules or papules seldom exceed 1 cm in diameter (Fig. 18.26). Their rough surface is sometimes better felt than seen.

Complications

Transition to a squamous cell carcinoma, although rare, should be suspected if a lesion enlarges, ulcerates or bleeds. Luckily such tumours seldom metastasize. A 'cutaneous horn' is a hard keratotic protrusion based on an actinic keratosis, a squamous cell papilloma or a viral wart (Fig. 18.27).

Differential diagnosis

There is usually no difficulty in telling an actinic keratosis from a seborrhoeic wart, a viral wart (p. 201), a keratoacanthoma, an intraepidermal carcinoma or a squamous cell carcinoma.

Investigations

A biopsy is needed if there is concern over malignant change.

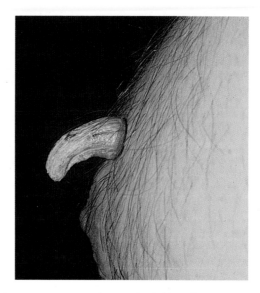

Fig. 18.27 Cutaneous horn with a bulbous fleshy base.

Histology

Alternating zones of hyper- and parakeratosis overlie a thickened or atrophic epidermis. The normal maturation pattern of the epidermis may be lost and occasional pleomorphic keratinocytes may be seen. Solar elastosis is seen in the superficial dermis.

Treatment

Freezing with liquid nitrogen or carbon dioxide snow is simple and effective. Curettage is best for large lesions and cutaneous horns. Multiple lesions, including subclinical ones, can be treated with 5-fluorouracil cream (Formulary 1, p. 338) after specialist advice. The cream is applied once or twice daily until there is a marked inflammatory response in the treated area. This takes about 3 weeks and only then should the applications be stopped. Healing is rapid and most patients are very pleased with their 'new' smooth skin. Severe discomfort from the treatment may be alleviated by the short-term application of a local steroid. 5-Fluorouracil cream is more effective for keratoses on the face than on the arms. Alternatively, less effective but causing less inflammation, 5-fluorouracil cream can be applied on just one or two days a week for 8 weeks. Recently, 3% sodium diclofenac made up in a hyaluronan gel has come on the market with a product licence to treat actinic

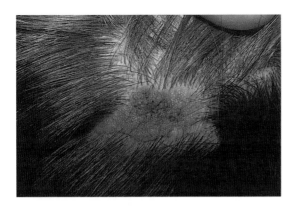

Fig. 18.28 Sebaceous naevus of the scalp.

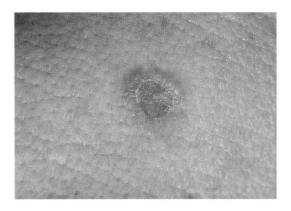

Fig. 18.29 Early basal cell carcinoma with rolled opalescent edge and central crusting.

keratoses but it is too early to judge its efficacy. Photo-dynamic therapy (p. 325), using aminolaevulinic acid hydrochloride followed by blue light, is effective but requires specialist facilities. Lesions that do not respond should be regarded with suspicion, and biopsied.

Sebaceous naevi (Fig. 18.28)

A flat hairless area at birth, usually in the scalp, these naevi become yellower and more raised at puberty. Basal cell carcinomas appear on some in adult life.

Malignant epidermal tumours

Basal cell carcinoma (rodent ulcer)

This is the most common form of skin cancer. It crops up most commonly on the faces of the middle-aged or elderly. Lesions invade locally but, for practical purposes, never metastasize.

Cause

Prolonged sun exposure is the main factor so these tumours are most common in white people living near the equator. They may also occur in scars caused by X-rays, vaccination or trauma. Photosensitizing pitch, tar and oils can act as cocarcinogens with ultraviolet radiation. Previous treatment with arsenic, once present in many 'tonics', predisposes to multiple basal cell carcinomas, often after a lag of many years.

Multiple basal cell carcinomas are found in the naevoid basal cell carcinoma syndrome (Gorlin's syndrome) where they may be associated with pal-

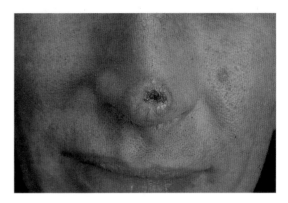

Fig. 18.30 Basal cell carcinoma with marked telangiectasia and ulceration.

moplantar pits, jaw cysts and abnormalities of the skull, vertebrae and ribs. The syndrome is inherited as an autosomal dominant trait and recent studies indicate that the genetic abnormality lies on chromosome 9q.

Presentation

Nodulo-ulcerative. This is the most common type. An early lesion is a small glistening translucent skin-coloured papule that slowly enlarges. Central necrosis, although not invariable, leaves an ulcer with an adherent crust and a rolled pearly edge (Fig. 18.29). Fine telangiectatic vessels often run across the tumour's surface (Fig. 18.30). Without treatment such lesions may reach 1–2 cm in diameter in 5–10 years.

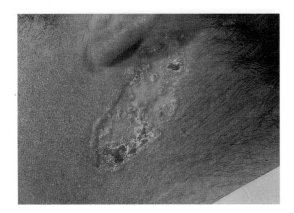

Fig. 18.31 Cicatricial basal cell carcinoma.

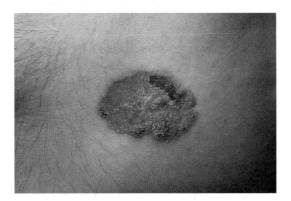

Fig. 18.32 Persistent scaly plaque—the whipcord edge gives away the diagnosis of a superficial basal cell carcinoma.

Cystic. The lesion is at first like the nodular type, but later cystic changes predominate and the nodule becomes tense and more translucent, with marked telangiectasia.

Cicatricial (morphoeic). These are slowly expanding yellow or white waxy plaques with an ill-defined edge. Ulceration and crusting, followed by fibrosis, are common, and the lesion may look like an enlarging scar (Fig. 18.31).

Superficial (multicentric). These arise most often on the trunk. Several lesions may be present, each expanding slowly as a pink or brown scaly plaque with a fine 'whipcord' edge (Fig. 18.32). Such lesions can grow to more than 10 cm in diameter.

Pigmented. Pigment may be present in all types of basal cell carcinoma causing all or part of the tumour

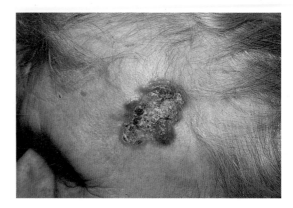

Fig. 18.33 A pigmented tumour on the temple. The opalescent rim points to the diagnosis of a basal cell carcinoma.

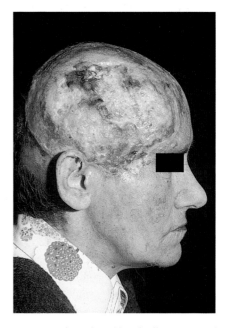

Fig. 18.34 A grossly neglected basal cell carcinoma already invading underlying bone.

to be brown or have specks of brown or black within it (Fig. 18.33).

Clinical course

The slow but relentless growth destroys tissue locally. Untreated, a basal cell carcinoma can invade underlying cartilage or bone (Fig. 18.34) or damage important structures such as the tear ducts.

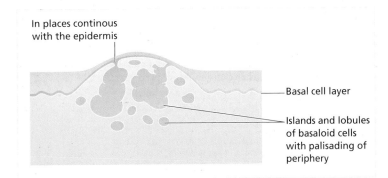

In places continous
with the epidermis

Basal cell layer

Islands and lobules
of basaloid cells
with palisading of
periphery

Fig. 18.35 Histology of nodular basal
cell carcinoma.

Histology

Small, darkly blue staining basal cells grow in well-
defined aggregates which invade the dermis (Fig. 18.35).
The outer layer of cells is arranged in a palisade. Numerous mitoses and apoptotic bodies are seen. In the
cicatricial type the islands of tumour are surrounded
by fibrous tissue.

Differential diagnosis

A nodular basal cell carcinoma may be confused with
an intradermal melanocytic naevus, a squamous cell
carcinoma, a giant molluscum contagiosum (p. 209)
or a keratoacanthoma. Pigmented basal cell carcinomas should be distinguished from seborrhoeic warts
and malignant melanomas. A cicatricial basal cell
carcinoma may mimic morphoea (p. 129) or a scar. A
superficial basal cell carcinoma may be confused with
an intraepidermal carcinoma, with psoriasis (Chapter 5) or with nummular eczema (p. 89).

Treatment

There is no single treatment of choice for all basal cell
carcinomas. Treatment should be tailored to the type
of tumour, its site and the age and general health of
the patient. Published guidelines are very useful (see
Further reading).

In general, excision, with 0.5 cm of surrounding
normal skin, is the treatment of choice for discrete
nodular and cystic tumours in patients under 60 years.
Cicatricial tumours, with their ill-defined edges,
and lesions near vital structures, should be excised
by specialist surgeons. Mohs' micrographic surgical

technique is highly effective; it includes careful histological checks in all planes of tissue excised during the
operation (see p. 323). Mohs' surgery is also becoming the treatment of choice for large (> 1 cm) tumours
and for those on cosmetically important sites, such as
the nose, and for tumours in certain anatomical areas,
such as the inner canthus and the nasolabial folds.
Radiotherapy is also effective; it is seldom used now
for biopsy-proven lesions in patients under 70 years,
but is helpful when surgery is contraindicated. Cryotherapy, curettage and cautery and photodynamic
therapy are sometimes useful for superficial lesions
(p. 325). Sometimes palliative treatment with curettage
and cautery may be preferable to aggressive treatment
for elderly patients in poor health; nowadays there
is seldom justification for doing nothing. The 5-year
cure rate for all types of basal cell carcinoma is over
95%, but regular follow-up is necessary to detect
local recurrences when they are small and remediable.

LEARNING POINTS

1 Catch lesions early: small ones are easy to
get rid of; larger ones can eat into cartilage
or bone.
2 Do not sit and watch doubtful lesions near
the eye.

Squamous cell carcinoma

This is a common tumour in which malignant keratinocytes show a variable capacity to form keratin.

Cause

These tumours often arise in skin damaged by long-term ultraviolet radiation and also by X-rays and infrared rays. Other carcinogens include pitch, tar, mineral oils and inorganic arsenic (see Basal cell carcinoma). Certain rare genetic disorders, with defective DNA repair mechanisms, such as xeroderma pigmentosum (p. 304), lead to multiple squamous and basal cell carcinomas, and to malignant melanoma; this illustrates the importance of altered DNA in the pathogenesis of malignancy. The DNA of the human papilloma virus (p. 201) can be integrated into the nuclear DNA of keratinocytes and cause malignant transformation. Immunosuppression and ultraviolet radiation predispose to this.

Multiple self-healing squamous cell carcinomas are found in the autosomal dominant trait described by Ferguson-Smith. The abnormal gene lies on chromosome 9q.

Clinical presentation and course

Tumours may arise as thickenings in an actinic keratosis or, *de novo*, as small scaling nodules; rapidly growing anaplastic lesions may start as ulcers with a granulating base and an indurated edge (Fig. 18.36). Squamous cell carcinomas are common on the lower lip (Fig. 13.36) and in the mouth. Tumours arising in areas of previous X-radiation or thermal injury, chronic draining sinuses, chronic ulcers, chronic inflammation or Bowen's disease are the most likely to metastasize. Tumours arising in non-exposed sites, such as the perineum and sole of foot and on the ear and lip, have a lesser malignant potential but may metastasize. Squamous cell carcinomas arising in sun-exposed areas and in actinic keratoses seldom metastasize. Tumours more than 2 cm in diameter are twice as likely to recur and metastasize compared with smaller tumours. Metastatic potential is also high in tumours greater than 4 mm in depth or invading to the subcutaneous tissue, in poorly differentiated tumours; in tumours with perineural involvement; and in those arising in the immunosuppressed.

Histology

Keratinocytes disrupt the dermo-epidermal junction and proliferate irregularly into the dermis. Malignant

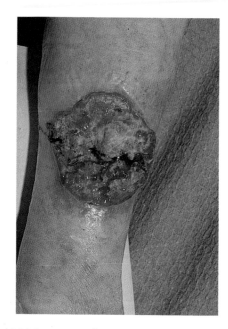

Fig. 18.36 Squamous cell carcinoma. Not a venous ulcer—too high up the leg, too raised, and no signs of venous insufficiency.

cells usually retain the capacity to produce keratin (Fig. 18.37).

Treatment

After the diagnosis has been confirmed by biopsy, the tumour should be excised with a 0.5-cm border of normal skin. Mohs' micrographic surgery is useful for high-risk tumours. Radiotherapy is effective but should be reserved for the frail and the elderly.

Malignant melanoma

Malignant melanoma attracts a disproportionate amount of attention because it is so often lethal. The public now knows more about its increasing incidence and dangers.

Incidence

The incidence in white people in the UK and USA is doubling every 10 years. In Scotland and northern parts of the USA the incidence is now about 10 per 100 000 per year, with females being affected more often than males. There is a higher incidence in white

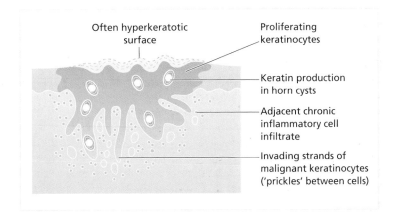

Often hyperkeratotic surface

Proliferating keratinocytes

Keratin production in horn cysts

Adjacent chronic inflammatory cell infiltrate

Invading strands of malignant keratinocytes ('prickles' between cells)

Fig. 18.37 The histology of a squamous cell carcinoma.

people living near the equator than in temperate zones and there the female preponderance is lost. The highest incidence, more than 40 per 100 000 per year, is seen in white people living in Australia and New Zealand. The tumour is rare before puberty and in black people, Asians and Orientals and when it does occur in these races it is most often on the palms, soles or mucous membranes.

Cause

Genetic. Malignant melanomas are most common in white people with blond or red hair, many freckles and a fair skin that tans poorly. Those of Celtic origin are especially susceptible. Ten to 15% of melanomas are familial (occur in families where two or more first-degree relatives have a melanoma). Molecular defects in both tumour suppressor genes and oncogenes have been linked to these melanomas; the one attracting most interest at present lies on chromosome 9p and encodes a tumour suppressor gene designated p16, also known as *CDKN2A*. Melanoma may affect several members of a single family in association with atypical (dysplastic) naevi (p. 259).

Sunlight. Both the incidence and mortality increase with decreasing latitude. Tumours occur most often, but not exclusively, on exposed skin.

Pre-existing melanocytic naevi. The risk of developing a malignant melanoma is highest in those with atypical naevi, congenital melanocytic naevi or many banal melanocytic naevi. A pre-existing naevus is seen histologically in about 30% of malignant melanomas.

Clinical features

Eighty per cent of invasive melanomas are preceded by a superficial and radial growth phase, shown clinically as the expansion of an irregularly pigmented macule or plaque (Fig. 18.38). Most are multicoloured mixtures of black, brown, blue, tan and pink. Their margins are irregular with reniform projections and notches. Malignant cells are at first usually confined to the epidermis and uppermost dermis, but eventually invade more deeply and may metastasize (Fig. 18.38).

There are four main types of malignant melanoma.
1 *Lentigo maligna melanoma* occurs on the exposed skin of the elderly. An irregularly pigmented, irregularly shaped macule (a lentigo maligna) may have been enlarging slowly for many years as an *in situ* melanoma before an invasive nodule (the lentigo maligna melanoma) appears (Fig. 18.39).
2 *Superficial spreading melanoma* is the most common type in Caucasoids. Its radial growth phase shows varied colours and is often palpable (Figs 18.40 and 18.41). A nodule coming up within such a plaque signifies deep dermal invasion and a poor prognosis (Table 18.4).
3 *Acral lentiginous melanoma* occurs on the palms and soles and, although rare in Caucasoids, is the most common type in Chinese and Japanese people. The invasive phase is again signalled by a nodule coming up within an irregularly pigmented macule or patch.
4 *Nodular melanoma* (Fig. 18.42) appears as a pigmented nodule with no preceding *in situ* phase. It is the most rapidly growing and aggressive type.

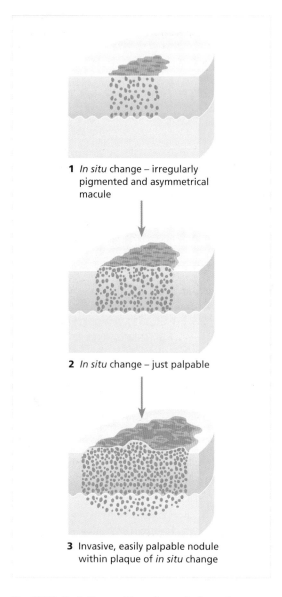

1 *In situ* change – irregularly pigmented and asymmetrical macule

2 *In situ* change – just palpable

3 Invasive, easily palpable nodule within plaque of *in situ* change

Fig. 18.38 Radial intraepidermal growth phase of melanoma (1 and 2) precedes vertical and invasive dermal growth phase (3).

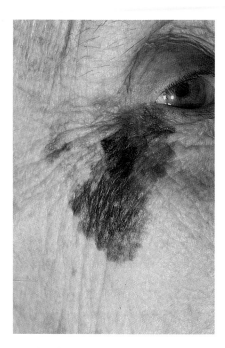

Fig. 18.39 This elderly patient, her friends and family doctor, had ignored for too long the slowly spreading macule of a lentigo maligna: now she has a frankly invasive melanoma within it (the darker area).

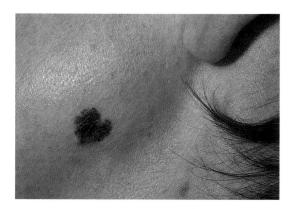

Fig. 18.40 Superficial spreading melanoma of the jawline. Small, and still curable at this stage.

Melanomas can also described by their colour, site and degree of spread.

• *Totally amelanotic melanomas* (Fig. 18.43) are rare and occur especially on the soles of the feet. Flecks of pigment can usually be seen with a lens.

• *Subungual melanomas* are painless areas of pigmentation expanding under the nail and onto the nail fold.

• *Metastatic melanoma* has spread to surrounding skin, regional lymph nodes or to other organs. At this stage it can rarely be cured.

Staging

The most popular staging systems for melanoma are the TNM classification (Europe) and the American

Table 18.4 Staging systems for melanoma.

TNM stage	AJCC stage	Breslow thickness (mm)	5-year survival (%)
I	Ia	Up to 0.75	95
	Ib	0.76–1.5	85
II	IIa	1.51–4.0	65
III	IIb	> 4.0	45
	III	Nodal disease	40
IV	IV	Metastatic disease	< 10

TNM, tumour, node, metastasis; AJCC, American Joint Committee on Cancer.

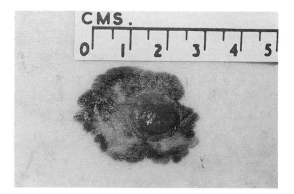

Fig. 18.41 This shows the hallmarks of a malignant melanoma with its asymmetry, irregular borders and variations in colour. The pink amelanotic nodule signifies deep dermal invasion.

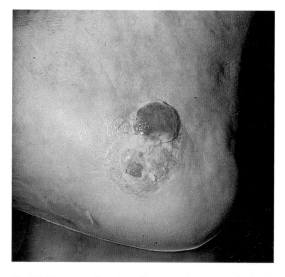

Fig. 18.43 An amelanotic malignant melanoma on the heel of an elderly person. Always obtain histology even if you think it is just a pyogenic granuloma or an atypical wart.

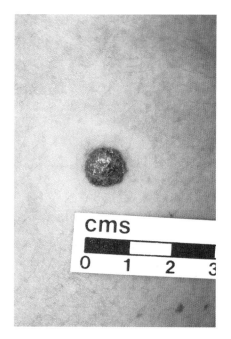

Fig. 18.42 A nodular malignant melanoma: just beginning to ulcerate.

Joint Committee on Cancer (AJCC) system in the USA (Table 18.4). They provide a useful guide to prognosis (see also Table 18.5).

Histology

- *Lentigo maligna.* Numerous atypical melanocytes, many in groups, are seen along the basal layer extending downwards in the walls of hair follicles.
- *Lentigo maligna melanoma.* Dermal invasion occurs, with a breach of the basement membrane region. *In situ* changes are seen in the adjacent epidermis.
- *Superficial spreading melanoma* in situ. Large epithelioid melanoma cells permeate the epidermis.
- *Superficial spreading melanoma.* The dermal nodule may be composed of epithelioid cells, spindle cells or naevus-like cells. *In situ* changes are seen in the adjacent epidermis.

Table 18.5 Prognostic indicators in malignant melanoma.

Indicator	Significance
Depth of primary tumour	Breslow < 0.75 mm, 5-year survival 95% 0.76–1.5 mm, 5-year survival 85% 1.51–4.0 mm, 5-year survival 65% > 4.0 mm, 5-year survival 45%
Sex	Females do better than males
Age	Prognosis worsens after 50 years of age, especially in males
Site	The prognosis is poor for tumours on trunk, upper arms, neck and scalp
Ulceration	Signifies a poor prognosis
Clinical stage	Prognosis worsens with advancing stage (see Table 18.4)

- *Acral lentiginous melanoma* in situ. Atypical melanocytes are seen in the base of the epidermis and permeating the mid epidermis.
- *Acral lentiginous melanoma*. Melanoma cells invade the dermis. *In situ* changes are seen in the adjacent epidermis.
- *Nodular melanoma*. The tumour comprises epithelioid, spindle and naevoid cells and there is no *in situ* melanoma in the adjacent epidermis.

Microstaging

The histology (Fig. 18.44) can be used to assess prognosis. Breslow's method is to measure, with an ocular micrometer, the vertical distance from the granular cell layer to the deepest part of the tumour. Clark's method is to assess the depth of penetration of the melanoma (Fig. 18.45) in relation to the different

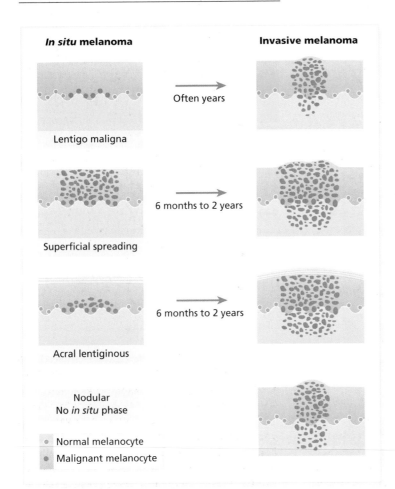

Fig. 18.44 Histology of the different types of melanoma.

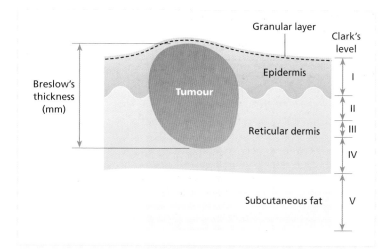

Fig. 18.45 Schematic representation of Breslow's and Clark's methods of microstaging malignant melanoma.

layers of the dermis. The thicker and more penetrating a lesion, the worse is its prognosis (see below).

Differential diagnosis

This includes a melanocytic naevus, seborrhoeic keratosis, pigmented actinic keratosis, pigmented basal cell carcinoma and sclerosing haemangioma; all are discussed in this chapter. A malignant melanoma can also be confused with a subungual or peri-ungual haematoma (see Fig. 13.21). A history of trauma helps here, as may paring. 'Talon noir' (Fig. 18.46) is a pigmented petechial area on the heel following minor trauma from ill-fitting training shoes. An amelanotic melanoma is most often confused with a pyogenic granuloma and with a squamous cell carcinoma.

Prognosis

The prognostic indicators, and their significance, are listed in Table 18.5. They have been established by following up large numbers of patients who have undergone appropriate surgical treatment (see below).

Treatment

Surgery. Surgical excision, with minimal delay, is required. An excision biopsy, with a 2-mm margin of clearance laterally, and down to the subcutaneous fat, is recommended for all suspicious lesions. If the histology confirms the diagnosis of malignant melanoma then wider excision, including the wound

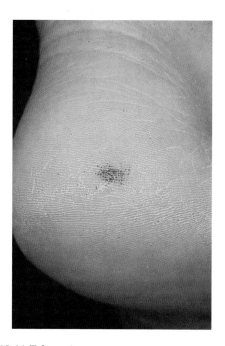

Fig. 18.46 Talon noir.

of the excision biopsy, should be performed as soon as possible. A minimum of 0.5 cm clearance for in situ melanomas and 1 cm clearance is required for all invasive melanomas. Nowadays many surgeons excise 1 cm of normal skin around the tumour (or wound) for every millimetre of tumour thickness, up to 3 mm (Fig. 18.47). The maximum clearance is thus 3 cm of normal skin and, depending on the site, primary closure—without grafting—is often possible. There is

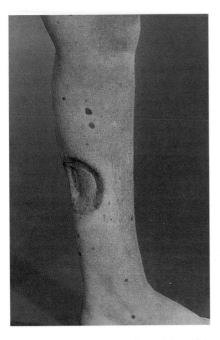

Fig. 18.47 Such a wide excision and unsightly graft is no longer acceptable for a thin good-prognosis melanoma. Note the many atypical moles.

no convincing evidence that excision margins wider than 3 cm confer any greater survival advantage. Tissue is removed down to, but not including, the deep fascia.

Elective regional node dissection may benefit patients with tumours of intermediate thickness (1.5–4.0 mm). The role of sentinel node biopsy in detecting occult metastases is currently being investigated in patients with melanomas greater than 1 mm thick, with the aim of carrying out elective dissection of the local nodes in positive cases, avoiding this significant procedure when the sentinel node is not involved. The sentinel node, the first and often nearest local node in the lymphatic drainage of the tumour, is detected by a blue dye and a radiolabelled colloid injected intradermally around the tumour before excision. The detection of a positive sentinel node does correlate with prognosis but, as yet, it remains to be shown that patients benefit from subsequent wide dissection of the nodes in the local basin or other adjuvant treatment (e.g. α-interferon) after a positive sentinel node is found.

Immunological treatments. Surgery cures most patients with early melanoma, but its effect on survival lessens as the disease advances. Many ongoing trials are investigating the role of immunotherapy (e.g. with melanoma-specific antigens) as an adjunct to surgery in patients with poor prognostic (e.g. TNM stages II and III) melanomas. Low dose α-interferon appears to improve the disease-free survival time and high-dose regimens may improve overall survival rates. The results of randomized control studies of adjunctive treatment with various melanoma vaccines are awaited with interest.

Chemotherapy. Although rarely curative, chemotherapy may be palliative in 25% of patients with stage III melanoma.

Paget's disease of the nipple (Fig. 18.48)

A well-defined red scaly plaque spreads slowly over and around the nipple. It is caused by the invasion of the epidermis by cells from an underlying intraductal carcinoma of the breast (Paget cells). The condition is unilateral, whereas eczema usually affects both nipples. A skin biopsy should be carried out first and if the diagnosis is confirmed mastectomy will be

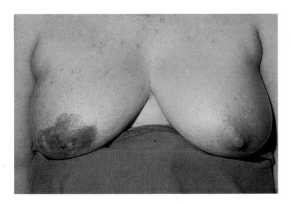

Fig. 18.48 Be alert to the possibility of Paget's disease if a red plaque affects only one nipple, and alters its normal architecture.

Table 18.6 Common vascular naevi.

Malformations
Present at birth. Do not involute ('salmon' patch is exception)
1 Capillary ('salmon' patch and 'port-wine' stain)
2 Arterial
3 Venous
4 Combined

Haemangiomas (sometimes called angiomatous naevi)
Usually appear after birth. More common in females, 50–60% on head and neck. Involute by 5–9 years after initial proliferation
1 Superficial (capillary)
2 Deep (cavernous)
3 Mixed

necessary. Extramammary Paget's disease affects sites bearing apocrine glands (p. 161) and is caused by an underlying ductal carcinoma of these.

Tumours of the dermis

Benign

Developmental abnormalities of blood vessels

These are either present at birth or appear soon after. They can be classified clinically (Table 18.6) but there is no good clinicohistological correlation. A capillary malformation is composed of a network of capillaries in the upper and mid dermis. A capillary cavernous haemangioma has multiple ectatic channels of varying calibre distributed throughout the dermis and even the subcutaneous fat.

Malformations

'Salmon' patches ('stork bites')

These common malformations, present in about 50% of all babies, are caused by dilated capillaries in the superficial dermis. They are dull red, often telangiectatic macules, most commonly on the nape of the neck ('erythema nuchae'), the forehead and the upper eyelids. Nuchal lesions may remain unchanged, but patches in other areas usually disappear within a year.

'Port-wine' stains

These are also present at birth and are caused by dilated dermal capillaries. They are pale, pink to purple macules, and vary from the barely noticeable to the grossly disfiguring. Most occur on the face or trunk. They persist, and in middle age may darken and become studded with angiomatous nodules (Fig. 18.49). Occasionally a port-wine stain of the trigeminal area (Fig. 18.50) is associated with a vascular malformation of the leptomeninges on the same side, which may cause epilepsy or hemiparesis (the Sturge–Weber syndrome), or with glaucoma.

Excellent results have been obtained with careful —and time-consuming—treatment with a 585-nm flashlamp-pumped pulsed dye laser (p. 327). Treatment sessions can begin in babies and anaesthesia is not always necessary. If a trial patch is satisfactory, 40–50 pulses can be delivered in a session and the procedure can be repeated at 3-monthly intervals. On the other hand, some adults become very adept at using cosmetic camouflage (see Fig. 1.6).

Combined vascular malformations of the limbs

A large port-wine stain of a limb may be associated with overgrowth of all the soft tissues of that limb with or without bony hypertrophy. There may be underlying venous malformations (Klippel–Trenaunay syndrome), arteriovenous fistulae (Parkes Weber syndrome) or mixed venous–lymphatic malformations.

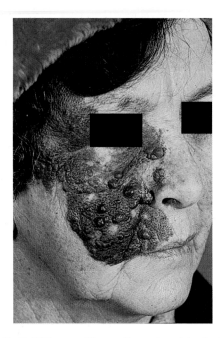

Fig. 18.49 Lifelong capillary malformation of the cheek showing no tendency to resolve. Note port-wine appearance of the upper pole, contrasting with the nodular elements elsewhere.

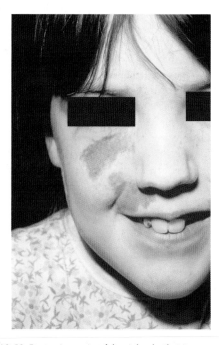

Fig. 18.50 Port-wine stain of the right cheek. No neurological problems in this patient.

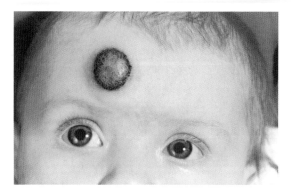

Fig. 18.51 Classical strawberry naevus, occurred and enlarged rapidly shortly after birth. (Courtesy of Dr M.J. Tidman, The Royal Infirmary of Edinburgh, Edinburgh, UK.)

Haemangiomas

Capillary cavernous haemangioma (strawberry naevus)

Strawberry naevi appear within a few weeks of birth, and grow for a few months, forming a raised compressible swelling with a bright red surface (Fig. 18.51). Spontaneous regression then follows; the surface whitens centrally (Fig. 18.52) and regression is complete by the age of 5 years in 50% of children and in 90% by the age of 9, leaving only an area of slight atrophy. Bleeding may follow trauma, and ulceration is common in the napkin (diaper) area.

Observation and encouragement is the management of choice for the great majority. Serial photographs of the way they clear up in other children help parents to accept this. Firm pressure may be needed to stop bleeding. If lesions interfere with feeding, or with vision, or if giant lesions sequestrate platelets (the Kasabach–Merritt syndrome), high doses of systemic steroids should be considered; they are most successful in the proliferative phase. Prednisolone (2–4 mg/kg/day) is given as a single dose in the morning and the dosage tapered to zero after 1 month. Ophthalmological help should be sought for all growing periocular haemangiomas; intralesional steroids have proved effective. Sometimes pulsed tuneable dye lasers are used for treating large lesions in infancy. Rarely, plastic surgery is necessary for a few large and unsightly haemangiomas that fail to improve spontaneously or to regress with the above measures.

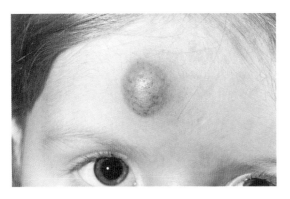

Fig. 18.52 The same strawberry naevus, as shown in Fig. 18.51, showing the whitening of the surface which is a sign of spontaneous remission.

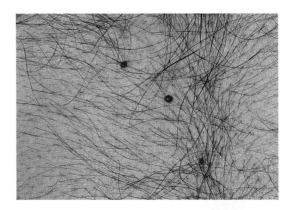

Fig. 18.53 Campbell de Morgan spots (cherry angiomas) of the chest.

Campbell de Morgan spots (cherry angiomas)

These benign angiomas are common on the trunks of the middle-aged and elderly. They are small bright red papules and of no consequence (Fig. 18.53).

Lymphangiomas

The most common type is lymphangioma circum-scriptum which appears as a cluster of vesicles resembling frog spawn. If treatment is needed, excision has to be wide and deep as dilated lymphatic channels and cisterns extend to the subcutaneous tissue.

Glomus tumours

These are derived from the cells surrounding small arteriovenous shunts. Solitary lesions are painful and most common on the extremities and under the nails. Multiple lesions are seldom painful and may affect other parts of the body. Painful lesions can be removed; others may be left.

Pyogenic granulomas

These badly named lesions are in fact common benign acquired haemangiomas, often seen in children and young adults. They develop at sites of trauma, over the course of a few weeks, as bright red raised, sometimes pedunculated and raspberry-like lesions which bleed easily (Fig. 18.54).

The important differential diagnosis is from an amelanotic malignant melanoma and, for this reason,

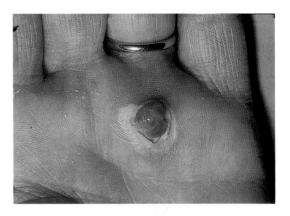

Fig. 18.54 Pyogenic granuloma of the palm: soggy after elastoplast dressing and bleeding easily.

the histology should always be checked. A pyogenic granuloma shows leashes of vessels of varying calibre covered by a thin, often ulcerated, epidermis.

Lesions should be removed by curettage under local anaesthetic with cautery to the base. Rarely, this is followed by recurrence or an eruption of satellite lesions around the original site.

Other benign dermal tumours

Dermatofibromas (histiocytomas)

These benign tumours are firm discrete usually solitary dermal nodules (Fig. 18.55), often on the extrem-

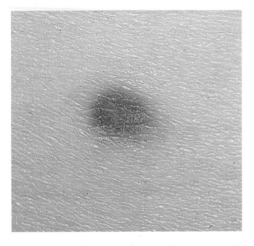

Fig. 18.55 A 0.5-cm diameter dermatofibroma—typically these lesions feel larger than they look. Its depressed surface became more obvious when the surrounding skin was pinched.

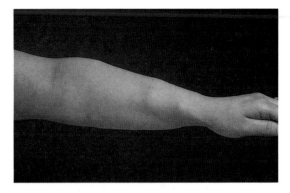

Fig. 18.56 Multiple lipomas.

ities of young adults. The lesions have an 'iceberg' effect in that they feel larger than they look. The overlying epidermis is often lightly pigmented and dimples when the nodule is squeezed. Some lesions seem to follow minor trauma or an insect bite. Histologically, the proliferating fibroblasts merge into the sparsely cellular dermis at the margins. A straightforward lesion may be left alone but, if there is any diagnostic doubt, it should be excised.

Neurofibromas

Although solitary tumours occur occasionally, multiple neurofibromas are most common and are usually seen as part of the inherited condition of neurofibromatosis. The clinical features of the tumour are described on p. 301.

Neuroma

This rare benign tumour is usually solitary. It may appear spontaneously but is seen most often as a result of nerve injury at the site of trauma or a surgical wound. There is nothing specific about the appearance of the skin-coloured dermal nodule but the tumour is frequently painful, even with gentle pressure. ENGLAND is a useful acronym for painful tumours (Eccrine spiradenoma, Neuroma, Glomus tumour, Leiomyoma, Angiolipoma, Neurofibroma (rarely) and Dermatofibroma (rarely)).

Keloid

This is an overgrowth of dense fibrous tissue in the skin, arising in response to trauma, however trivial. The tendency to develop keloids is genetically inherited. Keloids are common in Negroids and may be familial. Keloid formation is encouraged by infection, foreign material and by wounds (including surgical ones) especially those not lying along the lines of least tension or the skin creases. Even in Caucasoids, keloids are seen often enough on the presternal area, the neck, upper back and deltoid region of young adults to make doctors think twice before removing benign lesions there. Silicone sheeting and intralesional steroid injections are helpful but treatment should be given early, preferably for developing lesions.

Lipomas

Lipomas are common benign tumours of mature fat cells in the subcutaneous tissue. There may be one or many (Fig. 18.56) and lipomas are rarely a familial trait. They are most common on the proximal parts of the limbs but can occur at any site. They have an irregular lobular shape and a characteristic soft rubbery consistency. They are rarely painful. They need to be removed only if there is doubt about the diagnosis or if they are painful or unsightly.

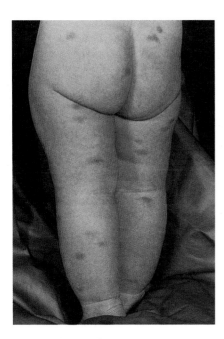

Fig. 18.57 Juvenile type of mastocytosis.

Mastocytosis (urticaria pigmentosa)

This term describes the various conditions in which the skin, and occasionally other tissues, contains an excess of mast cells. All types are characterized by a tendency for the skin to wheal after being rubbed. The main types are as follow.

• *Mastocytoma*. Usually presents as a solitary pink or brown itchy papule which wheals on rubbing. There are no systemic features.

• *Juvenile mastocytosis*. This is the most common type. Numerous pink or brown papules develop over the trunk and limbs (Fig. 18.57). There is no systemic involvement, and the condition is often mistaken for multiple melanocytic naevi.

• *Diffuse cutaneous mastocytosis*. This is rare and seen mostly in infants, being characterized by persistent dermographic wheals that appear after minor friction. The skin is diffusely infiltrated with mast cells, producing a thickened appearance like pigskin. The bone marrow, liver and spleen may be involved. Flushing is common. Death from massive histamine release is a real risk. Spontaneous improvement usually occurs.

• *Adult type*. Pink or pink-brown telangiectatic macules appear in early adult life and can spread to cover the whole body. The liver, spleen and bone are involved

in up to 20% of cases but systemic features such as headaches, flushing and palpitations are unusual.

Malignant

Kaposi's sarcoma

This malignant tumour of proliferating capillaries and lymphatics may be multifocal. There are two types: the classical, and that associated with immunosuppression. Human herpesvirus type 8 (HHV8) has been isolated from, and linked to, both types.

Classical Kaposi's sarcoma is seen most often in Africans and in elderly Jews of European origin. The tumours are usually on the feet and ankles but may be seen on the hands and on cold parts of the skin (e.g. the ears and nose). Initially they are dark blue to purple macules progressing to tumours and plaques which ulcerate and fungate. The rate of spread is variable but often slow. Tumours may metastasize to lymph nodes and spread to internal organs; oedema of the legs may be severe.

These tumours are very sensitive to radiotherapy which is the treatment of choice during the early stages; chemotherapy, with chlorambucil or vinblastine, helps when there is systemic involvement. Life expectancy is 5–9 years.

Kaposi's sarcoma and immunosuppression (see Figs 14.32–14.34). Smaller and more subtle (e.g. bruise-like) lesions may occur in an immunodeficient host. This tumour has recently become well known because of its association with AIDS (p. 211) caused by the human immunodeficiency virus (HIV-1). Lesions of AIDS-related Kaposi's sarcoma can appear anywhere but are most common on the upper trunk and head and neck. The initial bruise-like lesions tend to follow tension lines; they become raised, increasingly pigmented and evolve into nodules and plaques. Lesions frequently arise on the oral mucous membranes. Interestingly, HIV-positive intravenous drug abusers do not develop Kaposi's sarcoma as often as do HIV-positive homosexuals. The prognosis of AIDS patients with Kaposi's sarcoma is poor as most will develop opportunistic infections and the life expectancy in this situation is around 1 year. Single lesions respond to radiotherapy, cryotherapy or intralesional vinblastine; systemic treatment with α-interferon has helped some with multiple lesions.

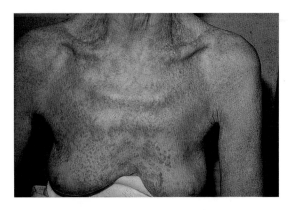

Fig. 18.58 Poikiloderma vasculare atrophicans may be a precursor of the tumour stage of CTCL.

Lymphomas and leukaemias

Skin involvement falls into two broad categories:
1 Disorders which arise in the skin or preferentially involve it. These include:
- T-cell lymphoma (mycosis fungoides);
- Sézary syndrome; and
- lymphoma associated with HIV infection.

2 Those arising extracutaneously, but which sometimes involve the skin. These include:
- Hodgkin's disease;
- B-cell lymphoma; and
- leukaemia.

Cutaneous T-cell lymphoma (CTCL; sometimes called mycosis fungoides)

This lymphoma of skin-associated helper T lymphocytes usually evolves slowly. There are three clinical phases: the patch, plaque and tumour stages, with involvement of lymph nodes and other tissues occurring late in the disease.

The *patch stage* (formerly termed 'premycotic' to denote an early phase of mycosis fungoides) may last for years (see Fig. 6.9). Most commonly it consists of scattered, barely palpable, erythematous, slightly pigmented, sharply marginated scaly patches rather like psoriasis or seborrhoeic dermatitis. Often they have a bizarre outline (e.g. arciform, or horseshoe-shaped) and, on close inspection, atrophy with surface wrinkling is usually evident. Their distribution is usually asymmetrical. Less commonly, the patch stage can be a widespread poikiloderma, with atrophy, pigmentation and telangiectasia (Fig. 18.58). As the lymphoma develops, some patches become indurated and palpable: *the plaque stage*. Some then turn into frank tumours which may become large (occasionally like mushrooms, hence the term 'mycosis fungoides') and

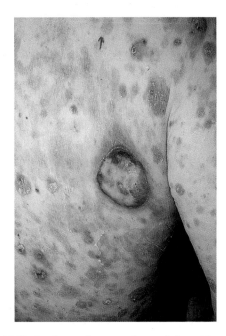

Fig. 18.59 An ulcerated tumour of mycosis fungoides against a background of plaques.

ulcerate (Fig. 18.59). The patch stage of CTCL may be difficult to diagnose clinically, but the plaque and tumour stages are usually characteristic. The first two phases of the disease may occupy 20 years or more, but the tumour stage is often short, with spread and death usually within 3 years.

The Sézary syndrome is also a CTCL caused by a proliferation of helper T lymphocytes. Generalized skin erythema and oedema is associated with pruritus and lymphadenopathy. Abnormal T lymphocytes, with large convoluted nuclei, are found circulating in the blood ('Sézary cells').

Histology

The histological hallmarks of plaque stage CTCL are:
• intraepidermal lymphocytic microabscesses (Pautrier microabscesses);
• a band of lymphoid cells in the upper dermis, infiltrating the epidermis; and
• atypical lymphocytes.

The histology of the patch stage poses more problems and may differ little from dermatitis. Immunophenotyping and T-cell receptor gene rearrangement studies (p. 19) are not always helpful in reaching a definitive diagnosis. Many biopsies, over several years, may be needed to prove that a suspicious rash is indeed an early stage of CTCL.

Differential diagnosis

The patch and plaque stages may be mistaken for psoriasis or parapsoriasis (Chapter 5), seborrhoeic dermatitis (p. 87) or tinea corporis (p. 216). However, they respond poorly to treatment for these disorders; the bizarre shapes of the patches and their asymmetrical distribution often raise suspicion. In the early stages skin scrapings may be needed to exclude tinea.

Treatment

Moderately potent or potent local steroids, and UVB treatment, may provide prolonged palliation in the patch stage. In the plaque stage, PUVA, oral retinoids and α-interferon are helpful. If lesions become more indurated, electron beam therapy may be used. Topical nitrogen mustard paint has also been used with success in both patch and plaque stages. Individual tumours respond well to low-dose radiotherapy. Systemic chemotherapy is disappointing.

Extracutaneous lymphomas

Hodgkin's disease

This is of interest to dermatologists because it may present with severe generalized pruritus (p. 291).

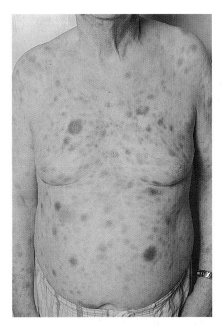

Fig. 18.60 Immunopathology showed that these nodules were caused by a B-cell lymphoma. (Courtesy of Dr E.C. Benton, The Royal Infirmary of Edinburgh, Edinburgh, UK.)

Patients with unexplained pruritus must be examined for lymphadenopathy and hepatosplenomegaly. Only rarely does Hodgkin's disease affect the skin directly, as small nodules and ulcers.

Leukaemia

Rarely, the first sign of leukaemia is a leukaemic infiltrate in the skin. Clinically, this shows as plum-coloured plaques or nodules or, less often, a thickening and rugosity of the scalp (cutis verticis gyrata). More often, the rashes associated with leukaemia are non-specific red papules ('leukaemids'). Other non-specific manifestations include pruritus, herpes zoster, acquired ichthyosis and purpura.

B-cell lymphomas

B-lymphocytic lymphomas presenting with skin lesions are rare. They appear as scattered plum-coloured nodules (Fig. 18.60). Histologically, a B-cell lymphoma infiltrates the lower dermis in a nodular or diffuse manner. Immunophenotyping shows a monoclonal expansion of B lymphocytes. Treatment is with radio-therapy and systemic chemotherapy.

Other malignant tumours

Dermatofibrosarcoma protuberans

Dermatofibrosarcoma protuberans is a slowly growing malignant tumour of fibroblasts, arising usually on the upper trunk. At first it seems like a dermatofibroma or keloid but, as it slowly expands, it turns into a plaque of red or bluish nodules with an irregular protuberant surface. It seldom metastasizes. It should be removed with extra wide margins, and even then will sometimes recur.

Cutaneous metastases

About 3% of patients with internal cancers have cutaneous metastases. They usually arise late and indicate a grave prognosis, but occasionally a solitary cutaneous metastasis is the first sign of the occurrence of a tumour.

The most common cutaneous metastases come from breast cancer. The skin of the breast is also most often involved by the direct extension of a tumour. This may show up as a sharply demarcated and firm area of erythema (carcinoma erysipeloides), firm telangiectatic plaques and papules (carcinoma telangiectoides) or as skin like orange peel (*peau d'orange*) caused by blocked and dilatated lymphatics. Carcinoma of the breast may also send metastases to the scalp causing patches of alopecia (Fig. 18.61), or to other areas as firm and discrete dermal nodules.

Other common primaries metastasizing to the skin are tumours of the lung, gastrointestinal tract, uterus, prostate and kidney. The most frequent sites for secondary deposits are the umbilicus and the scalp.

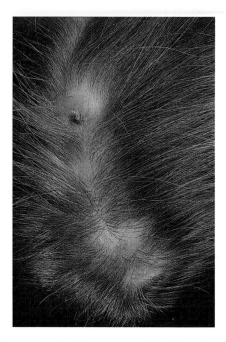

Fig. 18.61 Several scalp metastases arising from a breast carcinoma.

Further reading

Australian Cancer Network (1997) *Guidelines for the Management of Cutaneous Melanoma*. Stone Press, Epping.

Cox, N.H., Eedy, D.J. & Morton, C.A. (1999) Guidelines for the management of Bowen's disease. *British Journal of Dermatology* **141**, 633–641.

Fung, M.A., Murphy, M.J., Hoss, D.M. and Grant-Kels, J.M. (2002) Practical evaluation and management of cutaneous lymphoma. *Journal of the American Academy of Dermatology* **46**, 325–357.

Motley, R., Kersey, P. & Lawrence, C. (2002) Multiprofessional guidelines for the management of the patient with primary cutaneous squamous cell carcinoma. *British Journal of Dermatology* **146**, 18–25.

Roberts, D.L.L., Anstey, A.V., Barlow, R.J. *et al.* (2002) UK guidelines for the management of cutaneous melanoma. *British Journal of Dermatology* **146**, 7–17.

Telfer, N.R., Colver, G.B. & Bowers, P.W. (1999) Guidelines for the management of basal cell carcinoma. *British Journal of Dermatology* **141**, 415–423.

The skin in systemic disease

Only selected aspects of this huge subject can be covered here. In the first part of this chapter, the skin changes seen in particular diseases (e.g. sarcoidosis) or groups of diseases (e.g. internal malignancies) are described. The second part covers some individual skin conditions that can be associated with a wide range of internal disorders (e.g. pyoderma gangrenosum). Finally, although pregnancy is not a disease, for convenience its skin manifestations are listed here too.

The skin and internal malignancy

Obvious skin signs can be seen if a tumour invades the skin, or sends metastases to it; but there are other more subtle ways in which tumours can affect the skin. Sometimes they act physiologically, causing, for example, the acne seen with some adrenal tumours, flushing in the carcinoid syndrome, and jaundice with a bile duct carcinoma. These cast-iron associations need no further discussion here. However, the presence of some rare but important conditions should alert the clinician to the possibility of an underlying neoplasm.

1 *Acanthosis nigricans* is a velvety thickening and pigmentation of the major flexures. Setting aside those cases caused by obesity (Fig. 19.1), by diabetes and characterized by insulin resistance, or by drugs such as nicotinic acid used to treat hyperlipidaemia, the chances are high that a tumour is present, usually within the abdominal cavity.

2 *Erythema gyratum repens* is a shifting pattern of waves of erythema covering the skin surface and looking like the grain on wood.

3 *Acquired hypertrichosis lanuginosa* ('malignant down') is an excessive and widespread growth of fine lanugo hair.

4 *Necrolytic migratory erythema* is a figurate erythema with a moving crusted edge. When present, usually with anaemia, stomatitis, weight loss and diabetes, it signals the presence of a glucagon-secreting tumour of the pancreas.

5 *Bazex syndrome* is a papulosquamous eruption of the fingers and toes, ears and nose, seen with some tumours of the upper respiratory tract.

6 *Dermatomyositis*, other than in childhood (p. 125).

7 *Generalized pruritus*. One of its many causes is an internal malignancy, usually a lymphoma (p. 291).

8 *Superficial thrombophlebitis*. The migratory type has traditionally been associated with carcinomas of the pancreas.

9 *Acquired ichthyosis*. This may result from a number of underlying diseases (see p. 43) but it is always important to exclude malignancy, especially lymphomas, as the cause.

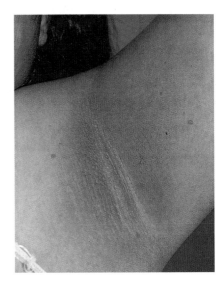

Fig. 19.1 Acanthosis nigricans—in this case caused by obesity.

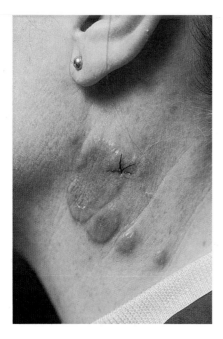

Fig. 19.2 Acute febrile neutrophilic dermatosis (Sweet's syndrome).

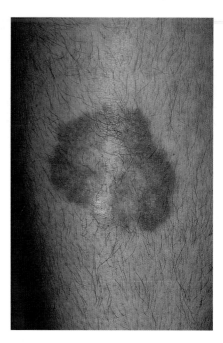

Fig. 19.3 Necrobiosis lipoidica: shiny yellowish patch with marked telangiectasia.

10 *Genetic conditions.* One example is the Muir–Torre syndrome in which sebaceous adenomas are accompanied by surprisingly unaggressive visceral malignancies.

11 *Acute febrile neutrophilic dermatosis* (Sweet's syndrome; Fig. 19.2). The classic triad found in association with the red oedematous plaques consists of fever, a raised erythrocyte sedimentation rate (ESR) and a raised blood neutrophil count. The most important internal association is with myeloproliferative disorders.

12 *Others.* Pachydermoperiostosis is a coarsening and thickening of the skin seen in association with severe clubbing. It can be inherited as an autosomal dominant trait, or be a result of the standard causes of clubbing which include conditions such as bronchial carcinoma.

The skin and diabetes mellitus

The following are more common in those with diabetes than in others.

1 *Necrobiosis lipoidica.* Less than 1% of diabetics have necrobiosis, but most patients with necrobiosis will have diabetes. The remaining few should have a glucose tolerance test followed by regular urine tests as some will become diabetic later. The lesions appear as one or more discoloured areas on the fronts of the shins (Fig. 19.3); they are shiny, atrophic and brown-red or slightly yellow. The underlying blood vessels are easily seen through the atrophic skin and the margin may be erythematous or violet. Minor knocks can lead to slow-healing ulcers; biopsy can do the same. No treatment is reliably helpful.

2 *Granuloma annulare.* The cause of granuloma annulare is not known and dermatologists still debate whether or not there is a genuine association with diabetes. If it exists at all, the association applies only to a few adults with extensive lesions. Children with standard lesions on the hands may need a single urine check for sugar but no more elaborate tests. Clinically, the lesions of granuloma annulare often lie over the knuckles and are composed of dermal nodules fused into a rough ring shape (Fig. 19.4). On the hands the lesions are skin-coloured or slightly pink; elsewhere a purple colour may be seen. Although a biopsy is seldom necessary, the histology shows a diagnostic palisading granuloma, like that of necrobiosis lipoidica. Lesions tend to go away over the

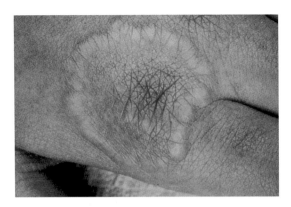

Fig. 19.4 Granuloma annulare.

course of a year or two. Stubborn ones respond to intralesional triamcinolone injections.

3 *Diabetic dermopathy.* In about 50% of Type I diabetics, multiple small (0.5–1 cm in diameter) slightly sunken brownish scars can be found on the limbs, most obviously over the shins.

4 *Candidal infections* (p. 38).

5 *Staphylococcal infections* (p. 190).

6 *Vitiligo* (p. 246).

7 *Eruptive xanthomas* (p. 289).

8 *Stiff thick skin* (diabetic sclerodactyly or cheiro-arthropathy) on the fingers and hands, demonstrated by the 'prayer sign' in which the fingers and palms cannot be opposed properly (Fig. 19.5).

9 *Atherosclerosis* with ischaemia or gangrene of feet.

10 *Neuropathic foot ulcers.*

The skin in sarcoidosis

About one-third of patients with systemic sarcoidosis have skin lesions; it is also possible to have cutaneous sarcoidosis without systemic abnormalities. The most important skin changes are as follows.

1 *Erythema nodosum* (see Fig. 8.10). This occurs in the early stages of sarcoidosis, especially in young women.

2 *Scar sarcoidosis.* Granulomatous lesions arising in longstanding scars should raise suspicions of sarcoidosis.

3 *Lupus pernio.* Dusky infiltrated plaques appear on the nose and fingers, often in association with sarcoidosis of the upper respiratory tract.

4 *Papular, nodular and plaque forms* (Fig. 19.6). These brownish-red, violaceous, or hypopigmented papules and plaques are indolent although often symptom-free. Sometimes they are annular. They vary in number, size and distribution. Intralesional and topical corticosteroids are sometimes helpful and hydroxychloroquine (Formulary 2, p. 351) has been used successfully. Chronic lesions respond poorly to any line of treatment short of systemic steroids, which are usually best avoided if involvement is confined to the skin.

The skin in liver disease

Some of the associated abnormalities are the following.

1 *Pruritus.* This is related to obstructive jaundice and may precede it (p. 291).

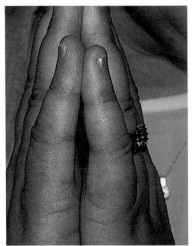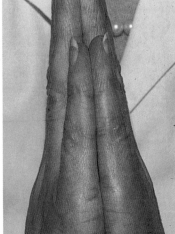

Fig. 19.5 Diabetic cheiropathy—the prayer sign. Poor finger apposition in the diabetic hand (on the left) compared with the normal one (on the right).

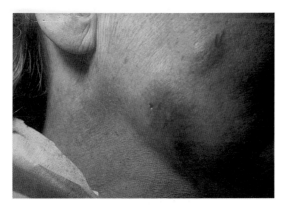

Fig. 19.6 Sarcoidosis: plum-coloured plaques on the cheek.

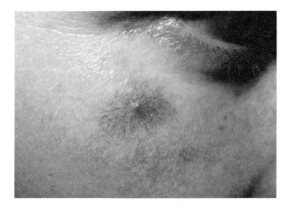

Fig. 19.7 Solitary spider naevus showing the central feeding vessel. No underlying liver disease in this case.

2 *Pigmentation*. With bile pigments and sometimes melanin (Chapter 17).
3 *Spider naevi* (Fig. 19.7). These are often multiple in chronic liver disease (p. 133).
4 *Palmar erythema* (p. 133).
5 *White nails*. These associate with hypoalbuminaemia.
6 *Porphyria cutanea tarda* (p. 287).
7 *Xanthomas*. In primary biliary cirrhosis (p. 289).
8 *Hair loss and generalized asteatotic eczema* may occur in alcoholics with cirrhosis who have become zinc deficient.

The skin in renal disease

The main changes are the following.
1 *Pruritus* and a generally dry skin.
2 *Pigmentation*. A yellowish sallow colour and pallor from anaemia.

3 *Half-and-half nail*. The proximal half is white and the distal half is pink or brownish.
4 *'Perforating disorders'*. Small papules in which collagen or elastic fibres are being extruded through the epidermis.
5 *'Pseudoporphyria'* (p. 289).
6 *The skin changes of the conditions leading to renal disease*. For example, leucocytoclastic vasculitis (p. 102), connective tissue disorders (Chapter 10), Fabry's disease (p. 291).

Graft-vs.-host disease

Marrow grafting is now used for several disorders including aplastic anaemia and leukaemia. Immunologically competent donor lymphocytes, however, may cause problems by reacting against host tissues, especially the skin, liver and gut.

Acute graft-vs.-host (GVH) disease appears within 4 weeks. Fever accompanies malaise and a worsening morbilliform rash, which may progress to a generalized desquamation or even toxic epidermal necrolysis. Chronic GVH disease occurs later: its skin changes are variable but may be like those of lichen planus or a pigmented scleroderma. The skin changes may be severe enough to need treatment with systemic prednisolone and azathioprine, PUVA or cyclosporin A.

Malabsorption and malnutrition

Some of the most common skin changes are listed in Table 19.1.

The porphyrias

There are at least seven enzymes in the metabolic pathway that leads to the synthesis of haem. There are also seven different types of porphyria, each being caused by a deficiency of one of these enzymes, and each having its own characteristic pattern of accumulation of porphyrin and porphyrin precursors. Some of these cause the photosensitivity (to ultraviolet radiation of wavelength 400 nm, which is capable of penetrating through window glass) that is the cardinal feature of the cutaneous porphyrias.

The different types can be separated on clinical grounds, aided by the biochemical investigation of

Table 19.1 Skin changes in malabsorption and malnutrition.

Condition	Skin changes
Malnutrition	Itching Dryness SymmetriFcal pigmentation Brittle nails and hair
Protein malnutrition (kwashiorkor)	Dry red-brown hair Pigmented 'cracked skin'
Iron deficiency	Pallor Itching Diffuse hair loss Koilonychia Smooth tongue
Vitamin A (retinol) deficiency	Dry skin Follicular hyperkeratoses Xerophthalmia
Vitamin B_1 (aneurin) deficiency	Beri-beri oedema
Vitamin B_2 (riboflavine) deficiency	Angular stomatitis Smooth purple tongue Seborrhoeic dermatitis-like eruption
Vitamin B_6 (pyridoxine) deficiency	Ill-defined dermatitis
Vitamin B_7 (niacin) deficiency	Pellagra with dermatitis, dementia and diarrhoea Dermatitis on exposed areas, pigmented
Vitamin C deficiency (scurvy)	Skin haemorrhages especially around follicular keratoses containing coiled hairs Bleeding gums Oedematous 'woody' swellings of limbs in the elderly

urine, faeces and blood. Only five varieties will be mentioned here.

Congenital erythropoietic porphyria

This is very rare, caused by mutations in the uroporphyrinogen cosynthase gene, and inherited as an autosomal recessive trait. Severe photosensitivity is noted soon after birth, and leads to blistering, scarring and mutilation of the exposed parts, which become increasingly hairy. The urine is pink and the teeth are brown, although fluorescing red under Wood's light. A haemolytic anaemia is present. Treatment is unsatisfactory but must include protection from, and avoidance of, sunlight. Gene therapy may be possible in the future. The hairy appearance, discoloured teeth and the tendency to avoid daylight may have given rise to legends about werewolves.

Erythrohepatic protoporphyria (erythropoietic protoporphyria)

In this more common, autosomal dominant condition, caused by mutations in the ferrochelatase gene, a less severe photosensitivity develops during childhood. A burning sensation occurs within minutes of exposure to sunlight. Soon the skin becomes swollen and crusted vesicles sometimes appear, leading to pitted scars. Liver disease and gallstones occur. In addition to sun avoidance and the use of sunscreens (Formulary 1, p. 330), beta-carotene may be given orally.

Cutaneous hepatic porphyria (porphyria cutanea tarda)

There are two types: a sporadic type (accounting for 80% of cases) and a type inherited as an autosomal

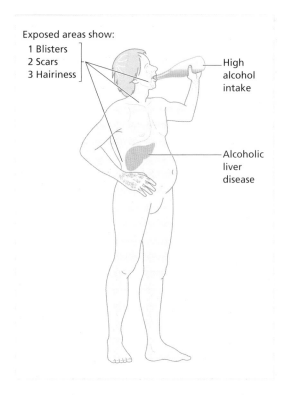

Exposed areas show:
1 Blisters
2 Scars
3 Hairiness

High alcohol intake

Alcoholic liver disease

Fig. 19.8 Cutaneous hepatic porphyria (porphyria cutanea tarda).

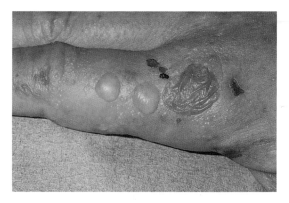

Fig. 19.9 Blisters, milia and erosions on the side of a finger.

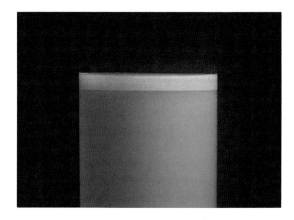

Fig. 19.10 Cutaneous hepatic porphyria. Coral-red fluorescence of urine under Wood's light denoting excessive uroporphyrins (chloroform extraction).

dominant trait (20%). Both are characterized by low hepatic uroporphyrinogen decarboxylase activity. The sporadic type is usually seen in men, but rarely in women, who have damaged their livers by drinking too much alcohol but may also occur in women taking oestrogens. Recently it has been shown that some cases are caused by a previous hepatitis C virus infection. Blisters, erosions and milia form on the exposed parts of the face, and on the backs of the hands (Figs 19.8 and 19.9), in response to sunlight or to minor trauma. These areas become scarred and hairy. The urine is pink and fluoresces a bright coral-pink under Wood's light (p. 33) as a result of excessive uroporphyrins (Fig. 19.10). Treatment is based on avoiding alcohol and oestrogens, but other measures are usually needed too, including regular venesection or very low-dose hydroxychloroquine therapy (e.g. 100 mg twice weekly) under specialist supervision. Higher doses cause toxic hepatitis in these patients.

Acute intermittent porphyria

This condition, inherited as an autosomal dominant trait as a result of mutations of the porphobilinogen deaminase gene, is most common in Scandinavia. Skin lesions do not occur. Attacks of abdominal pain, accompanied by neuropsychiatric symptoms and the passage of dark urine, are sometimes triggered by drugs (especially barbiturates, griseofulvin, oestrogens and sulphonamides).

Variegate porphyria

This disorder, inherited as an autosomal dominant trait, and a result of mutations of the protoporphyrinogen oxidase gene, is particularly common in South Africa. It shares the skin features of porphyria cutanea tarda and the systemic symptoms and drug provocation of acute intermittent porphyria.

'Pseudoporphyria'

This term is used when skin changes like those of cutaneous hepatic porphyria occur without an underlying abnormality of porphyrin metabolism. It is seen in a few patients on haemodialysis, and can be induced by some drugs—notably frusemide (furosemide) and non steroidal anti-inflammatory drugs. The overuse of sun beds is another possible cause.

Some metabolic disorders

Amyloidosis

Amyloid is a protein that can be derived from several sources, including immunoglobulin light chains and probably keratins. It is deposited in the tissues under a variety of circumstances and is then usually in combination with a P component derived from the plasma. Systemic amyloidosis of the type that is secondary to chronic inflammatory disease, such as rheumatoid arthritis or tuberculosis, tends not to affect the skin. In contrast, skin changes are prominent in primary systemic amyloidosis, and also in the amyloid associated with multiple myeloma. Skin blood vessels infiltrated with amyloid rupture easily, causing 'pinch purpura' to occur after minor trauma. The waxy deposits of amyloid, often most obvious around the eyes, may also be purpuric. Distinct from the systemic amyloidoses are localized deposits of amyloid. These are uncommon and usually take the form of macular areas of rippled pigmentation, or of plaques made up of coalescing papules. Both types are itchy.

Mucinoses

The dermis becomes infiltrated with mucin in certain disorders.
1 *Myxoedema*. In the puffy hands and face of patients with hypothyroidism.
2 *Pretibial myxoedema*. Pink or flesh-coloured mucinous plaques are seen on the lower shins, together with marked exophthalmos, in some patients with hyperthyroidism. They may also occur after the thyroid abnormality has been treated.

3 *Scleromyxoedema*. A diffuse thickening and papulation of the skin may occur in connection with an immunoglobulin G (IgG) monoclonal paraproteinaemia.
4 *Follicular mucinosis*. In this condition, the infiltrated plaques show a loss of hair. Some cases are associated with a lymphoma.

Xanthomas

Deposits of fatty material in the skin and subcutaneous tissues (xanthomas) may provide the first clue to important disorders of lipid metabolism.

Primary hyperlipidaemias are usually genetic. They fall into six groups, classified on the basis of an analysis of fasting blood lipids and electrophoresis of plasma lipoproteins. All, save type I, carry an increased risk of atherosclerosis—in this lies their importance and the need for treatment.

Secondary hyperlipidaemia may be found in a variety of diseases including diabetes, primary biliary cirrhosis, the nephrotic syndrome and hypothyroidism.

The clinical patterns of xanthoma correlate well with the underlying cause. The main patterns and their most common associations are shown in Table 19.2.

Phenylketonuria

Phenylketonuria is a rare metabolic cause of hypopigmentation. Its prevalence is about 1 in 25 000. It is inherited as an autosomal recessive trait, the abnormal gene lying on chromosome region 12q22-q24, and is caused by a deficiency of the liver enzyme phenylalanine hydroxylase, which catalyses the hydroxylation

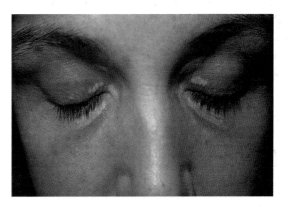

Fig. 19.11 Xanthelasma: flat yellow lesions on the eyelids, often with normal blood lipids.

Table 19.2 Xanthomas: clinical appearance and associations.

Type	Clinical appearance	Types of hyperlipidaemia (Frederickson classification) and associated metabolic abnormalities
Xanthelasma palpebrarum (Fig. 19.11)	Soft yellowish plaques on the eyelids	None or type II, III or IV
Tuberous xanthomas (Fig. 19.12)	Firm yellow papules and nodules, most often on points of knees and elbows	Types II, III and secondary
Tendinous xanthomas	Subcutaneous swellings on fingers or by Achilles tendon	Types II, III and secondary
Eruptive xanthomas	Sudden onset, multiple small yellow papules Buttocks and shoulders	Types I, IV, V and secondary (usually to diabetes)
Plane xanthomas (Fig. 19.13)	Yellow macular areas at any site Yellow palmar creases	Type III and secondary
Generalized plane xanthomas	Yellow macules lesions over wide areas	Myeloma

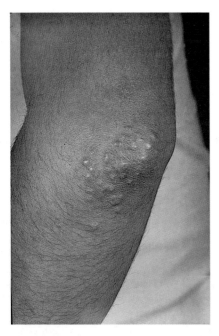

Fig. 19.12 Tuberous xanthoma on the points of the elbows—a mixture of nodules and papules.

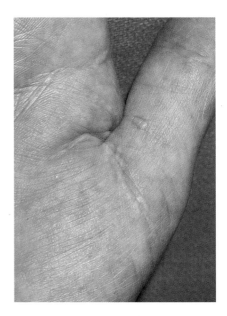

Fig. 19.13 Plane xanthoma with yellow palmar creases.

of phenylalanine to tyrosine. This leads to the accumulation of phenylalanine, phenylpyruvic acid and their metabolites.

Affected individuals have fair skin and hair. They often develop eczema, usually of atopic type, and may be photosensitive. The accumulation of phenylalanine and its metabolites damages the brain during the phase of rapid development just before and just after birth. Mental retardation, epilepsy and extrapyramidal manifestations such as athetosis and mental retardation may then occur.

Oculocutaneous albinism can usually be distinguished by its eye signs. The Guthrie test, which detects raised blood phenylalanine levels, is carried out routinely at birth in most developed countries.

A low-phenylalanine diet should be started as soon as possible to prevent further neurological damage.

Alkaptonuria

In this rare recessively inherited disorder, based on a homogentisic acid oxidase deficiency, dark urine may be seen in childhood, and in adult life pigment may be deposited in various places including the ears and sclera. Arthropathy may occur.

Fabry's disease (angiokeratoma corporis diffusum)

A deficiency of the enzyme α-galactosidase A is found in this sex-linked disorder (chromosome region Xq21.3–22); abnormal amounts of glycolipid are deposited in many tissues as a result. The skin lesions are grouped, almost black, small telangiectatic papules especially around the umbilicus and pelvis. Progressive renal failure occurs in adult life. Most patients have attacks of excruciating unexplained pain in their hands. Some female carriers have skin changes, although these are usually less obvious than those of affected males. Similar skin lesions may be seen in lysosomal storage disorders such as fucosidosis.

Generalized pruritus

Pruritus is a symptom with many causes, but not a disease in its own right. Itchy patients fall into two groups: those whose pruritus is caused simply by surface causes (e.g. eczema, lichen planus and scabies), which seldom need much investigation; and the others, who may or may not have an internal cause for their itching, such as the following.
1 *Liver disease.* Itching signals biliary obstruction. It is an early symptom of primary biliary cirrhosis. Cholestyramine often helps cholestatic pruritus, possibly by promoting the elimination of bile salts.
2 *Chronic renal failure.* Urea itself seems not to be responsible for this symptom, which plagues about one-third of patients undergoing renal dialysis.

3 *Iron deficiency.* Treatment with iron may help the itching.
4 *Polycythaemia.* The itching here is usually triggered by a hot bath; it has a curious pricking quality and lasts about an hour.
5 *Thyroid disease.* Itching and urticaria may occur in hyperthyroidism. The dry skin of hypothyroidism may also be itchy.
6 *Diabetes.* Generalized itching may be a rare presentation of diabetes.
7 *Internal malignancy.* The prevalence of itching in Hodgkin's disease may be as high as 30%. It may be unbearable, yet the skin often looks normal. Pruritus may occur long before other manifestations of the disease. Itching is uncommon in carcinomatosis.
8 *Neurological disease.* Paroxysmal pruritus has been recorded in multiple sclerosis and in neurofibromatosis. Brain tumours infiltrating the floor of the fourth ventricle may cause a fierce persistent itching of the nostrils.
9 The skin of the elderly may itch because it is too dry.

The search for a cause has to be tailored to the individual patient, and must start with a thorough history and physical examination. The presence of a 'butterfly sign' (Fig. 19.14) sometimes suggests an internal cause for the itching. Unless a treatable cause is found, therapy is symptomatic and consists of sedative antihistamines, and the avoidance of rough clothing, overheating and vasodilatation, including that brought on by alcohol. UVB may help the itching associated with chronic renal, and perhaps liver disease. Local

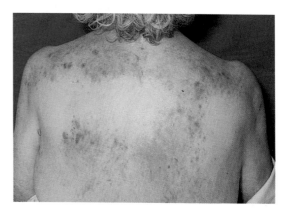

Fig. 19.14 An example of the butterfly sign. This lady could not reach her upper back but could scratch her skin everywhere else. In other patients, the spared area is shaped more like a butterfly.

applications include calamine and mixtures containing small amounts of menthol or phenol (Formulary 1, p. 330). Sometimes lubricating the skin with emollients helps.

Pyoderma gangrenosum

An inflamed nodule or pustule breaks down centrally to form an expanding ulcer with a polycyclic or serpiginous outline, and a characteristic undermined bluish edge (Fig. 19.15). The condition is not bacterial in origin but its pathogenesis, presumably immunological, is not fully understood. It may arise in the absence of any underlying disease, but tends to associate with the following conditions.

1 Ulcerative colitis.
2 Conditions causing polyarthritis, including rheumatoid arthritis (Fig. 19.16)
3 Crohn's disease (Fig. 19.17).
4 Monoclonal gammopathies.
5 Leukaemia (with a bullous form of pyoderma).

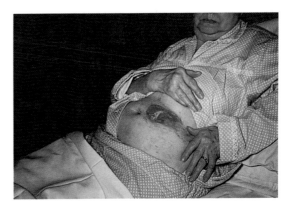

Fig. 19.16 This longstanding ulcer was pyoderma gangrenosum secondary to the patient's rheumatoid arthritis. (Courtesy of Dr G.W. Beveridge, The Royal Infirmary of Edinburgh, Edinburgh, UK.)

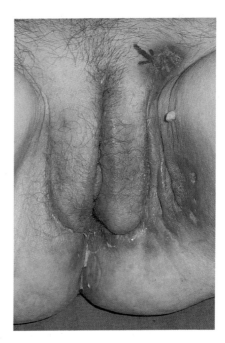

Fig. 19.17 Another manifestation of Crohn's disease: grossly oedematous vulva with interconnecting sinuses. Biopsy at the site arrowed showed a granulomatous histology.

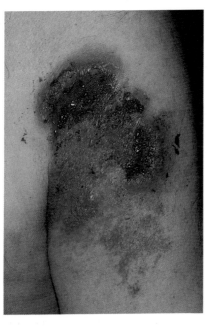

Fig. 19.15 Pyoderma gangrenosum: a plum-coloured lesion with a typical cribriform appearance.

Lesions may be single or multiple. If gut disease is present then control of this will help the pyoderma. Otherwise the condition responds to systemic steroids but not to antibiotics, and lesions heal leaving papery scars.

The skin changes of pregnancy

Physiological

A darkening of the nipples, genitals, and of a line down the centre of the abdominal wall, is often accompanied by a generalized increase in skin pigmentation. Sebum excretion may increase. Spider naevi and palmar erythema are both common in pregnancy, and are caused by high oestrogen levels. Stretch marks and skin tags are common too.

Dermatoses of pregnancy

Itching is common in pregnancy, usually for obvious reasons such as scabies, but sometimes in association with mild cholestasis. The terminology of the more striking itchy dermatoses of pregnancy has always been confusing. We now prefer to divide them into only three main categories.

1 *Pruritic urticarial papules and plaques of pregnancy* (PUPP) (Fig. 19.18). This usually starts in the third trimester. The urticated lesions favour the abdomen, particularly in association with stretch marks. The cause of PUPP is not known, but it is not associated with danger to the unborn child, and clears after the child is born. Treatment is symptomatic.

2 *Prurigo of pregnancy.* The development of many excoriated papules, which are not urticated, starts rather earlier than PUPP. It also caries no threat to the unborn child and clears after the child is born.

3 *Pemphigoid gestationis* is rare, and triggered by HLA differences between the mother and the fetus. However, the autoantibodies are directed at the same antigens as those of ordinary pemphigoid (p. 111). The condition may start at any time during pregnancy, or even just after childbirth, tending to start earlier in subsequent pregnancies. The itchy urticarial plaques, often annular, go on to blister. Immunofluorescence differentiates the condition from PUPP. Systemic corticosteroids are usually required, and there may be a risk of premature delivery.

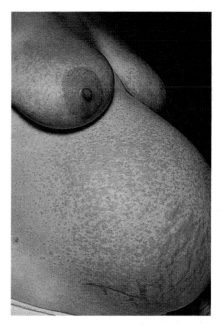

Fig. 19.18 Pruritic urticarial papules and plaques in late pregnancy.

Effect of pregnancy on other dermatoses

Candidiasis is common in pregnancy and genital warts can become unusually luxuriant. Podophyllin should be avoided for the latter as it may be toxic to the fetus. The effects of pregnancy on common disorders, such as atopic eczema, acne and psoriasis, are unpredictable in any individual patient, but there is an overall trend towards improvement.

Further reading

Braverman, I.M. (1998) *Skin Signs of Systemic Disease*, 3rd edn. W.B. Saunders, Philadelphia, PA.

Kroumpouzas, G. and Cohen, L.M. (2001) Dermatoses of pregnancy. *Journal of the American Academy of Dermatology* 45, 1–19.

Provost, T.T. & Flynn, J.A. (2001) *Cutaneous Medicine: Cutaneous Manifestations of Systemic Disease.* B.C. Decker, Ontario.

Savin, J.A., Hunter, J.A.A. & Hepburn, N.C. (1997) *Skin Signs in Clinical Medicine: Diagnosis in Colour.* Mosby-Wolfe, London.

20 The skin and the psyche

Most people accept that there are strong links between skin disease and the emotions, but only a few skin disorders, such as dermatitis artefacta, have emotional factors as their direct cause. The relationships between the mind and the skin are usually subtler and more complex than this. Nevertheless, patients with skin disorders do have a higher prevalence of psychiatric abnormalities than the general population, although specific personality profiles and disorders can seldom be tied to specific skin diseases. Similarly, it is still not clear how, or even how often, psychological factors trigger, worsen or perpetuate such everyday problems as atopic eczema or psoriasis.

Each school of psychiatry has its own theories on the subject, but their explanations do not satisfy everyone. Do people really damage their skin to satisfy guilt feelings? Does their skin 'weep' because they have themselves suppressed weeping? Until more is known, it may be wise to adopt a simpler and more pragmatic approach, in which interactions between the skin and psyche are divided into two broad groups:

• emotional reactions to the presence of skin disease, real or imagined; and
• the effects of emotions on skin disease (Fig. 20.1).

Reactions to skin disease

The presence of disfiguring skin lesions can distort the emotional development of a child: some become withdrawn, others become aggressive, but many adjust well. The range of reactions to skin disease is therefore wide. At one end lies indifference to grossly disfiguring lesions and, at the other, lies an obsession with skin that is quite normal. Between these extremes are reactions ranging from natural anxiety over ugly

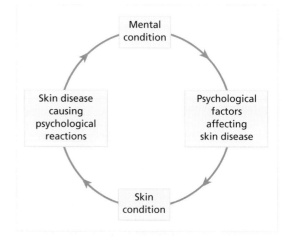

Fig. 20.1 Mind–skin interactions.

skin lesions to disproportionate worry over minor blemishes.

A chronic skin disease such as psoriasis can undoubtedly spoil the lives of those who suffer from it. It can interfere with work, and with social activities of all sorts including sexual relationships, causing sufferers to feel like outcasts. The heavy drinking of so many men with severe psoriasis is one result of these pressures. An experienced dermatologist will be on the lookout for depression and the risk of suicide, as up to 10% of patients with psoriasis have had suicidal thoughts. However, these reactions do not necessarily correlate with the extent and severity of the eruption as judged by an outside observer. Who has the more disabling problem: someone with 50% of his body surface covered in psoriasis, but who largely ignores this and has a happy family life and a productive job, or one with 5% involvement whose social life is ruined by it? The concept of 'body image' is useful here.

Body image

All of us think we know how we look, but our ideas may not tally with those of others. The nose, face, hair and genitals tend to rank high in a person's 'corporeal awareness', and trivial lesions in those areas can generate much anxiety. The facial lesions of acne, for example, can lead to a huge loss of self-esteem.

Dermatological delusional disease

Dysmorphophobia

This is the term applied to distortions of the body image. Minor and inconspicuous lesions are magnified in the mind to grotesque proportions.

Dermatological 'non-disease'

This is a form of dysmorphobia. The clinician can find no skin abnormality, but the distress felt by the patient leads to anxiety, depression or even suicide. Such patients are not uncommon. They expect dermatological solutions for complaints such as hair loss, or burning, itching and redness of the face or genitals. The dermatologist, who can see nothing wrong, cannot solve matters and no treatment seems to help. Such patients are reluctant to see a psychiatrist although some may suffer from a monosymptomatic hypochondriacal psychosis.

Other delusions

These patients sustain single hypochondriacal delusions for long periods, in the absence of other recognizable psychiatric disease. Some are eccentric and live in social isolation. Some believe that they have syphilis, AIDS or skin cancer. In dermatology, many of these patients have the delusion that their skin is infested with parasites.

Delusions of parasitosis (Fig. 20.2)

This term is better than 'parasitophobia', which implies a fear of becoming infested. Patients with delusions of parasitosis are unshakably convinced that they are already infested. No rational argument can convince them that they are not; the pest control agencies that they have called in, and their medical advisers therefore must both be wrong. Symptoms include odd sensations of crawling and biting, and patients often bring to the clinic a box of specimens of the 'parasite' at different stages of its supposed life cycle. These must be examined microscopically but usually turn out to be fragments of skin, hair, clothing, haemorrhagic crusts or unclassifiable debris. The skin changes may include gouge marks and scratches, but it is convenient to consider these patients separately from those with dermatitis artefacta.

These patients become angry if doubts are cast on their ideas, or if they are referred to a psychiatrist. How could treatment for mental illness possibly be expected to kill parasites? Family members may share their delusions and much tact is needed to secure any cooperation with treatment. Direct confrontations are best avoided; sometimes it may be best simply to treat with psychotropic drugs, explaining that these may be able to help some of the symptoms.

The delusions of a few of these patients are based on an underlying depression or schizophrenia, and of a further few on organic problems such as vitamin deficiency or cerebrovascular disease. These disorders must be treated on their own merits. However, most patients suffer from monosymptomatic hypochondriacal delusions, which can often be suppressed by treatment with drugs, accepting that these will be needed long-term. Otherwise, the outlook for resolution is poor. Pimozide was once the most popular treatment for this condition but high doses carry cardiac risks. If pimozide is used, an electrocardiogram (ECG) should be performed before starting treatment and the drug should not be given to those with a prolonged Q-T interval or with a history of cardiac dysrhythmia. Patients on pimozide in excess of 16 mg daily need periodic ECG checks. Tardive dyskinesia may develop and persist despite withdrawal of the drug. Risperidone, olanzapine and sulpiride are reasonable, and perhaps safer, alternatives. Some patients gain insight and relief. Others hint that their parasites still persist although this no longer disables them.

Dermatitis artefacta

Here the skin lesions are caused and kept going by the patient's own actions, but parasites are not held to be to blame. Patients with dermatitis artefacta deny self-trauma but, naturally, if treatment is left to them to carry out, their problems do not improve. Lesions will

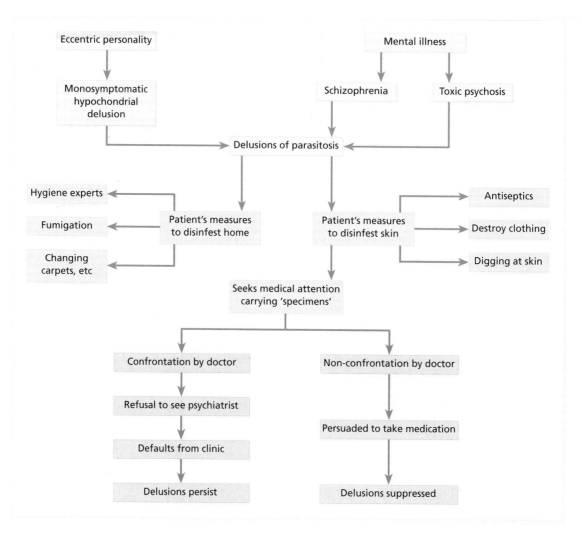

Fig. 20.2 Delusions of parasitosis—the sequence of events.

heal under occlusive dressings, but this does not alter the underlying psychiatric problems, and lesions may recur or crop up outside the bandaged areas. Different types of dermatitis artefacta are listed in Table 20.1.

The lesions favour accessible areas, and do not fit with known pathological processes. The diagnosis is often difficult to make, but an experienced clinician will suspect it because there are no primary lesions and because of the bizarre shape or grouping of the lesions, which may be rectilinear or oddly grouped (Fig. 20.3). Areas damaged by burning (Fig. 20.4), corrosive chemicals (Fig. 20.5), or by digging have their own special appearance.

Table 20.1 Types of dermatitis artefacta.

Type	Personality
Minor habits, e.g. excoriated acne	Relatively normal
More obvious lesions	Hysterical or neurotic (secondary gain)
Bizarre	Psychotic
Malingering	Criminal

More subtle changes are seen in 'dermatological pathomimicry', in which patients reproduce or aggravate their skin disease by deliberate contact with materials to which they know they will react.

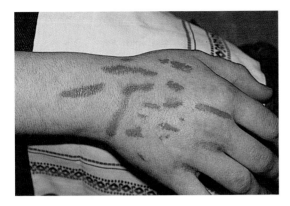

Fig. 20.3 Obvious dermatitis artefacta: back your own judgement against the patient's here.

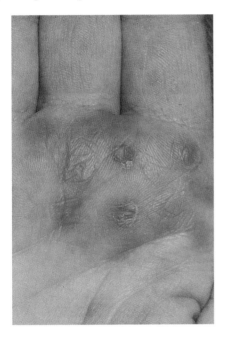

Fig. 20.4 A lighted cigarette was responsible for this appearance.

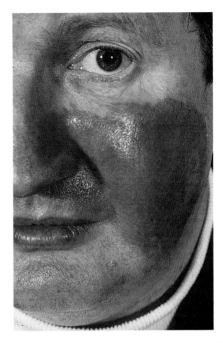

Fig. 20.5 Dermatitis artefacta: denials of self-trauma did not convince us that this was caused by any other skin disease.

LEARNING POINTS

1 Do not reward a delusion with a treatment for scabies.
2 Direct confrontations with patients with dermatitis artefacta or delusions of parasitosis may make you feel better, but do little for them.

Apart from frank malingerers, the patients are often young women with some medical knowledge, perhaps a nurse. Some form of 'secondary gain' from having skin lesions may be obvious. The psychological problems may be superficial and easily resolved, but sometimes psychiatric help is needed and the artefacts are part of a prolonged psychiatric illness. A few patients respond to banal treatments if given the chance to save face. Direct confrontation and accusations are usually best avoided, and the condition may last for some years.

Neurotic excoriations

Patients with neurotic excoriations differ from those with other types of dermatitis artefacta in that they admit to picking and digging at their skin. This habit affects women more often than men and is most active at times of stress. The clinical picture is mixed, with crusted excoriations and pale scars, often with a hyperpigmented border, lying mainly on the face, neck, shoulders and arms (Fig. 20.6). The condition may last for years and psychiatric treatment is seldom successful.

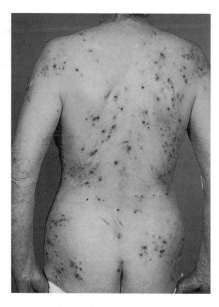

Fig. 20.6 Unusually extensive neurotic excoriations.

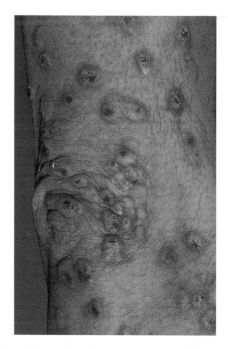

Fig. 20.7 The excoriated lesions of prurigo nodularis.

Acne excoriée

Here the self-inflicted damage is based to some extent on the lesions of acne vulgaris, which may in themselves be mild, but become disfiguring when dug and squeezed to excess. The patients are usually young girls who may leave themselves with ugly scars. A psychiatric approach is often unhelpful and a daily ritual of attacking the lesions, helped by a magnifying mirror, may persist for years.

Localized neurodermatitis (lichen simplex)

This term refers to areas of itchy lichenification, perpetuated by bouts of scratching in response to stress. The condition is not uncommon and can occur on any area of skin. In men, lesions are often on the calves; in women, they favour the nape of the neck where the redness and scaling look rather like psoriasis. Some examples of persistent itching in the anogenital area are caused by lichen simplex there.

Patients with localized neurodermatitis develop scratch responses to minor itch stimuli more readily than controls. Local therapy does not alter the underlying cause, but topical steroids, sometimes only the most potent ones, ameliorate the symptoms. Occlusive bandaging of suitable areas clears only those lesions that are covered.

Nodular prurigo (Fig. 20.7) may be a variant on this theme as manifested in atopic subjects, who scratch and rub remorselessly at their extremely itchy nodules.

Hair-pulling habit

Trichotillomania is too dramatic a word for what is usually only a minor comfort habit in children, ranking alongside nail-biting and lip-licking. Perhaps the term should be dropped in favour of 'hair-pulling habit'. It is usually of little consequence, and children who twist and pull their hair, often as they are going to sleep, seldom have major psychiatric disorders. The habit often goes away most quickly if it is ignored. However, more severe degrees of hair-pulling are sometimes seen in disturbed adolescents and in those with learning difficulties; then the outlook for full regrowth is less good, even with formal psychiatric help.

The diagnosis can usually be made on the history, but some parents do not know what is going on. The bald areas do not show the exclamation-mark hairs of alopecia areata, or the scaling and inflammation of scalp ringworm. The patches are irregular in outline and hair loss is never complete. Those hairs that remain are bent or broken, and of variable length.

Dermatoses precipitated or perpetuated by emotional factors

Popular candidates for inclusion in this group of diseases are psoriasis, urticaria, atopic eczema, pompholyx, discoid eczema, alopecia areata, lichen simplex and lichen planus. Fancy rather than fact still rules here, but a scientific basis for these effects is gradually being established. For example, in psoriasis, stress increases the neuropeptide content of lesions, with a concomitant drop in the activity of enzymes that degrade neuropeptides, especially mast-cell chymase. In addition, the blood concentrations of certain neuromediators, especially β-endorphin, changes during exacerbations. Yet an aura of doubt lingers on—for a variety of reasons. The concept of stress is not a simple one, and the terms in which it is discussed are sometimes used rather vaguely. Each type of stress may well provoke its own pattern of response. For this reason many investigators have preferred to record damaging life events rather than to speculate about the presence of stress itself. However, there are problems with this approach too, as a barrage of minor daily annoyances may well be more important than major life events. Every dermatologist will have seen apparent examples of associations between external stress and exacerbations of most of these conditions, but proof that stress causes them is hard to find. Some studies suggest that even hyperhidrosis of the palms and soles, once thought to be an accentuated response to stress, has no relationship to chronic anxiety at all. No one questions that stress can cause sweating of the palms, but some studies suggest that chronic hyperhidrosis of the palms and soles, once thought to be simply an accentuated response to stress, has no relationship to chronic anxiety at all.

Further reading

Elmer, K.B., George, R.M. & Peterson, K. (2000) Therapeutic update: use of risperidone for the treatment of monosymptomatic hypochondriacal psychosis. *Journal of the American Academy of Dermatology* **43**, 683–686.

Gupta, M.A. & Gupta, K. (1996) Psychodermatology: an update. *Journal of the American Academy of Dermatology* **34**, 1030–1046.

Koo, J.Y. & Pham, C.T. (1992) Psychodermatology: practical guidelines on pharmacotherapy. *Archives of Dermatology* **128**, 381–388.

Koo, J.Y., Do, J.H. & Lee, C.S. (2000) Psychodermatology. *Journal of the American Academy of Dermatology* **43**, 848–853.

Picardi, A., Abeni, D., Melchi, C.F., Puddu, P. & Pasquini, P. (2000) Psychiatric morbidity in dermatological outpatients: an issue to be recognized. *British Journal of Dermatology* **143**, 983–991.

21 Other genetic disorders

The human genome consists of 23 pairs of chromosomes carrying an estimated 30 000 genes. The pairs of matching chromosomes as seen at colchicine-arrested metaphase are numbered in accordance with their size. A centromere divides each chromosome into a shorter (p) and a longer (q) arm.

Any individual's chromosomal make-up (karyotype) can be expressed as their total number of chromosomes plus their sex chromosome constitution. A normal male therefore is 46XY. A shorthand notation exists for recording other abnormalities such as chromosome translocations and deletions.

The precise location of any gene can be given by naming the chromosome, the arm of the chromosome (p or q), and the numbers of the band and subband of the chromosome, as seen with Giemsa staining, on which it lies. One of the genes important for atopy, for instance, lies on chromosome 11q13, i.e. on the long arm of chromosome 11 at band 13.

Several techniques can be used to identify the position of a gene.

1 A clue maybe offered by finding that some affected individuals have chromosomal deletions or unbalanced translocations, suggesting that the gene in question lies on the abnormal segments.

2 *Linkage analysis*. Genes are linked if they lie close together on the same chromosome; they will then be inherited together. The closer together they are, the less is the chance of their being separated by crossovers, one to six of which, depending on length, occur on each chromosome at meiosis. Each member of an affected family has to be examined both for the presence of the trait to be mapped, and also for a marker, usually a DNA probe, which has already been mapped. If linkage is established then the two loci will be close on the same chromosome. The probability of the results of such a study representing true linkage can be expressed as a logarithm of the odds (Lod) score. A

score of three or more suggests that the linkage is likely to be genuine.

3 *Somatic cell hybridization*. A hybrid made by fusing a human cell with a mouse cell will at first have two sets of chromosomes. Later human chromosomes are lost randomly until a stable state is reached. Those cells that produce a particular human protein must contain the relevant chromosome. A panel of such hybrid cells can be created which differ in their content of human chromosomes. By comparing these, the chromosomal site of the relevant gene can be deduced.

4 In situ *hybridization*. A cloned sequence of DNA, if made single-stranded by heat, will anneal to its complementary sequence on a chromosome. Radioactive or fluorescent labelling can be used to indicate its position there.

Non-Mendelian genetics

Traditional genetics has also been extended by the introduction of several new non-Mendelian concepts of importance in dermatology. These include the following.

1 *Mosaicism*. A mosaic is a single individual made up of two or more genetically distinct cell lines. The concept is important in several skin disorders including incontinentia pigmenti (p. 305) and segmental neurofibromatosis (p. 302). The mutation of a single cell in a fetus (a postzygotic mutation) may form a clone of abnormal cells. In the epidermis these often adopt a bizarre pattern of lines and whorls—Blaschko's lines, named after the dermatologist who recorded them in linear epidermal naevi in 1901.

2 *Contiguous gene deletions*. Complex phenotypes occur when several adjacent genes are lost. In this way,

for example, X-linked ichthyosis may associate with hypogonadism or anosmia.

3 *Genomic imprinting* means that genes may differ in their effect depending on the parent from which they are inherited. Genes from the father seem especially important in psoriasis, and from the mother in atopy (p. 82).

4 *Uniparental disomy* occurs when both pairs of genes are derived from the same parent so that an individual lacks either a maternal or a paternal copy. In this way a disorder usually inherited as a recessive trait can arise even though only one parent is a carrier.

Inheritance is important in many of the conditions discussed in other chapters and this has been highlighted in the sections on aetiology. This chapter includes some genetic disorders not covered elsewhere.

Neurofibromatosis

This relatively common disorder affects about 1 in 3000 people and is inherited as an autosomal dominant trait. There are two main types: von Recklinghausen's neurofibromatosis (*NF1*; which accounts for 85% of all cases) and bilateral acoustic neurofibromatosis (*NF2*); these are phenotypically and genetically distinct.

Cause

The *NF1* gene has been localized to chromosome 17q11.1. It is unusually large (300 kb) and many different mutations within it have now been identified. The *NF1* gene is a tumour suppressor gene, the product of which, neurofibromin, interacts with the product of the *RAS* proto-oncogene. This may explain the susceptibility of *NF1* patients to a variety of tumours. The inheritance of *NF1* is as an autosomal dominant trait but about one-half of index cases have no preceding family history.

The inheritance of *NF2* is also autosomal dominant. Mapping to chromosome 22q12.2 followed the observation of changes in chromosome 22 in meningiomas as these tumours may be seen in *NF2*. This gene also normally functions as a tumour-suppressor gene, the product of which is known as schwannomin.

Clinical features

The physical signs include the following.

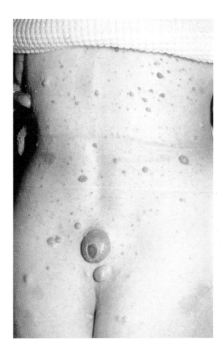

Fig. 21.1 Neurofibromatosis: one large but benign neurofibroma has ulcerated over the sacrum. Several *café au lait* patches are visible.

Von Recklinghausen's neurofibromatosis (NF1)

• Six or more *café au lait* patches (light brown oval macules; Fig. 21.1), usually developing in the first year of life.

• Axillary freckling (Fig. 21.2) in two-thirds of affected individuals.

• Variable numbers of skin neurofibromas, some small and superficial, others larger and deeper, ranging from flesh-coloured to pink, purple or brown (Fig. 21.1). Most are dome-like nodules, but others are irregular raised plaques. Some are firm, some soft and compressible through a deficient dermis ('button-hole' sign); others feel 'knotty' or 'wormy'. Neurofibromas may not appear until puberty and become larger and more numerous with age.

• Small circular pigmented hamartomas of the iris (Lisch nodules; Fig. 21.3), appear in early childhood.

Nearly all NF1 patients meet the criteria for diagnosis by the age of 8 years, and all do so by 20 years. The usual order of appearance of the clinical features is *café au lait* macules, axillary freckling, Lisch nodules and neurofibromas.

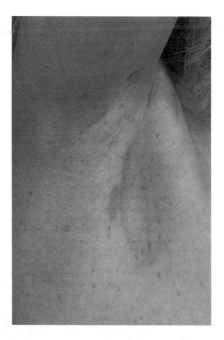

Fig. 21.2 Freckling of the axilla and a *café au lait* patch—both markers of neurofibromatosis.

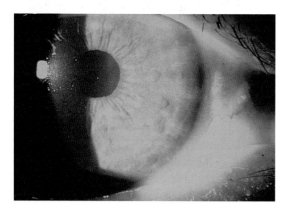

Fig. 21.3 Lisch nodules: best seen with a slit-lamp.

Bilateral acoustic neurofibromatosis (*NF2*)

- Bilateral acoustic neuromas.
- Few, if any, cutaneous manifestations.
- No Lisch nodules.

Diagnosis

The *café au lait* marks, axillary freckling and Lisch nodules should be looked for, as they appear before the skin neurofibromas. A segmental form of NF1 is caused by a postzygotic mutation. Isolated neurofibromas are not uncommon in individuals without neurofibromatosis and are of little consequence unless they are painful.

Complications

Von Recklinghausen's neurofibromatosis

A neurofibroma will occasionally change into a neurofibrosarcoma. Other associated features may include kyphoscoliosis, mental deficiency, epilepsy, renal artery stenosis and an association with phaeochromocytoma. Forme fruste variants occur, e.g. segmental neurofibromatosis.

Bilateral acoustic neurofibromatosis

Other tumours of the central nervous system may occur, especially meningiomas and gliomas.

Management

Ugly or painful lesions, and any suspected of undergoing malignant change, should be removed. The chance of a child of an affected adult developing the disorder is 1 in 2—parents should be advised about this.

Tuberous sclerosis

This uncommon condition, with a prevalence of about 1 in 12 000 in children under 10 years, is also inherited as an autosomal dominant trait, with variable expressivity even within the same family. As fertility is reduced, transmission through more than two generations is rare.

Cause

Mutations at two different loci can, independently, cause clinically identical tuberous sclerosis. The product of one gene (*TSC1*), lying at 9q34, is hamartin; that encoded by the other gene (*TSC2*) is tuberin. Both are associated *in vivo*, and probably act in the same biological pathways as tumour suppressors. *TSC1* gene mutations are responsible for a minority of cases and are under-represented in sporadic cases.

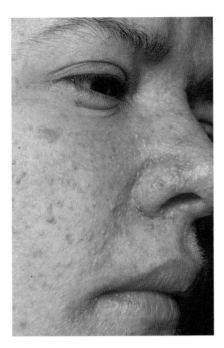

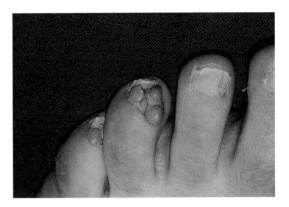

Fig. 21.5 The peri-ungual fibromas of tuberous sclerosis are found in adult patients.

Fig. 21.4 Tuberous sclerosis. Adenoma sebaceum, understandably, was referred to the acne clinic.

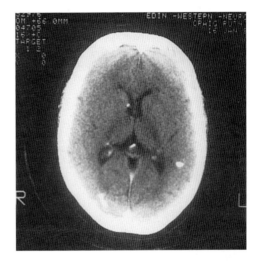

Fig. 21.6 Computed tomography scan of a patient with tuberous sclerosis. Modern imaging techniques can sometimes show cortical tubers (white) even when the skin changes are minimal.

Clinical features

The skin changes include the following.
• *Small oval white patches* ('ash leaf macules') occur in 80% of those affected. These are important as they may be the only manifestation at birth.
• *Adenoma sebaceum* occur in 85% of those affected. They develop at puberty as pink or yellowish acne-like papules on the face, often around the nose (Fig. 21.4).
• *Peri-ungual fibromas* occur in 50% of patients. These develop in adult life as small pink sausage-like lesions emerging from the nail folds (Fig. 21.5).
• *Connective tissue naevi* ('shagreen patches') are seen in 40% of patients. Cobblestone, somewhat yellow plaques often arise in the skin over the base of the spine.

Other features may include:
• epilepsy (in 75% of patients);
• mental retardation (in 50% of patients);
• ocular signs, including retinal phakomas and pigmentary abnormalities (in 50% of patients);
• hyperplastic gums;

• gliomas along the lateral walls of the lateral ventricles (80% of cases) and calcification of the basal ganglia; and
• renal and heart tumours.

Diagnosis and differential diagnosis

Any baby with unexplained epilepsy should be examined with a Wood's light (p. 33) to look for ash leaf macules. Skull X-rays and computer assisted tomography scans (Fig. 21.6) help to exclude involvement of the central nervous system and kidneys.

The lesions of adenoma sebaceum (a misnomer, as histologically they are angiofibromas) may be mistaken for acne.

Management

Affected families need genetic counselling. Apparently unaffected parents with an affected child will wish to know the chances of further children being affected. Before concluding that an affected child is the result of a new mutation, the parents should be examined with a Wood's light and by an ophthalmologist to help exclude the possibility of genetic transmission from a subtly affected parent. As the gene defects become established, prenatal screening of DNA should indicate those at risk.

Adenoma sebaceum improves cosmetically after electrodessication, dermabrasion or destruction by laser but tends to recur.

Xeroderma pigmentosum

Xeroderma pigmentosum is a heterogeneous group of autosomal recessive disorders, characterized by the defective repair of DNA after its damage by ultraviolet radiation. The condition is rare affecting about 5 per million in Europe.

Cause

Ultraviolet light damages DNA by producing covalent linkages between adjacent pyrimidines. These distort the double helix and inhibit gene expression. Cells from xeroderma pigmentosum patients lack the ability of normal cells to repair this damage.

DNA repair is a complex process using a large number of genes that encode a variety of interacting products that locate and prepare damaged sites for excision and replacement. It is not surprising therefore that many genetic defects can lead to a similar clinical picture. The genes for seven main types of xeroderma pigmentosum have now been identified.

Clinical features

There are many variants but all follow the same pattern.

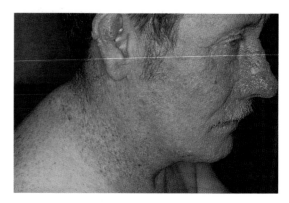

Fig. 21.7 Xeroderma pigmentosum: obvious freckling on neck. Scars on nose mark the spots where tumours have been removed.

- The skin is normal at birth.
- Multiple freckles, roughness and keratoses on exposed skin appear between the ages of 6 months and 2 years (Fig. 21.7). Photosensitivity increases thereafter.
- The atrophic facial skin shows telangiectases and small angiomas.
- Many tumours develop on light-damaged skin: these include basal cell carcinomas, squamous cell carcinomas, keratoacanthomas and malignant melanomas. Many patients die before the age of 20 years.
- Eye problems are common and include photophobia, conjunctivitis and ectropion.
- The condition may be associated with microcephaly, mental deficiency, dwarfism, deafness and ataxia (De Sanctis–Cacchione syndrome).

Diagnosis

This becomes evident on clinical grounds, although variants with minor signs may cause difficulty. The DNA repair defect can be detected in a few laboratories after the ultraviolet irradiation of cultured fibroblasts or lymphocytes from the patient.

Treatment

Skin cancers can be prevented by strict avoidance of sunlight, the use of protective clothing, wide-brimmed hats and of reflectant sunscreens and dark glasses. If possible, patients should not go out by day. Early and complete removal of all tumours is essential. Radio-therapy should be avoided.

Incontinentia pigmenti

This rare condition is an X-linked dominant disorder, usually lethal before birth in males. The gene for familial cases has been mapped to Xq28 and that for the more severe sporadic cases to Xp11. The bizarre patterning of the skin is caused by random X-inactivation (Lyonization). The lines of affected and normal skin represent clones of cells in which either the abnormal or normal X chromosome is active.

Clinical features

There are three stages in the evolution of the skin signs.
1 *Vesicular*. Linear groups of blisters occur more on the limbs than trunk.
2 *Warty*. After a few weeks the blisters dry up and the predominant lesions are papules with a verrucous hyperkeratotic surface.
3 *Pigmented*. A whorled or 'splashed' macular pigmentation, ranging from slate-grey to brown, replaces the warty lesions. Its bizarre patterning is a strong diagnostic pointer.

Occasionally, the vesicular and warty stages occur *in utero*; warty or pigmented lesions may therefore be the first signs of the condition. There is also a variant in which pale rather than dark whorls and streaks are seen.

Associated abnormalities are common. One-quarter of patients have defects of their central nervous system, most commonly mental retardation, epilepsy or microcephaly. Skull and palatal abnormalities may also be found. Delayed dentition, and even a total absence of teeth, are recognized features. The incisors may be cone- or peg-shaped. Ocular defects occur in one-third of patients, the most common being strabismus, cataract and optic atrophy.

Differential diagnosis

Diagnosis is usually made in infancy when bullous lesions predominate so the differential diagnosis includes bullous impetigo (p. 190), candidiasis (p. 38),

and the rarer linear immunoglobulin A (IgA) bullous disease of childhood (p. 113) and epidermolysis bullosa (p. 116).

Investigations

There is frequently an eosinophilia in the blood. Biopsy of an intact blister reveals an intraepidermal vesicle filled with eosinophils.

Management

This is symptomatic and includes measures to combat bacterial and candidial infection during the vesicular phase. Family counselling should be offered.

Ehlers–Danlos syndrome

Eleven subtypes are now recognized and this complicated subject has earned its own scientific group, which continuously updates classification and molecular biology.

Cause

All varieties of the Ehlers–Danlos syndrome are based on abnormalities in the formation or modification of collagen and the extracellular matrix, but are not necessarily a result of mutations in the collagen genes themselves. Established defects include lysyl hydroxylase deficiency, abnormalities in pro-alpha-1 (V) collagen chains, mutations in type III collagen genes, a deficiency of procollagen protease, and a fibronectin defect.

Clinical features

- Hyperelasticity of the skin.
- Hyperextensibility of the joints.
- Fragility of skin and blood vessels.
- Easy bruising.
- Curious ('cigarette paper') scars.

Complications

These depend on the type. They include subluxation of joints, varicose veins in early life, an increased liability to develop hernias, kyphoscoliosis, aortic aneurysms and ruptured large arteries, and intraocular haemorrhage. Affected individuals may be born prematurely as a result of the early rupture of fragile fetal membranes.

Diagnosis and treatment

The diagnosis is made on the clinical features and family history. The frequent skin lacerations and prominent scars may suggest child abuse. The diagnosis and type can sometimes be confirmed by enzyme studies on isolated fibroblasts. There is no effective treatment but genetic counselling is needed.

Pseudoxanthoma elasticum

This is the classical inherited connective tissue disorder affecting the elastic structures in the body—most obviously in the skin, blood vessels and eyes.

Cause

It has recently been found that both the dominantly and recessively inherited types are a result of mutations in a gene (on chromosome 16p13.1) encoding for a transmembrane transporter protein, which is a member of the ABC transporters superfamily. It is still not clear how this causes the disease.

Pathology

The elastic fibres in the mid-dermis become swollen and fragmented; their calcification is probably a secondary feature. The elastic tissue of blood vessels and of the retina may also be affected.

Clinical features

The skin of the neck and axillae, and occasionally of other body folds, is loose and wrinkled. Groups of small yellow papules give these areas a 'plucked chicken' appearance (Fig. 21.8). Breaks in the retina show as angioid streaks, which are grey poorly defined areas radiating from the optic nerve head. Arterial involvement may lead to peripheral, coronary or cerebral arterial insufficiency.

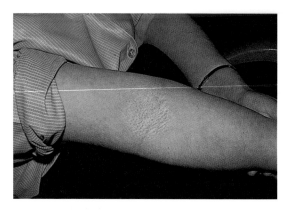

Fig. 21.8 The 'plucked chicken' appearance of pseudoxanthoma in the antecubital fossa.

> **LEARNING POINT**
>
> In all genodermatoses, the decision to have children, or not, must lie with the family concerned. Make sure they have all of the facts before them.

Complications

The most important are hypertension, recurrent gut haemorrhages, ischaemic heart disease and cerebral haemorrhage.

Diagnosis and treatment

The diagnosis is made clinically and confirmed by the histology. There is no effective treatment.

Further reading

Harper, J. (1996) *Inherited Skin Disorders: the Genodermatoses.* Butterworth-Heinemann, Oxford.

Matthew, C. (2001) Postgenomic technologies: hunting the genes for common disorders. *British Medical Journal* 122, 1031–1034.

Moss, C. & Savin, J.A. (1995) *Dermatology and the New Genetics.* Blackwell Science, Oxford.

Rees, J.L. (2000) Genetics, past and present, and the rise of systems dermatology. *British Journal of Dermatology* 143, 41–46.

Drug eruptions

Almost any drug can cause a cutaneous reaction, and many inflammatory skin conditions can be caused or exacerbated by drugs. A drug reaction can reasonably be included in the differential diagnosis of most skin diseases.

Mechanisms

These are many and various (Table 22.1), being related both to the properties of the drug in question and to a variety of host factors. Indeed, pharmaceutical companies study genes to predict responders and non-responders, and to detect patients who may be unable to metabolize a drug normally. For example, drug-induced lupus erythematosus occurs more commonly among 'slow acetylators' who take hydralazine. However, not all adverse drug reactions have a genetic basis; the excess of drug eruptions seen in the elderly may reflect drug interactions associated with their high medication intake.

Non-allergic drug reactions

Not all drug reactions are based on allergy. Some are a result of overdosage, others to the accumulation of drugs, or to unwanted pharmacological effects, e.g. stretch marks from systemic steroids (Fig. 22.1). Other reactions are idiosyncratic (an odd reaction peculiar to one individual), or a result of alterations of ecological balance (see below).

Cutaneous reactions can be expected from the very nature of some drugs. These are normal but unwanted responses. Patients show them when a drug is given in a high dose, or even in a therapeutic dose. For example, mouth ulcers frequently occur as a result of the cytotoxicity of methotrexate. Silver-based preparations, given for prolonged periods, can lead to a

Table 22.1 Some mechanisms involved in drug reactions.

Pharmacological
Caused by overdosage or failure to excrete or metabolize
Cumulative effects
Altered skin ecology
Allergic
   IgE-mediated
   Cytotoxic
   Immune complex-mediated
   Cell-mediated
Idiosyncratic
Exacerbation of pre-existing skin conditions

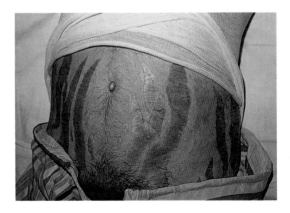

Fig. 22.1 Gross striae caused by systemic steroids.

slate-grey colour of the skin (argyria). Acute vaginal candidiasis occurs when antibiotics remove the normal resident bacteria from the female genital tract and so foster colonization by yeasts. Dapsone or rifampicin, given to patients with lepromatous leprosy, may cause erythema nodosum leprosum as the immune response to the bacillus is re-established.

Non-allergic reactions are often predictable. They affect many, or even all, patients taking the drug at a sufficient dosage for a sufficient time. Careful studies before marketing should indicate the types of reaction that can be anticipated.

Allergic drug reactions

Allergic drug reactions are less predictable. They occur in only a minority of patients receiving a drug and can do so even with low doses. Allergic reactions are not a normal biological effect of the drug and usually appear after the latent period required for an immune response. Chemically related drugs may cross-react.

Fortunately, allergic drug reactions present in only a limited number of forms, namely urticaria and angioedema, vasculitis, erythema multiforme, or a morbilliform erythema. Rarer allergic reactions include bullae, erythroderma, pruritus, toxic epidermal necrolysis and the hypersensitivity syndrome reaction. This syndrome includes the triad of fever, rash (from morbilliform to exfoliative dermatitis) and internal involvement (hepatitis, pneumonitis, nephritis and haematological abnormalities).

Presentation

Some drugs and the reactions they can cause

Experience helps here, together with a knowledge of the reactions most likely to be caused by individual drugs, and also of the most common causes of the various reaction patterns. Any unusual rash should be suspected of being a drug reaction, and approached along the lines listed in Table 22.2.

Antibiotics

Penicillins and sulphonamides are among the drugs most commonly causing allergic reactions. These are often morbilliform (Fig. 22.2), but urticaria and erythema multiforme are common too. Viral infections are often associated with exanthems, and many rashes are incorrectly blamed on an antibiotic when, in fact, the virus was responsible. Most patients with infectious mononucleosis develop a morbilliform rash if

Table 22.2 The six vital questions to be asked when a drug eruption is suspected.

1 Can you exclude a simple dermatosis (such as scabies or psoriasis) and the known skin manifestations of an underlying disorder (e.g. systemic lupus erythematosus)?
2 Does the rash itself suggest a drug eruption (e.g. urticaria, erythema multiforme)?
3 Does a past history of drug reactions correlate with current prescriptions?
4 Was any drug introduced a few days before the eruption appeared?
5 Which of the current drugs most commonly cause drug eruptions (e.g. penicillins, sulphonamides, thiazides, allopurinol, phenylbutazone, etc.)?
6 Does the eruption fit with a well-recognized pattern caused by one of the current drugs (e.g. an acneiform rash from lithium)?

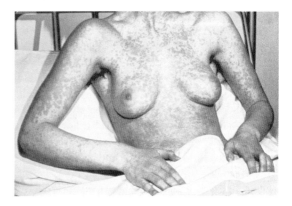

Fig. 22.2 Symmetrical erythematous maculopapular rash as a result of ampicillin.

ampicillin is administered. Penicillin is a common cause of severe anaphylactic reactions, which can be life-threatening. Minocycline can accumulate in the tissues and produce a brown or grey colour in the mucosa, sun-exposed areas or at sites of inflammation, as in the lesions of acne. Minocycline can rarely cause the hypersensitivity syndrome reaction, hepatitis, worsen lupus erythematosus, or elicit a transient lupus-like syndrome.

Penicillamine

Like penicillin itself, this can cause morbilliform eruptions or urticaria, but the drug has also been incriminated as a cause of haemorrhagic bullae at sites of trauma, of the extrusion of elastic tissue through the skin, and of pemphigus.

Oral contraceptives

Reactions to these are less common now that their hormonal content is small. The hair fall that may follow stopping the drug is like that seen after pregnancy (telogen effluvium; p. 168). Chloasma, hirsutism, erythema nodosum, acne and photosensitivity are other reactions.

Gold

This frequently causes rashes. Its side-effects range from pruritus to morbilliform eruptions, to curious papulosquamous eruptions such as pityriasis rosea or lichen planus. Erythroderma, erythema nodosum, hair fall and stomatitis may also be provoked by gold.

Steroids

Cutaneous side-effects from systemic steroids include a ruddy face, cutaneous atrophy, striae (Fig. 22.1), hirsutism, an acneiform eruption and a susceptibility to cutaneous infections, which may be atypical.

Anticonvulsants

There may be cross-reactivity between phenytoin, carbamazepine and phenobarbitol. Skin reactions are common and include erythematous, morbilliform, urticarial and purpuric rashes. Toxic epidermal necrolysis, erythema multiforme, exfoliative dermatitis, the hypersensitivity syndrome reaction and a lupus erythematosus-like syndrome are rare. A phenytoin-induced pseudolymphoma syndrome has also been described in which fever and arthralgia are accompanied by generalized lymphadenopathy and hepatosplenomegaly and, sometimes, some of the above skin signs. Long-term treatment with phenytoin may cause gingival hyperplasia (Fig. 22.3) and coarsening of the features as a result of fibroblast proliferation.

Highly active antiretroviral drugs

The long-term use of highly active antiretroviral drugs (HAART) has been commonly associated with lipodystrophy, producing a gaunt facies with sunken cheeks.

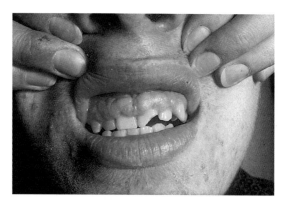

Fig. 22.3 Gingival hyperplasia caused by long-term phenytoin treatment.

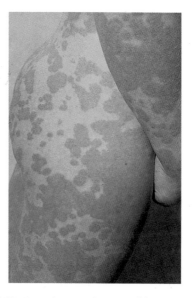

Fig. 22.4 Toxic erythema with urticarial features.

Some common reaction patterns and drugs which can cause them

Toxic (reactive) erythema

This vague term describes the most common type of drug eruption, looking sometimes like measles or scarlet fever, and sometimes showing prominent urticarial Fig. 22.4) or erythema multiforme-like elements. Itching and fever may accompany the rash. Culprits include antibiotics (especially ampicillin), sulphonamides and related compounds (diuretics and hypoglycaemics), barbiturates, phenylbutazone and para-aminosalicylate (PAS).

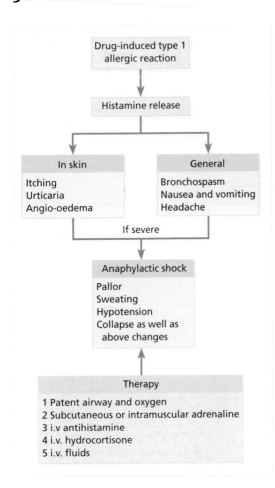

Fig. 22.5 The cause, clinical features and treatment of anaphylaxis.

Urticaria (Chapter 8)

Many drugs may cause this but salicylates are the most common, often working non-immunologically as histamine releasers. Antibiotics are also often to blame. Insect repellents and nitrogen mustards can cause urticaria on contact. Urticaria may be part of a severe and generalized reaction (anaphylaxis) that includes bronchospasm and collapse (Fig. 22.5).

Allergic vasculitis (Chapter 8)

The clinical changes range from urticarial papules, through palpable purpura, to necrotic ulcers. Erythema nodosum may occur. Sulphonamides, phenylbutazone,

indomethacin (indometacin), phenytoin and oral contraceptives are among the possible causes.

Erythema multiforme (Chapter 8)

Target-like lesions appear mainly on the extensor aspects of the limbs, and bullae may form. In the Stevens–Johnson syndrome, the patients are often ill and the mucous membranes are severely affected. Sulphonamides, barbiturates, lamotrigine and phenylbutazone are known offenders.

Purpura

The clinical features are seldom distinctive apart from the itchy brown petechial rash on dependent areas that is characteristic of carbromal reactions. Thrombocytopenia and coagulation defects should be excluded (Chapter 11). Thiazides, sulphonamides, phenylbutazone, sulphonylureas, barbiturates and quinine are among the drugs reported to cause purpura.

Bullous eruptions

Some of the reactions noted above can become bullous. Bullae may also develop at pressure sites in drug-induced coma.

Eczema

This is not a common pattern and occurs mainly when patients sensitized by topical applications are given the drug systemically. Penicillin, sulphonamides, neomycin, phenothiazines and local anaesthetics should be considered.

Exfoliative dermatitis

The entire skin surface becomes red and scaly. This can be caused by drugs (particularly phenylbutazone, PAS, isoniazid and gold), but can also be caused by widespread psoriasis and eczema.

Fixed drug eruptions

Round, erythematous or purple, and sometimes bullous plaques recur at the same site each time the drug

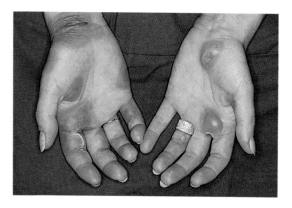

Fig. 22.6 Fixed drug eruption—an unusually severe bullous reaction.

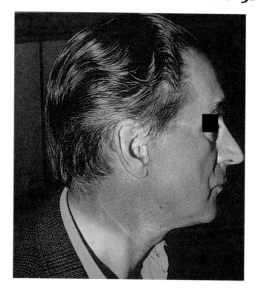

Fig. 22.7 Note sparing of skin creases and area shielded by spectacle frames in this patient with photorelated hyperpigmentation from a phenothiazine drug.

is taken (Fig. 22.6). Pigmentation persists between acute episodes. The glans penis seems to be a favoured site. The causes of fixed drug eruptions in any country follow the local patterns of drug usage there; but these change as old drugs drop out of use and are replaced by new ones with an unknown potential for causing this type of reaction. For example, in the UK, three of the four most common causes of fixed drug eruptions in 1970 (barbiturates, phenolphthalein and oxyphenbutazone) are no longer common causes. Paracetamol is currently the most common offender in the UK; trimethoprim-sulfa leads the list in the USA. Nonsteroidal anti-inflammatory drugs (NSAIDs; including aspirin), antibiotics, systemic antifungal agents and psychotropic drugs lie high on the list of other possible offenders.

Acneiform eruptions

Lithium, iodides, bromides, oral contraceptives, androgens or glucocorticosteroids, antituberculosis and anticonvulsant therapy may cause an acneiform rash (Chapter 12).

Lichenoid eruptions

These resemble lichen planus (Chapter 6), but not always very closely as mouth lesions are uncommon and as scaling and eczematous elements may be seen. Consider antimalarials, NSAIDs, gold, phenothiazines and PAS.

Toxic epidermal necrolysis (p. 115)

In adults, this 'scalded skin' appearance is usually drug-induced (e.g. sulphonamides, barbiturates, phenylbutazone, oxyphenbutazone, phenytoin, carbamazepine, lamotrigine or penicillin).

Hair loss

This is a predictable side-effect of acitretin and cytotoxic agents, an unpredictable response to some anticoagulants, and sometimes seen with antithyroid drugs. Diffuse hair loss may occur during, or just after, the use of an oral contraceptive.

Hypertrichosis

This is a dose-dependent effect of diazoxide, minoxidil and cyclosporin A.

Pigmentation (see also p. 252)

Chloasma (p. 251) may follow an oral contraceptive plus sun exposure. Large doses of phenothiazines impart a blue-grey colour to exposed areas (Fig. 22.7); heavy metals can cause a generalized browning;

clofazimine makes the skin red; mepacrine turns the skin yellow; and minocycline turns leg skin a curious greenish grey colour that suggests a bruise.

Photosensitivity

This is dealt with in Chapter 16. Always exclude the common drug causes (thiazides, tetracyclines, phenothiazines, sulphonamides or psoralens).

Xerosis

The skin can become rough and scaly in patients receiving oral retinoids, nicotinic acid or lithium.

Exacerbation of pre-existing skin conditions

Psoriasis and acne are good examples of this. Psoriasis may be made worse by giving β-blockers, antimalarials, terbinafine or lithium. Glucocorticoids, progesterone, androgens, anticonvulsants, bromides, iodidies and lithium may exacerbate acne.

Course

The different types of reaction vary so much that a brief summary is not possible. If a reaction occurs during the first course of treatment, it characteristically begins late, often about the ninth day, or even after the drug has been stopped. In such cases, it has taken that lag time to induce an immune reaction. In previously exposed patients the common morbilliform allergic reaction starts 2–3 days after the administration of the drug. The speed with which a drug eruption clears depends on the type of reaction and the rapidity with which the drug is eliminated.

Differential diagnosis

The differential diagnosis ranges over the whole subject of dermatology depending on which disease is mimicked. For instance, toxic erythema reactions can look very like measles, pityriasis rosea or even secondary syphilis. The general rule is never to forget the possibility of a drug eruption when an atypical rash is seen. Six vital questions should be asked (Table 22.2).

Treatment

The first approach is to withdraw the suspected drug, accepting that several drugs may need to be stopped at the same time. This is not always easy as sometimes a drug is necessary and there is no alternative available. At other times the patient may be taking many drugs and it is difficult to know which one to stop. The decision to stop or continue a drug depends upon the nature of the drug, the necessity of using the drug for treatment, the availability of chemically unrelated alternatives, the severity of the reaction, its potential reversibility, and the probability that the drug is actually causing the reaction.

Assessment depends upon clinical detective work (Table 22.2). Judgements must be based on probabilities and common sense. Every effort must be made to correlate the onset of the rash with prescription records. Often, but not always, the latest drug to be introduced is the most likely culprit. Prick tests and *in vitro* tests for allergy are still too unreliable to be of value. Re-administration, as a diagnostic test, is usually unwise except when no suitable alternative drug exists.

Non-specific therapy depends upon the type of eruption. In urticaria, antihistamines are helpful. In some reactions, topical or systemic corticosteroids can be used, and applications of calamine lotion may be soothing.

Anaphylactic reactions require special treatment (Fig. 22.4) to ensure that the airway is not compromised (e.g. oxygen, assisted respiration or even emergency tracheostomy). One or more injections of adrenaline (epinephrine) (1 : 1000) 0.3–0.5 mL should be given subcutaneously or intramuscularly in adults before the slow (over 1 min) intravenous injection of chlorphenamine maleate (10–20 mg diluted in syringe

---

LEARNING POINTS

1 This whole chapter is a warning against polypharmacy. Do your patients really need all the drugs they are taking?
2 If you suspect a drug eruption, keep on going back to the history.
3 Watch out for eruptions from new drugs.
4 Avoid provocation tests unless there are very strong indications for them.

with 5–10 mL of blood). Although the action of intravenous hydrocortisone (100 mg) is delayed for several hours it should be given to prevent further deterioration in severely affected patients. Patients should be observed for 6 h after their condition is stable, as late deterioration may occur. If an anaphylactic reaction is anticipated, patients should be taught how to self-inject adrenaline, and may be given a salbutamol inhaler to use at the first sign of the reaction.

To re-emphasize, the most important treatment is to stop the responsible drug. Desensitization, seldom advisable or practical, may rarely be carried out when therapy with the incriminated drug is essential and when there is no suitable alternative (e.g. with some anticonvulsants, antituberculous and antileprotic drugs). An expert, usually a physician with considerable experience of the drug concerned, should supervise desensitization.

Further reading

Bruinsma, W.A. (1990) *A Guide to Drug Eruptions: the European File of Side-effects in Dermatology*, 5th edn. The Files of Medicines, Oosthuizen, the Netherlands.

Knowles, S., Shapiro, L. & Shear, N.H. (1999) Drug eruptions in children. *Advances in Dermatology* **14**, 399–415.

Knowles, S.R., Uetrecht, J. & Shear, N.H. (2000) Idiosyncratic drug reactions: the reactive metabolite syndromes. *Lancet* **356**, 1587–1591.

Litt, J.Z. (2001) *Drug Eruption Reference Manual, 8th edn, 2002*. Parthenon, London.

Vervoet, D. & Durham, S. (1998) Adverse reactions to drugs. *British Medical Journal* **316**, 1511–1514.

Wolkenstein, P. & Revuz, J. (2000) Toxic epidermal necrolysis. *Dermatology Clinics* **3**, 485–495.

23 Medical treatment

An accurate diagnosis, based on a proper history and examination (Chapter 3), must come before a rational line of treatment can be chosen; even when a firm diagnosis has been reached, each patient must be treated as an individual. For some, no treatment may even be the best treatment, especially when the disorder is cosmetic or if the treatment would be worse than the condition itself. A patient with minimal vitiligo, for example, may be helped more by careful explanation and reassurance than by prescriptions.

If a diagnosis cannot be reached, the doctor has to decide whether a specialist opinion is needed, or whether it is best to observe the rash, perhaps treating it for a while with a bland application. In either case, the indiscriminate use of topical steroids or other medications, in the absence of a working diagnosis, often confuses the picture and may render the future diagnosis more difficult.

However, a firm diagnosis can usually be made, and a sensible course of treatment can be planned, but even then results are often better when patients understand their disease and the reasons behind their treatment. The cause and nature of their disease should be explained carefully, in language they can understand, and they must be told what can realistically be expected of their treatment. False optimism or undue pessimism, by patients or doctors, leads only to an unsound relationship. Too often patients become discontented, not because they do not know the correct diagnosis but because they have not been told enough about its cause or prognosis. Even worse, they may have little idea of how to use their treatment and what to expect of it; poor compliance often follows poor instruction. If the treatment is complex, instruction sheets are helpful; they reinforce the spoken word and answer unasked questions.

The principal steps in diagnosis and management are:

> **LEARNING POINT**
>
> One correct diagnosis is worth a hundred therapeutic trials.

- history;
- examination;
- investigations;
- diagnosis;
- explanation of the condition, its cause and prognosis;
- choice of treatment and instructions about it;
- discussion of expectations; and
- follow-up, if necessary.

Therapeutic options

Some of the treatments used in dermatology are listed in Table 23.1.

Table 23.1 Therapeutic options in dermatology.

Drugs	Topical
	Systemic
Physical	Surgical
	excision
	curettage
	Electrodessication
	Cryotherapy
	Radiotherapy
	Phototherapy
	Laser therapy

314

Topical vs. systemic therapy

The great advantage of topical therapy is that the drugs are delivered directly to where they are needed, at an optimum concentration for the target organ. Systemic side-effects from absorption are less than those expected from the same drug given systemically: with topical treatment, vital organs such as the marrow, liver and kidneys are exposed to lower drug concentrations than is the skin. However, topical treatment is often messy, time-consuming and incomplete, and takes time to apply, whereas systemic treatment is clean and quick and its effect is uniform over the entire skin surface. Cost must also be considered.

Some drugs can only be used topically (e.g. gamma benzene hexachloride for scabies and mupirocin for bacterial infections), while others only work systemically (e.g. dapsone for dermatitis herpetiformis and griseofulvin for fungal infections).

When a choice exists, and both possibilities are equally effective, then local treatment is usually to be preferred. Most cases of mild pityriasis versicolor, for example, respond to topical antifungals alone so systemic itraconazole is not the first treatment of choice.

Topical treatment

Percutaneous absorption

A drug used on the skin must be dissolved or suspended in a vehicle (base). The choice of the drug and of the vehicle are both important and depend on the diagnosis and the state of the skin. For a drug to be effective topically, it must pass the barrier to diffusion presented by the horny layer (Chapter 2). This requires the drug to be transferred from its vehicle to the horny layer, from which it will diffuse through the epidermis into the papillary dermis. Passage through the horny layer is the rate-limiting step.

The transfer of a drug from its vehicle to the horny layer depends on its relative solubility in each (measured as the 'partition coefficient'). Movement across the horny layer depends both upon the concentration gradient and on restricting forces (its 'diffusion constant'). In general, non-polar substances penetrate more rapidly than polar ones. A rise in skin temperature and in hydration, both achieved by covering a treated area with polyethylene occlusion, encourages penetration.

Some areas of skin present less of a barrier than do others. Two extreme examples are palmar skin, with its impermeable thick horny layer, and scrotal skin, which is thin and highly permeable. The skin of the face is more permeable than the skin of the body. Body fold skin is more permeable than nearby unoccluded skin. In humans, absorption through the hair follicles and sweat ducts is of little significance and the amount of hair on the treated site is no guide to its permeability.

In many skin diseases, the horny layer becomes abnormal and loses some of its barrier function. The abnormal nucleated (parakeratotic) horny layers of psoriasis and chronic eczema, although thicker than normal, have lost much of their protective qualities. Water loss is increased and therapeutic agents penetrate more readily. Similarly, breakdown of the horny layer by chemicals (e.g. soaps and detergents) and by physical injury will allow drugs to penetrate more easily.

In summary, the penetration of a drug through the skin depends on the following factors:
- its concentration;
- the base;
- its partition coefficient;
- its diffusion constant;
- the thickness of the horny layer;
- the state, including hydration, of the horny layer; and
- temperature.

Active ingredients

These include corticosteroids, tar, dithranol, antibiotics, antifungal and antiviral agents, benzoyl peroxide, retinoic acid and many others (Formulary 1, p. 328). The choice depends on the action required, and prescribers should know how each works. As topical steroids are the mainstay of much local dermatological therapy, their pharmacology is summarized in Table 23.2.

Vehicles (bases)

Most vehicles are a mixture of powders, water and greases (usually obtained from petroleum). Figure 23.3 shows that blending these bases together produces preparations that retain the characteristics of each of their components.

Table 23.2 The pharmacology of topical steroid applications.

Active constituents	Include hydrocortisone and synthetic halogenated derivatives Halogenation increases activity
Bases	Available as solutions, lotions, creams, ointments, sprays, mousses and tapes
Penetration	Readily penetrate via the horny layer and appendages Form a reservoir in the horny layer Polyethylene occlusion and high concentrations increase penetration
Metabolism	Some minor metabolism in epidermis and dermis (e.g. hydrocortisone converts to cortisone and other metabolites) Leave skin via dermal vascular plexus and enter general metabolic pool of steroids Further metabolism in liver
Excretion	As sulphate esters and glucuronides
Actions	Anti-inflammatory 1 Vasoconstrict 2 Decrease permeability of dermal vessels 3 Decrease phagocytic migration and activity 4 Decrease fibrin formation 5 Decrease kinin formation 6 Inhibit phospholipase A_2 activity and decrease products of arachidonic acid metabolism 7 Depress fibroblastic activity 8 Stabilize lysosomal membranes Immunosuppressive Antigen–antibody interaction unaffected but inflammatory consequences lessened by above mechanisms and by inhibiting cytokines (e.g. IFN-γ, GM-CSF, IL-1,2,3 and TNF-α) Lympholytic Decrease epidermal proliferation
Side-effects	1 Thinning of epidermis 2 Thinning of dermis 3 Telangiectasia and striae (caused by 1 and 2; Figs 23.1 and 23.2) 4 Bruising (caused by 2 and vessel wall fragility) 5 Hirsutism 6 Folliculitis and acneiform eruptions 7 May worsen or disguise infections (bacterial, viral and fungal) 8 Systemic absorption (rare but may be important in infants, when applied in large quantities under polyethylene pants) 9 Tachyphylaxis—lessening of clinical effect with the same preparation 10 Rebound—worsening, sometimes dramatic on withdrawing treatment
Uses	Eczema, psoriasis in some instances (facial, flexural, and palms/soles) Many non-infective, inflammatory dermatoses

GM-CSF, granulocyte macrophage colony-stimulating factor; INF-γ, γ-interferon; IL, interleukin; TNF, tumour necrosis factor.

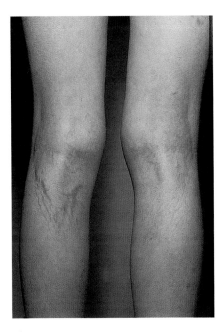

Fig. 23.1 Stretch marks behind the knee caused by the topical steroid treatment of atopic eczema.

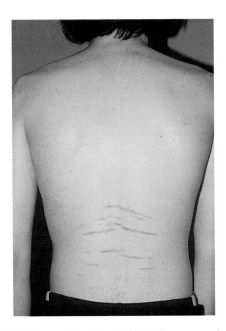

Fig. 23.2 Often attributed to Cushing's disease, or to local steroid therapy—but stretch marks across the back are common in normal fast-growing teenagers.

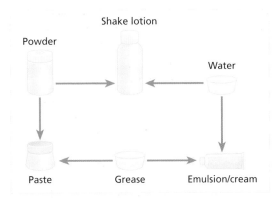

Fig. 23.3 The derivation of vehicles.

A vehicle should maximize the delivery of topical drugs but may also have useful properties in its own right. Used carelessly, vehicles may even do harm. Suggested indications are shown in Table 23.3. The choice of vehicle depends upon the action desired, availability, messiness, ease of application and cost.

Individual vehicles

Dusting powders are used in the folds to lessen friction between opposing surfaces. They may repel water (e.g. talc) or absorb it (e.g. starch); zinc oxide powder has an absorptive power midway between these extremes. Powders ought not be used in moist areas where they tend to cake and abrade.

Watery lotions evaporate and cool inflamed areas. This effect is hastened by adding an alcohol, but glycerol or arachis oil slow evaporation and retain skin moisture. Substances that precipitate protein (astringents; e.g. silver nitrate) lessen exudation.

Shake lotions are watery lotions to which powder has been added so that the area for evaporation is increased. These lotions dry wet weeping skin. When water has evaporated from the skin, the powder particles clump together and may become abrasive. This is less likely if an oil such as glycerol has been added.

Creams are used for their cooling, moisturizing and emollient effects. They are either oil-in-water emulsions [e.g. aqueous cream (UK), acid mantle cream (USA)] or water-in-oil emulsions [e.g. oily cream (UK), cold

Table 23.3 Vehicles and their properties.

Base	Used on	Effect	Points of note
Dusting powders	Flexures (may be slightly moist)	Lessen friction	If too wet clump and irritate
Alcohol-based applications (tinctures)	Scalp	Clean vehicle for steroid application	Cosmetically elegant, do not gum up hair May sting raw areas
Watery and shake lotions	Acutely inflamed skin (wet and oozing)	Drying, soothing and cooling	Tedious to apply Frequent changes (lessened by polyethylene occlusion) Powder in shake lotions may clump
Creams	Both moist and dry skin	Cooling, emollient and moisturizing	Short shelf life Fungal and bacterial growth in base Sensitivities to preservatives and emulsifying agents
Ointments	Dry and scaly skin	Occlusive and emollient	Messy to apply, soil clothing Removed with an oil
Pastes	Dry, lichenified and scaly skin	Protective and emollient	Messy and tedious to apply (linen or calico needed) Most protective if applied properly
Sprays	Weeping acutely inflamed skin Scalp	Drying, non-occlusive	Vehicle evaporates rapidly No need to touch skin to treat it
Gels	Face and scalp	Vehicle for steroids, salicylic acid and tretinoin	May sting when applied to inflamed skin Can be covered by make-up
Mousse	Scalp	Clean vehicle for steroid application	Doesn't matt the hair

cream (USA)]. Emulsifying agents are added to increase the surface area of the dispersed phase and that of any therapeutic agent in it.

Ointments are used for their occlusive and emollient properties. They allow the skin to remain supple by preventing the evaporation of water from the horny layer. There are three main types:
1 those that are water-soluble (macrogols, polyethylene glycols);
2 those that emulsify with water; and
3 those that repel water (mineral oils, and animal and vegetable fats).

Pastes are used for their protective and emollient properties and usually are made of powder added to a mineral oil or grease. The powder lessens the oil's occlusive effect.

Variations on these themes have led to the numerous topical preparations available today. Rather than

use them all, and risk confusion, doctors should limit their choice to one or two from each category. Table 23.3 summarizes the properties and uses of some common preparations.

Preservatives

Water-in-oil emulsions, such as ointments, require no preservatives. However, many creams are oil-in-water emulsions that permit contaminating organisms to spread in a continuous watery phase. These preparations therefore, as well as lotions and gels, require the incorporation of preservatives. Those in common use include the parahydroxybenzoic acid esters (parabens), chlorocresol, sorbic acid and propylene glycol. Some puzzling reactions to topical preparations are based on allergy to the preservatives they contain.

Methods of application

Ointments and creams are usually applied sparingly twice daily, but the frequency of their application will depend on many factors including the nature, severity and duration of the rash, the sites involved, convenience, the preparation (some new local steroids need only be applied once daily; Formulary 1, p. 332) and, most important, on common sense. In extensive eruptions, a tubular gauze cover keeps clothes clean and hampers scratching (see Fig. 7.19).

Three techniques of application are more specialized: immersion therapy by bathing, wet dressings (compresses) and occlusive therapy.

Bathing

Once-daily bathing helps to remove crusts, scales and medications. After soaking for about 10 min, the skin should be rubbed gently with a sponge, flannel or soft cloth; cleaning may be made easier by soaps, oils or colloidal oatmeal.

Medicated baths are occasionally helpful, the most common ingredients added to the bath water being bath oils, antiseptics and solutions of coal tar.

After cleaning, the most important function of a bath is hydration. The skin absorbs water and this can be held in the skin for some time if an occlusive ointment is applied after bathing.

Older patients may need help to get into a bath and should be warned about falling if the bath contains an oil or another slippery substance.

Wet dressings (compresses)

These are used to clean the skin or to deliver a topical medication. They are especially helpful for weeping, crusting and purulent conditions such as eczema, and are described more fully on p. 75. Five or six layers of soft cloth (e.g. cotton gauze) are soaked in the solution to be used; this may be tap water, saline, an astringent or antiseptic solution, and the compress is then applied to the skin. Open dressings allow the water to evaporate and the skin to cool. They should be changed frequently, e.g. every 15 min for 1 h.

Closed dressings are covered with a plastic (usually polyethylene) sheet; they do not dry out so quickly and are usually changed twice daily. They are espe-

Table 23.4 Minimum amount of cream (g) required for twice-daily application for 1 week.

Age	Whole body	Trunk	Both arms and legs
6 months	35	15	20
4 years	60	20	35
8 years	90	35	50
12 years	120	45	65
Adult (70 kg male)	170	60	90

cially helpful for debriding adherent crusts and for draining exudative and purulent ulcers.

Occlusive therapy

Sometimes steroid-sensitive dermatoses will respond to a steroid only when it is applied under a plastic sheet to encourage penetration. This technique is best reserved for the short-term treatment of stubborn localized rashes. The drawback of this treatment is that the side-effects of topical steroid treatment (Table 23.2) are highly likely to occur. The most important is systemic absorption if a large surface area of skin, relative to body weight, is treated (e.g. when steroids are applied under the polyethylene pants of infants).

Monitoring local treatment

One common fault is to underestimate the amount required. The guidelines given in Table 23.4 and Fig. 23.4 are based on twice daily applications. Lotions go further than creams, which go further than ointments and pastes.

Pump dispensers have recently become available for some topical steroids which allow measured amounts to be applied. Alternatively, 'fingertip units' (Fig. 23.5) can increase the accuracy of prescribing. As a guide,

> **LEARNING POINT**
>
> You know how much digoxin your patients are taking, but do you know how much of a topical corticosteroid they are applying? Keep a check on this.

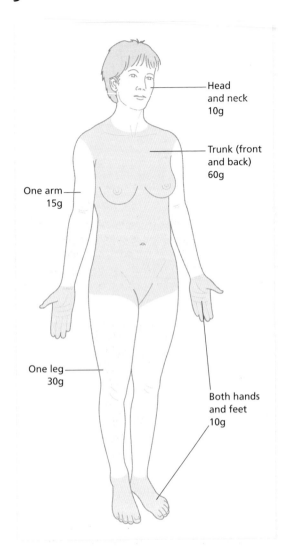

Fig. 23.4 The minimum amount of a cream required in 1 week by an adult applying it twice daily.

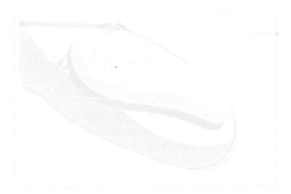

Fig. 23.5 A fingertip measures about 0.5 g ointment.

one fingertip unit in an adult male from a standard nozzle provides 0.5 g ointment.

Systemic therapy

Systemic treatment is needed if a skin condition is associated with systemic disease, or if the medicament of choice is inactive topically (e.g. griseofulvin). The principles of systemic therapy in dermatology are no different from those in other branches of medicine:

some drugs act specifically, others non-specifically. For example, antihistamines (H1 blockers) act specifically in urticaria, and non-specifically, by a sedative effect, on the most common skin symptom—itch.

Systemic disease coexists with skin disease in several ways (Chapter 19). Sometimes a systemic disease such as systemic lupus erythematosus may cause a rash; at other times, a skin disease causes a systemic upset. Examples of this are the depression that occurs in some patients affected with severe rashes, and high-output cardiac failure, which may occur in exfoliative dermatitis from the shunting of blood through the skin. A systemic upset caused by skin disease can be treated with drugs designed for such problems while the skin is being treated in other ways.

Further reading

Arndt, K.A. (1995) *Manual of Dermatologic Therapeutics*, 5th edn. Little, Brown, Boston, MA.

Flynn, G.L., Shah, V.P., Tenjarla, S.N. *et al.* (1999) Assessment of value and applications of *in vitro* testing of topical dermatological drug products. *Pharmacological Research* **16**, 1325–1330.

Greaves, M.W. & Gatti, S. (1999) The use of glucocorticoids in dermatology. *Journal of Dermatological Treatment* **10**, 83–91.

Shah, V.P., Behl, C.R., Flynn, G.L., Higuchi, W.I. & Schaefer, H. (1993) Principles and criteria in the development and optimization of topical therapeutic products. *Skin Pharmacology* **6**, 72–80.

24   Physical forms of treatment

The skin can be treated in many ways, including surgery, freezing, burning, ultraviolet radiation and lasers. Some broad principles will be discussed here.

Surgery

As our population ages, and becomes more concerned about appearances, requests for skin surgery are becoming more common. The distinction between traditional dermatological surgery and cosmetic surgery is blurring. There are few over the age of 50 years who do not have a benign tumour (Chapter 18) that they consider unsightly and wish to have removed. There are also many who are unhappy with a skin damaged by cumulative sun exposure (see p. 239), or concerned about medically trivial abnormalities on their face. To term the treatment of all these as 'cosmetic' seems harsh. Health care systems cannot cover the cost of treating all such problems but family doctors and dermatologists should be able to discuss with their patients any recent developments in phototherapy, laser treatment and specialized surgery that might help them. For example, doctors should be able to explain that diode lasers can remove unwanted hair permanently and without visible scarring, and the pros and cons of such treatment as well as supplying the names of specialists expert in it.

Skin biopsy

The indications for biopsy, and the techniques employed, are described in Chapter 3.

Excision

Excision under local anaesthetic, using an aseptic technique, is a common way of removing small

tumours (Figs 24.1 and 24.2). First, the lesion must be examined carefully and important underlying structures (e.g. the temporal artery) noted. If possible, the incision should run along the line of a skin crease, especially on the face. If necessary, charts or pictures of standard skin creases should be consulted

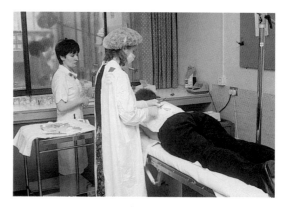

Fig. 24.1 No surgery is minor. Always use an aseptic technique, in proper surroundings, with appropriate help.

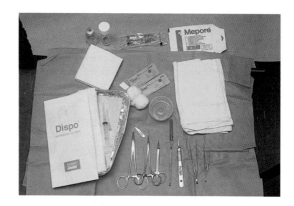

Fig. 24.2 Our standard pack is suitable for most skin surgery.

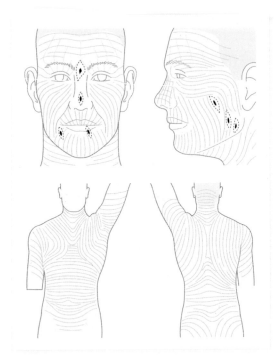

Fig. 24.3 Skin wrinkle figures are helpful in deciding the direction of wounds following skin surgery. Those performing dermatological surgery should have ready access to them.

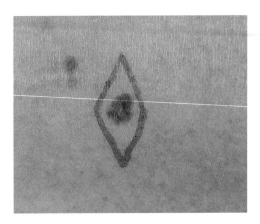

Fig. 24.4 Suspicious pigmented lesions should be removed with a 2-mm margin marked out in advance.

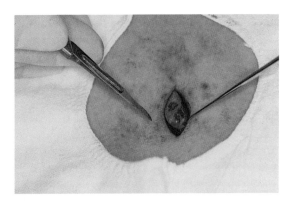

Fig. 24.5 A Gillies hook helps to remove an elliptical biopsy without damaging it.

(Fig. 24.3). After injection of the local anaesthetic [usually 1 or 2% lignocaine (lidocaine) with or without 1 in 200 000 adrenaline (epinephrine); see p. 37], the lesion is excised as an ellipse with a margin of normal skin, the width of which varies with the nature of the lesion and the site (Fig. 24.4). The scalpel should be held perpendicular to the skin surface and the incision should reach the subcutaneous fat. The ellipse of skin is carefully removed with the help of a skin hook (Fig. 24.5) or fine-toothed forceps. Larger wounds, and those where the scar is likely to stretch (e.g. on the back), are closed in layers with absorbable sutures (e.g. Dexon) before apposing the skin edges without tension using non-absorbable interrupted or continuous subcuticular sutures such as nylon or Prolene (see Further reading at end of this chapter for precise techniques of suturing). Stitches are removed from the face in 4–5 days and from the trunk and limbs in 7–14 days. Artificial sutures (e.g. Steri-Strip) may be used to take the tension off the wound edges after the stitches have been taken out.

Shave excision

Many small lesions are removed by shaving them off at their bases with a scalpel under local anaesthesia. This procedure is suitable only for exophytic tumours that are believed to be benign. Some cells at the base may be left and these, in the case of malignant tumours, would lead to recurrence.

Saucerization excision

This modified shave excision extends into the subcutaneous fat. It is used to remove certain small skin cancers and worrying melanocytic naevi. It leaves more scarring than a shave excision but the technique provides tissue that allows the dermatopathologist to determine if a tumour is invading and to measure

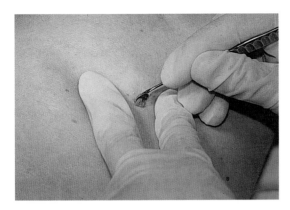

Fig. 24.6 Curettage beats excision if a seborrhoeic wart has to be removed. Stretching the skin helps to hold the lesion steady.

tumour thickness if the lesion is a melanoma. Furthermore, the technique may ensure complete removal more adequately than shave excision.

Curettage

Curettage under local anaesthetic is also used to treat benign exophytic lesions (e.g. seborrhoeic keratoses; Fig. 24.6) and, combined with electrodesiccation (see below), to treat some basal cell carcinomas. Its main advantage over purely destructive treatment is that histological examination can be carried out on the curettings. A sharp curette is used to scrape off the lesion and haemostasis is achieved by local haematinics, by electrocautery or electrodesiccation. The wound heals by secondary intention over 2–3 weeks, with good cosmetic results in most cases.

When a basal cell carcinoma is treated, the curette is scraped firmly and thoroughly along the sides and bottom of the tumour (the surrounding dermis is tougher and more resistant to curettage than the carcinoma) and the bleeding wound bed is then electrodesiccated aggressively. This stops bleeding and destroys a zone of tissue under and around the excised tumour to provide a tumour-free margin. The process is repeated once or twice at the same session to ensure that all of the tumour has been removed or destroyed. Only small basal cell carcinomas outside the skin folds should be treated in this way. The recurrence rates are relatively high for tumours in the nasolabial folds, over the inner canthi and on the nose, glabella and lips. The technique should not ordinarily be used for sclerosing basal cell carcinomas, invasive lesions larger than 1–2 cm, rapidly growing tumours or for those with micronodular features on histology.

Microscopically controlled excision (Mohs' surgery)

This form of surgery for malignant skin tumours is time-consuming and expensive, but the probability of cure is greater than with excision or curettage. First, the tumour is removed with a narrow margin. The excised specimen is then marked at the edges, mapped and, after rapid histological processing, is immediately examined in horizontal and vertical section. If the tumour extends to any margin, further tissue is removed from the appropriate place, based on the markings and mappings, and again checked histologically. This process is repeated until clearance has been proved histologically at all margins. The resulting wound can then be closed directly, covered with a split skin graft or allowed to heal by secondary intention.

Mohs' surgery is useful to treat:
• a basal cell carcinoma with a poorly defined edge;
• a sclerosing basal cell carcinoma (can suggest an enlarging scar clinically);
• a recurrent basal cell carcinoma;
• a basal cell carcinoma lying where excessive margins of skin cannot be sacrificed to achieve complete removal of the tumour (e.g. one near the eye);
• basal cell carcinomas in areas with a high incidence of recurrence such as the nose, glabella or nasolabial folds;
• some squamous cell carcinomas; and
• occasional malignant tumours other than basal and squamous cell carcinomas.

Flaps and grafts

These can be used to reconstruct a defect left by the wide excision of a tumour, or when a tumour is removed at a difficult site, e.g. the eyelid or tip of the nose (see Further reading at the end of this chapter as the techniques are beyond the scope of this book).

Electrosurgery

This is often combined with curettage, under local anaesthesia, to treat skin tumours. The main types are shown in Fig. 24.7.

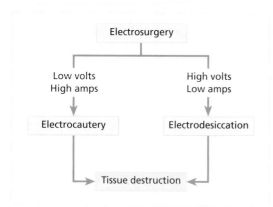

Fig. 24.7 Types of electrosurgery.

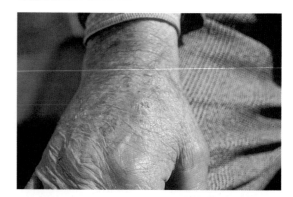

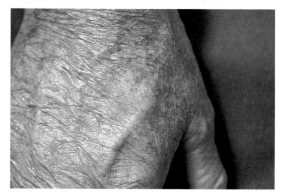

Fig. 24.9 Two freeze–thaw cycles with liquid nitrogen cleared this actinic keratosis. (Courtesy of Dr R. Dawber, The Churchill Hospital, Oxford, UK.)

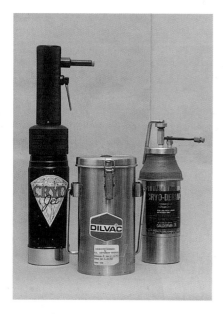

Fig. 24.8 Liquid nitrogen can be applied through a spray, or with a cotton wool bud direct from a vacuum flask (centre).

Cryotherapy

Liquid nitrogen (–196°C) is now used more often than carbon dioxide snow ('dry ice', –79°C). It is effective for viral warts, seborrhoeic keratoses, actinic keratoses and some superficial skin tumours (e.g. intraepidermal carcinoma and lentigo maligna). It is applied either on a cotton bud or with a special spray gun (Fig. 24.8). The lesion is frozen until it turns white, with a 1–2 mm halo of freezing around. Two freeze–thaw cycles kill tissue more effectively than one but are usually unnecessary for warts and some keratoses (Fig. 24.9). Patients should be warned to expect pain and possible blistering after treatment. Care should be taken when treating warts on fingers as digital nerve damage can occur after overenthusiastic freezing. Standard freeze–thaw times have been established for superficial tumours but temperature probes in and around deep tumours are needed to gauge the degree of freezing for their effective treatment. A crust, including the necrotic tumour, should slough off after about 2 weeks. Melanocytes (p. 242) are very sensitive to cold injury; hypopigmentation at a treated site is common and may be permanent.

Radiotherapy

Superficial radiation therapy (50–100 kV) can be used to treat biopsy-proven skin cancers in those over

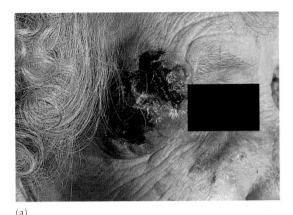

(a)

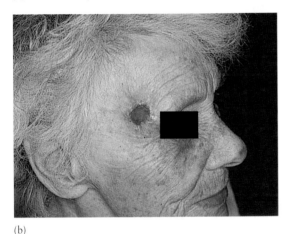

(b)

Fig. 24.10 (a) A 90-year-old, unfit for surgery, did well with radiotherapy for this massive basal carcinoma. (b) The reaction was healing well after a few weeks.

70 years old or who are too frail to tolerate surgery (Fig. 24.10). The usual dose is 3000 cGy, given in fractions over 5–10 days. The scars from radiotherapy worsen with time (Fig. 24.11), in contrast to surgical scars which improve. Nowadays radiotherapy is seldom used for inflammatory conditions.

Phototherapy

Ultraviolet radiation (UVR) helps some conditions (e.g. psoriasis, atopic dermatitis, nummular eczema, parapsoriasis, pityriasis lichenoides, pityriasis rosea, acne and cutaneous T-cell lymphoma; Table 16.4). For psoriasis, UVB (p. 58) may be given up to three times weekly, for 3–8 weeks, on its own or com-

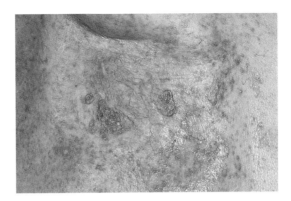

Fig. 24.11 Radiodermatitis with scarring, telangiectasia and hyperkeratosis.

bined with tar (Goeckerman) treatment or dithranol (anthralin; Ingram) treatment (Chapter 5). After tests to establish a starting dose, irradiance is increased by small increments, aiming to produce minimal erythema only after 24 h. Ultraviolet A is combined with psoralens in PUVA treatment (p. 59). Close supervision is needed because extreme phototoxicity from an overdose, from sunlight or concomitant use of tanning booths, has produced severe burns and even death. A careful record should also be kept of the cumulative UVR dose as the risk of developing skin cancers, including malignant melanoma, is increased when a patient has received a large cumulative dose.

Photodynamic therapy

Photodynamic therapy (PDT) is a new form of phototherapy used for skin cancers and precancers such as superficial basal cell carcinoma less than 2 mm thick (p. 266), intraepidermal carcinoma (p. 325), erythroplasia of Queyrat (p. 188) and actinic keratoses (p. 263). Selective tumour destruction is achieved by incorporating the photosensitizer in the target (malignant) tissue and then activating it with either a laser or non-laser light source. A promising combination is the naturally occurring porphyrin precursor, aminolaevulinic acid (ALA) and irradiation with a red light. The water-soluble ALA (20% in Unguentum M) is applied topically, under occlusion, to the tumour. After 4 h or so, when the ALA has been selectively absorbed by the tumour (Fig. 24.12), the area is exposed to the light for 15–60 min. The activated ALA converts molecular oxygen to cytotoxic singlet oxygen and free radicals, which in turn cause

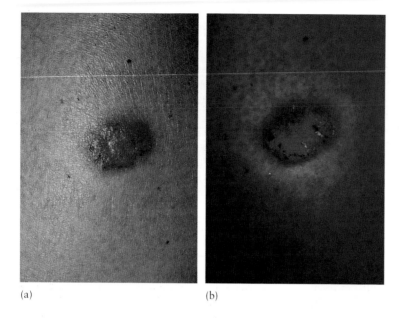

Fig. 24.12 A basal cell carcinoma (a), showing, by fluorescence, a selective uptake of ALA. (Courtesy of the Photobiology Unit, Ninewells Hospital, Dundee, UK.)

(a) (b)

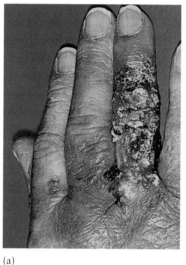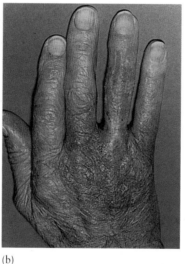

(a) (b)

Fig. 24.13 (a) Hyperkeratotic Bowen's disease on a finger. (b) Treated successfully with photodynamic therapy. This would have been an awkward site for surgery. (Courtesy of the Photobiology Unit, Ninewells Hospital, Dundee, UK.)

ischaemic necrosis of the tumour by damaging cell membranes, especially those in the walls of blood vessels. PDT is carried out in an outpatient setting and its potential advantages over standard treatments include:

• non-invasiveness;
• ability to treat many lesions at once;
• rarely causes ulceration and leads to a good cosmetic result;
• good patient acceptability; and
• useful for treating tumours on sites that present surgical difficulty, e.g. the taut skin of the finger (Fig. 24.13).

Laser therapy

Lasers (acronym for light amplification by the stimulated emission of radiation) are high-intensity coherent light sources of a specific wavelength. The photons are absorbed by a target chromophore (e.g. a tattoo pigment, melanin in hair, oxyhaemoglobin in blood vessels) and, depending on the energy, duration of the pulse of emission and the thermal relaxation time, cause local, sometimes microscopic, tissue destruction. Lasers are now being used to treat many skin lesions including capillary haemangiomas, tattoos, epidermal naevi, pigmented lesions, seborrhoeic keratoses, warts and tumours.

Since 1960, when T.H. Maiman won the Nobel Prize for inventing the first laser, technology has advanced rapidly and many types of laser are now available for clinical use. Most treatments can be carried out under local anaesthetic and as an outpatient. Port-wine stains can be treated successfully in children as well as in adults, using the flashlamp pulsed dye laser emitting light at 585 nm. Most tattoos can be removed by treatment with a Q-switched ruby laser (694 nm), a flashlamp pumped pulsed dye laser (510 nm) or an alexandrite laser (760 nm). Scarring should not be a problem. Benign but unsightly pigmented lesions such as *café au lait* marks, melasma, the naevus of Ota and senile lentigines can be greatly improved by treatment with the flashlamp pumped pulsed dye laser (510 nm) and the Q-switched neodymium: yttrium aluminium garnet (Nd:YAG) laser (532 nm). Unwanted hair can be permamently removed with a pulsed diode laser (800 nm) or with a Q-switched Nd:YAG laser emitting light at 1064 nm.

Rhinophyma, sebaceous gland hyperplasia, seborrhoeic keratoses, syringomas and many of the signs of chronic photodamage (e.g. rhytides, actinic cheilitis, actinic keratoses) can be helped by cutaneous resurfacing using CO_2 lasers emitting a wavelength of 10 600 nm (infrared) or a Q-switched erbium (Er): YAG laser emitting pulsed waves of 2940 nm in the near infrared, which is absorbed by water 10 times more efficiently than the pulsed CO_2 laser beam (Fig. 24.14). Good postoperative care is important, as the patient is left with what is essentially a partial thickness burn which heals by re-epithelialization from the cutaneous appendages. After profuse exudation for 24–48 h the treated area heals, usually in 5–10 days. Absolute contraindications for laser resurfacing include the use of isotretinoin within the previous year, concurrent

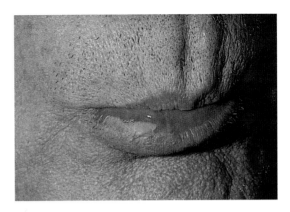

Fig. 24.14 Leukoplakia caused by chronic actinic damage—most suitable for laser resurfacing treatment.

bacterial or viral infection and any hint of ectropion. Dark skin (skin types V and V1; p. 233) should be treated with special care as pigmentary side-effects are common. Cutaneous laser resurfacing is more effective on the face than on the neck and extremities.

Laser treatments should be carried out only by fully trained specialists.

Further reading

Dover, J.S., Arndt, K.A., Dinehart, S.M., Fitzpatrick, R.E., Gonzales, E. & the Guidelines/Outcomes Committee. (1999) Guidelines of care for laser surgery. *Journal of the American Academy of Dermatology* **41**, 484–495.

Kalka, K., Merk, H. & Mukhtar, H. (2000) Photodynamic therapy in dermatology. *Journal of the American Academy of Dermatology* **42**, 389–413.

Ratner, D., Tse, Y., Goldman, M.P., Fitzpatrick, R.E. & Fader, D.J. (1999) Cutaneous laser resurfacing. *Journal of the American Academy of Dermatology* **41**, 365–389.

Topical treatments

Our selection has been determined by personal preferences and we accept that we have left out many effective remedies. However, the preparations listed here are those that we use most often. As a result some appear only in the UK column but not in the USA one,

and vice versa. To conform with current prescribing recommendations whenever possible we have listed these products under their active ingredients, with their proprietary names in brackets.

Type of preparation and general comments	UK preparation	USA
Emollients These are used to make dry scaly skin smoother. Most are best applied after a shower or bath	Soft white paraffin BP Emulsifying ointment BP Aqueous cream BP—can be used as a soap substitute Diprobase cream and ointment E45 range Oilatum range Unguentum M—a useful diluent: contains propylene glycol and sorbic acid, which may sensitize Neutrogena dermatological cream Aquadrate cream—contains urea Calmurid cream—contains urea	Petrolatum alba USP Vanacream—devoid of fragrances and many sensitizers Aquaphor –a hydrophilic petrolatum Plastibase—a hydrophilic polyglycol Eucerin—hydrophilic petrolatum containing water Oilatum range Neutrogena dermatological cream Curel Moisturel Lubraderm Carmol range—contains urea Tricream—cerimide-dominant barrier repair
Bath additives/shower gels These are a useful way of ensuring application to the whole skin. Most contain emollients which help with dry itchy skin. Others contain tar (see section on psoriasis) or antibacterials	Balneum range Emulsiderm—contains benzalkonium chloride Oilatum range Aveeno range Ster-Zac bath concentrate—contains antibacterial triclosan Hydromol bath emollient	Oilatum range Mineral oil bath emulsion (Keri Moisture Rich Shower and Bath Oil) Colloidal oatmeal (Aveeno Moisturizing Formula Bath)

Type of preparation and general comments	UK preparation	USA
Shampoos All contain detergents which help to remove debris and scales; some have added ingredients to combat psoriasis, seborrhoeic eczema and bacterial infections. Most work best if their lather is left on the scalp for 5 min before being rinsed off	**Containing tar** Alphosyl 2 in 1 Polytar range T-Gel Capasal—also contains salicylic acid **Others** Betadine—contains antibacterial povidone iodine Ceanel concentrate—contains cetrimide, undecenoic acid Selsun—contains selenium sulphide and can be used to treat pityriasis versicolor (p. 221) Nizoral—contains ketoconazole and is useful for seborrhoeic dermatitis and pityriasis versicolor Meted—contains salicylic acid and sulphur	**Containing tar** Pentrax shampoo Sebutone shampoo Denorex shampoo—tingles on scalp T-Gel Polytar range **Others** Selenium (Selsun shampoo) and can be used to treat pityriasis versicolor Ketoconazole (Nizoral shampoo) useful for seborrhoeic dermatitis and pityriasis versicolor Zinc pyrethione (Head and Shoulders, Zincon) Contains salicylic and sulfur (Meted, Sebulex) Fluocinonide (Caprex shampoo)
Cleansing agents These are used to remove debris and to combat infection. Some are astringents which precipitate protein and in doing so help to seal the moist surface of a weeping eczema or a stasis ulcer	Solution of sodium chloride 0.9% (Normasol)—used to clean wounds and ulcers Potassium permanganate (Permitabs—one tablet in 4 L water makes a 0.01% solution)—will stain clothing and skin Aluminium acetate lotion—use at 0.65% in water—is mildly astringent and used as wet dressing Silver nitrate—use at 0.5% in water—is astringent, stains skin brown Chlorhexidine/cetrimide (Hibicet Hospital Concentrate—dilute to 1 in 100)	Chlorhexidine 5% (Hibiclens) concentrate—use diluted to 1 in 100 (a 0.05% solution of chlorhexidine in water for skin disinfection) Cetaphil gentle skin cleanser (lipid-free) Benzalkonium chloride (Ionax line) Triclosan (Dial, Lever 2000)—deodorant, antibacterial Sulfacetamide/Sulfur (Plexon)—cleanser for rosacea
Barrier preparations These are used to protect the skin from irritants and are of value in the napkin (diaper) area and around stomas. Many contain the silicone, dimeticone. The choice of barrier creams for use at work depends upon individual circumstances: recommendations are not given here	Zinc and castor oil ointment BP Dimethicone and benzalkonium chloride (Conotrane) Dimethicone and cetrimide (Siopel) Dimethicone, calamine and zinc oxide (Vasogen)	Zinc oxide ointment Kerodex 51 (water-miscible) Kerodex 71 cream (water-repellant) Bentoquatum (Ivy Block Lotion) protective against toxicodendron (poison ivy allergy) Dermaguard spray Flexible collodion (film)

Continued p. 330

Type of preparation and general comments	UK preparation	USA
		Zinc oxide, lanolin, talc and vitamins A and D (Desitin ointment)
		Dimethicone (Diaper Guard Ointment)
		Anusol (zinc oxide plus pramoxine)
		Bag Balm (contains 8-hydroxyquinoline sulfate)

Depigmenting agents

These contain hydroquinone. The use of agents containing monobenzone causes permanent complete depigmentation	None in BNF but some preparations available without prescription from chemists/cosmetic counters	Hydroquinone 2–4% (Melanex topical solution—contains 3% hydroquinone, Solaquin forte—contains 4% hydroquinone and sunscreen, Glyquin—contains 10% glycolic acid and 4% hydroquinone)
		Hydroquinone (4%), tretinoin (0.05%) and fluocinonide (0.01%) (Tri-Luma)
		Monobenzene/monobenzyl ether of hydroquinone (Benaquin) (Caution: permanent depigmentation)

Camouflaging preparations

Blemishes which cannot be removed can often be made less obvious by covering them. Expert cosmetic advice may be needed to obtain the best colour match	Boots Covering Cream	Covermark range of products
	Covermark range	Dermablend
	Dermablend range	Powder Palette (Physician's Formula—Pierre Fabre) in green for correcting red blush of rosacea
	Keromask range	

Sunscreens and sunblocks

These help the light-sensitive but are not a substitute for sun avoidance and sensible protective clothing. The sun protection factor (SPF) is a measure of their effectiveness against UVB more than UVA, but those recommended here block UVA also	Cinnamate and oxybenzone (RoC Total Sunblock cream), Uvistat range	Cinnamates, benzophenones, and salicylates: Coppertone waterproof lines, Neutrogena sunblock lines, Presun active clear gel, Lubraderm daily UV lotion
	Titanium dioxide (Sun E45 range)	Avobenzone 3%, Homosalate 12%, Octyl methoxycinnamate 7.5%, Octocrylene 1.5%, Oxybenzone 6% (Solbar PF)
Allergic contact dermatitis from the sunscreen ingredients may be missed and the rash put down to a deterioration of the original photosensitivity	Cinnamate, oxybenzone and titanium dioxide (Sunsense Ultra)	Titanium dioxide (5% Ti-Screen Natural Moisturizing Titanium Dioxide Sunblock Lotion, 2.4% Neutrogena Natural Buff 50)
		Zinc oxide ointment
		Zinc Oxide 8%, Titanium dioxide 3% (Vanicream Sunscreen)

Antipruritics

Remember that these are of limited value: try to make a firm diagnosis which will lead to an effective line of treatment	Calamine lotion BP	Calamine lotion
	Oily Calamine lotion BP—contains arachis oil	Crotamiton (Eurax cream and lotion) also used to treat scabies

Type of preparation and general comments	UK preparation	USA
	Menthol (0.5%) or phenol (1.0%) in aqueous cream Crotamiton cream and lotion (Eurax)—also used to treat scabies Doxepin (Xepin cream)	Menthol and camphor (Sarna lotion) contains menthol and camphor Menthol, phenol and zinc oxide (Shamberg's lotion) Doxepin (Zonalon cream) Pramoxine (Prax, Pramegel) Benzocaine (Boil ease ointment, solarcaine)—caution: may sensitize
Antiperspirants The most effective preparations for excessive sweating in the armpits are those which contain aluminium chloride hexahydrate in an alcohol base. They also help palmar sweating but to a lesser extent	Aluminium chloride hexahydrate 20% (Anhydrol Forte solution or Driclor solution)	Aluminum chlorate 20% (Drysol) 12.5% (CertainDry Roll-On), 6.25% (Xerac-AC) Formaldehyde 10% solution (Lazerformaldehyde)—caution: may sensitize
Keratolytics These are used to counter an excessive production of keratin. Salicylic acid preparations should be used for limited areas only and not above 6%, as absorption and toxicity may follow their prolonged and extensive application, especially in infants	Salicylic acid, 2–4% in emulsifying ointment or soft white paraffin Urea preparations (see Emollients above) Propylene glycol, 20% in aqueous cream	Salicylic acid (5% Keralyt gel) Salicylic acid, 2–4% in emulsifying ointment or soft white paraffin Urea preparations (see Emollients) Propylene glycol (Epilyt)
Depilatories These are used to remove unwanted facial hairs. All are irritating	None in BNF but freely available over-the-counter	Sulfides (Magic Shaving Powder) Thioglycollates (Nair line, Neet line) Zip wax, Nair microwave wax—mechanical hair removal
Steroids Our selection here has had to be ruthless as so many brands and mixtures are now on the market. Conventionally, they are classified according to their potency. Your aim should be to use the least potent preparation which will cope with the skin disorder being treated. Side-effects and dangers are listed in Table 23.2 (p. 316) Nothing stronger than 1% hydrocortisone should be used on the face (except in special circumstances, e.g. discoid lupus erythematosus) or in infancy. Be	**Mildly potent** Hydrocortisone 0.5, 1.0, 2.5% preparations Fluocinolone acetonide (Synalar cream 1 in 10) **Moderately potent** Alclometasone diproprionate (Modrasone cream and ointment) Betamethasone valerate (Betnovate RD cream and ointment) Clobetasone butyrate cream and ointment (Eumovate)	**Mildly potent** Hydrocortisone 0.5, 1.0, 2.5% (numerous manufacturers) Desonide (Desowen, Tridesilon) Alclometasone (Aclovate) **Moderately potent** Betamethasone valerate (Valisone) Fluticasone (Cutivate) Hydrocortisone valerate (Westcort) Triamcinolone 0.025%, 0.1% (Kenalog, Aristocort, various manufacturers)

Continued p. 332

Type of preparation and general comments	UK preparation	USA
reluctant to prescribe more than 200 g of a mildly potent, 50 g of a moderately potent, or 30 g of a potent preparation per week for any adult for more than a month Most of the preparations listed are available as lotions, creams, oily creams, and ointments; your choice of vehicle will depend upon the condition under treatment (p. 317). Use twice daily except for Cutivate and Elocon, which are just as effective if used once a day	**Potent** Betamethasone valerate (Betnovate range including scalp application, Betacap scalp application, Bettamousse scalp application) Fluticasone propionate (Cutivate cream and ointment) Mometasone furoate (Elocon range) Hydrocortisone 17-butyrate (Locoid range) Fluocinolone acetonide (Synalar range) **Very potent** Clobetasol propionate (Dermovate range) Halcinonide (Halciderm cream) Diflucortolone valerate (Nerisone Forte range)	**Potent** Betamethasone dipropionate (Diprosone) Diflorasone (Elocon) Fluocinonide (Lidex) Desoximetasone (Topicort 0.025%) **Very potent** Clobetasol (Temovate) Halobetasol (Ultravate) Betamethasone dipropionate in enhanced vehicle (Diprolene) Diflorasone (Psorcon)

Steroid combinations

With antiseptics	**Mildly potent** Hydrocortisone and clioquinol (Vioform-hydrocortisone cream and ointment) **Potent** Betamethasone valerate and clioquinol (Betnovate-C cream and ointment) Hydrocortisone 17-butyrate with chlorquinaldol (Locoid-C cream and ointment) Fluocinolone acetonide with clioquinol (Synalar-C cream and ointment)	**Mildly potent** Clioquinol and hydrocortisone (1%) Iodoquinol 1% and hydrocortisone 1% (Vytone cream)
With antibiotics	**Mildly potent** Hydrocortisone and oxytetracycline (Terra-Cortril ointment) **Moderately potent and potent** Betamethasone valerate and neomycin (Betnovate-N cream and ointment) Fluocinolone acetonide and neomycin (Synalar-N cream and ointment)	**Mildly potent** Polysporin, neomycin, bacitracin, hydrocortisone 1% (Corticosporin)
With antifungals	**Mildly potent** Hydrocortisone and clotrimazole (Canesten HC cream) Hydrocortisone and miconazole (Daktacort cream and ointment) Hydrocortisone and econazole (Econacort)	**Very potent** Clotrimazole and betamethasone dipropionate (Lotrisone)

Type of preparation and general comments	UK preparation	USA
With antibacterials and antifungals	**Mildly potent** Hydrocortisone, chlorhexidine and nystatin (Nystaform HC cream and ointment) Hydrocortisone, oxytetracycline and nystatin (Terra-Cortril Nystatin cream) Hydrocortisone, benzalkonium, nystatin and dimeticone (a silicone) (Timodine cream) **Moderately potent** Clobetasone butyrate, oxytetracycline and nystatin (Trimovate cream) **Very potent** Clobetasol propionate, neomycin and nystatin (Dermovate NN cream and ointment)	**Moderately potent** Neomycin, nystatin, triamcinolone 0.1% (Mycolog II)
With tar	**Mildly potent only** Hydrocortisone, allantoin and coal tar extract (Alphosyl HC cream)	
With Calcipotriol	**Potent only** Betamethasone dipropionate (Dovobet ointment)	
With salicylic acid	**Potent only** Betamethasone dipropionate and salicylic acid (Diprosalic ointment—and scalp application)	

Preparations for use in the mouth

Useful mouth washes	Benzydamine solution (Difflam oral rinse)—an analgesic for painful inflammation in the mouth Chlorhexidine (Corsodyl mouth wash) Hexetidine solution (Oraldene) an antiseptic gargle	Cetylpyridinium (Cepacol antiseptic mouthwash) Listerine antiseptic mouthrinse (contains thymol, eucalyptol, methylsalicylate, menthol) 'All-purpose mouthwash'—different formulations—e.g. compounded as nystatin suspension 100 000 U/ml, 120 ml; diphenhydramine elixir 12.5 mg/5 ml, 480 ml; hydrocortisone powder 240 mg; sodium carboxymethylcellulose 2%, 720 ml

Continued p. 334

Type of preparation and general comments	UK preparation	USA
		'Magic mouthwash' —different formulations—e.g. compounded as equal parts Maalox (Magnesia and alumina oral suspension) and diphenhydramine elixer 12.5 mg/5 ml) —some also add dexamethasone
Topical steroids	Triamcinolone acetonide (Adcortyl in Orabase) a paste that adheres to mucous membranes Hydrocortisone pellets (Corlan pellets) to be dissolved slowly in mouth near the lesion—usually an aphthous ulcer	Triamcinolone acetonide (Kenalog in orabase)—a paste that adheres to mucous membranes Fluocinonide gel (Lidex gel) Clobetasol gel (Temovate gel)
For yeast infections	Miconazole (Daktarin oral gel) Amphotericin (Fungilin lozenges) Nystatin (Nystan oral suspension)	Clotrimazole (Mycelex troches) Nystatin oral suspension or pastilles (Nilstat, Mycostatin)
Topical immunomodulators Watch out for local infection. No information yet on development of skin cancer at exposed sites when treated for prolonged periods	Tacrolimus (Protopic ointment 0.03%, 0.1%) Pimecrolimus (Elidel cream 1%)	Tacrolimus (Protopic ointment 0.03%, 0.1%) Pimecrolimus (Elidel cream 1%)
Preparations for otitis externa Otitis externa, essentially an eczema, is often complicated by bacterial or yeast overgrowth—hence the combinations listed here	Aluminium acetate ear drops 8%—an effective astringent for the weeping phase: best applied on ribbon gauze Hydrocortisone with neomycin and polymyxin (Otosporin drops) Cotrimazole (Canesten solution)	Aluminium acetate ear drops 8%—an effective astringent for the weeping phase: best applied on ribbon gauze Hydrocortisone, neomycin and polymyxin (Corticosporin drops) Ciprofloxacin 0.2% and hydrocortisone 1% (Cipro HC Otic) Acetic acid 2% with or without hydrocortisone (VoSol/VoSol-HC)
Antibacterial preparations The ideal preparation should have high antibacterial activity, low allergenicity, and the drug should not be available for systemic use; this combination is hard to find. Some compromises are given here	Mupirocin (Bactroban cream and ointment) Fusidic acid (Fucidin ointment, cream or gel) Neomycin and gramicidin (Graneodin ointment) Polymyxin and Bacitracin (Polyfax ointment)	Mupirocin (Bactroban ointment) Nitrofurazone (Furacin ointment, cream or solution) Bacitracin (Baciguent ointment) Gentamicin (Garamycin ointment) Bacitracin and polymyxin (Polysporin ointment) Silver sulfadiazine 1% cream—various manufacturers
	To eliminate nasal carriage of staphylococci Mupirocin (Bactroban Nasal cream) Chlorhexidine and neomycin (Naseptin cream)	**To eliminate nasal carriage of staphylococci** Mupirocin (Bactroban ointment)

Type of preparation and general comments	UK preparation	USA
Antifungal preparations In our view imidazole, terbinafine, butenafine and amorolfine creams have now supplanted their messier, more irritant, and less effective rivals (e.g. Whitfield's ointment). They have the added advantage of combating yeasts as well as dermatophytes Systemic therapy will be needed for tinea of the scalp, of the nails, and of widespread or chronic skin infections which prove resistant to topical treatment	Clotrimazole (Canesten cream) Miconazole (Daktarin cream) Terbinafine (Lamisil cream) Amorolfine (Loceryl cream and nail lacquer) Tioconazole (Trosyl nail solution)—applied locally it may increase the success rate of griseofulvin. Used by itself it may also cure or improve some nails	Clotrimazole (Lotrimin cream and solution Miconazole (Micatin cream) Econazole (Spectazole cream) Terbinafine (Lamisil cream) Butenafine (Mentax cream) Ciclopirox (Loprox cream and lotion, Penlac nail lacquer) Naftifine (Naftin cream)
Antiviral preparations These have little part to play in the management of herpes zoster. However, if used early and frequently, they may help with recurrent herpes simplex infections	Aciclovir cream Idoxuridine in dimethyl sulphoxide (Herpid application)—absorption of dimethyl sulphoxide may cause a garlic-like taste	Penciclovir (Denavir cream) Acyclovir (Zovirax cream)
Wart treatments		
Palmoplantar warts	Salicylic acid and lactic acid (Salactol paint or Salatac and Cuplex gel) Salicylic acid (at 26%, Occlusal solution: at 50%, Verrugon ointment) Glutaraldehyde (Glutarol solution) Formaldehyde (Veracur gel)	Salicylic acid (Duofilm, Occlusal-HP) Salicylic acid plasters 40% Salicylic acid, 15% in karaya (Transversal)
Anogenital warts	Podophyllin resin (Podophyllin paint compound)—use with care (p. 205) Podophyllotoxin (Condyline solution) Imiquimod (Aldara cream)—an immunomodulator (p. 205)	Podophyllin resin, 15% (Podophyllin paint compound–use with care (p. 205) Podofilox (Condylox gel) Imiquimod (Aldara cream), (p. 205)
Preparations for treatment of scabies Poor results follow inefficient usage rather than ineffective preparations. We prefer Lyclear or precipitated sulphur in young children, and pregnant and lactating women. Written instructions are helpful (p. 230)	Permethrin (Lyclear Dermal Cream) Benzyl benzoate application (BP) Malathion (Quellada M liquid or Derbac-M liquid) Precipitated sulphur 6% in soft white paraffin Crotamiton (Eurax cream) for use if itching persists after treatment with more effective scabicides	Permethrin (Elimite cream) Lindane (Kwell lotion) Crotamiton (Eurax cream) for use if itching persists after treatment with more effective scabicides Precipitated sulphur 6% in soft white paraffin

Continued p. 336

Type of preparation and general comments	UK preparation	USA
Preparations for treatment of pediculosis Resistance to lindane has limited its usefulness for scalp lice. Lotions left on for a minimum of 12 h are perhaps more effective, although less convenient than shampoos	Malathion (Prioderm alcohol-based lotion or Derbac-M aqueous lotion or Quellada lotion) Permethrin (Lyclear Creme Rinse)	Malathione (Prioderm lotion and cream shampoo) Permethrin (Nix) Permethrin/Piperonyl butoxide (Rid) Benzyl benzoate solution 20–25% Precipitated sulphur 6% in Nivea Oil
Preparations for acne Active ingredient **Benzoyl peroxide** (an antibacterial agent) induces dryness during the first few weeks; this usually settles, even with continued use	Benzoyl peroxide (Panoxyl and Acetoxyl ranges) Potassium hydroxyquinoline (Quinoderm range)	Benzoyl peroxide (Panoxyl, Benzac, Desquam-X range 2.5, 5 and 10%) Sulfur (Sulphoxyl)
Retinoids Potent comedolytic agents, also used to reverse photoageing. May irritate. Must be avoided during pregnancy/lactation	Isotretinoin (Isotrex) Tretinoin (Retin-A preparations) Adapalene (Differin gel and cream)	Tretinoin (Retin-A preparations) Tazarotene (Tazarac gel 0.05 and 0.1%) Adapalene (Differin gel, lotion and cream)
Antibiotics	Clindamycin (Dalacin-T solution or roll-on) Erythromycin (Stiemycin solution) Erythromycin and zinc acetate (Zineryt)	Clindamycin (Cleocin-T solution and gel) Erythromycin 2% solution—various manufacturers Sulfacetamide (Klaron lotion) Clindamycin and benzoyl peroxide (Clinderm) Erythromycin and benzoyl peroxide (Benzamycin)
Abrasives	Aluminum oxide (Brasivol paste Nos 1 & 2)	Brasivol Facial Cleanser (fine, medium, rough)
Sulphur	2–10% sulphur in calamine lotion	2–10% sulphur in calamine lotion Sulfur creams (Liquimat, Fostril) Sulfur and resorcinol (Rezamid)
Azelaic acid and salicylic acid	Azelaic acid (Skinoren cream) Salicylic acid (Acnisal solution)	Azelaic acid (Azalex cream) Salicylic acid (Neutrogena clear pore gel, Clearasil stick, Stridex gel) Sulfur and sulfacetamide (Sulfacet-R)
Preparations for rosacea	Metronidazole (Metrogel or Zyomet gels)	Metronidazole gel, lotion, cream (Metrogel, Metrocream, Metrolotion, Noritate) Sulfur and Sulfacetamide (Sulfacet-R) Sulfacetamide (Klaron)

Type of preparation and general comments	UK preparation	USA
Preparations for psoriasis **Vitamin D derivatives** Calcipotriol (calcipotriene, USA) and tacalcitol. Avoid using in patients with disorders of calcium metabolism. May irritate initially	Calcipotriol (Dovonex cream, ointment and scalp solution). Maximum weekly doses: 6–12 years, 50 g; 12–16 years, 75 g; adults, 100 g Tacalcitol (Curatoderm ointment). Maximum daily dose for adults, 10 g. Not recommended for children	Calcipotriene (Dovonex cream, lotion, and ointment) Same as UK
Steroids Routine long-term treatment with potent or very potent steroids is not recommended. For indications (p. 57)		
Scalp applications	Betamethasone (Betnovate scalp application, Diprosalic scalp lotion—also contains salicylic acid) Fluocinolone (Synalar gel)	Clobetasol (Temovate scalp application, Olux mousse) Fluocinonide (Lidex solution) Fluocinonide in peanut oil (Dermasmoothe FS) Betamethasone valerate (Valisone lotion, Luxiq foam)
For use elsewhere Tar—steroid combinations are helpful	(*See* section on topical steroids above)	
Dithranol/anthralin Stains normal skin and clothing. May be irritant, therefore start with low concentration. For 30-minute regimen *see* p. 58	Dithrocream range Micanol range	Micanol 1% Dithrocreme 0.1, 0.25, 0.5, 1%
Retinoid Contraindicated in pregnancy and during lactation	Tazarotene (Zorac gel)	Tazarotene (Tazarec gel)
Tar These clean refined tar preparations are suitable for home use. Messier, although more effective, formulations exist but are best used in treatment centres		
Bath additives	Polytar emollient Psoriderm bath emulsion	Balnetar liquid
Applications	Alphosyl cream Carbo-Dome cream Psoriderm cream	Estar gel 5% PsoriGel 1.5% MG-217 2% ointment

Continued p. 338

Type of preparation and general comments	UK preparation	USA

Scalp applications
Salicylic acid
Used mostly for scalp psoriasis
Tar–salicylic acid combinations
	Alphosyl lotion
	Cocois ointment (*see* Keratolytics)
	Pragmatar cream—also contains
	  sulphur
	Gelcosal gel
		Neutrogena T Gel therapeutic
		  conditioner
		10% Liquor carbonis detergens in
		  Nivea oil
		Scalpicin Hypoallergenic Formula

Preparations for venous ulcers Regardless of topical applications, venous ulcers will heal only if local oedema is eliminated. Remember that the surrounding skin is easily sensitized. To choose treatment for an individual ulcer (p. 142)		

For cleansing	Saline, potassium permanganate
	  (*see* Cleansing agents above)
	Hydrogen peroxide solution (3%)
		Saline, potassium permanganate
		  (*see* Cleansing agents)
		Hydrogen peroxide solution (3%)

Antibacterial gauze dressings	Chlorhexidine (Bactigras tulle) Soframycin (Sofra-tulle)	

Other applications	Silver sulfadiazine—active against
	  Pseudomonas (Flamazine cream)
	Silver nitrate aqueous solution (0.5%)
	Cadexomer iodine (Iodosorb powder)
		Enzymes (Elase Ointment—contains
		  fibrinolysin and desoxyribonuclease;
		  Collagenase Santyl ointment—
		  contains collagenase)
		Silver sulfadiazine (Silvadene cream)
		Nitrofurazone (Nitrofurazone solution)
		Mupirocin (Bactroban Ointment)

Medicated bandages Beware of allergic contact reactions to parabens preservatives which are in most bandages	Zinc paste and calamine (Calaband) Zinc paste and ichthammol (Ichthopaste) Zinc oxide (Viscopaste PB7)	

Other dressings	Hydrocolloid (Granuflex, DuoDERM
	  Extra Thin)
	Calcium alginate (Kaltostat)
	Polyurethane foam (Tielle)
	Vapour-permeable film dressing
	  (Opsite)
	Activated charcoal with silver
	  (Actisorb silver)
	Dextranomer (Debrisan)
		Hydrocolloid (Duoderm)
		Vapour-permeable film dressing
		  (Opsite, Tegaderm)
		Hydrogel (Vigilon)
		Dextranomer (Debrisan)
		Calcium alginate

Miscellaneous		
5-Flourouracil The treatment of individual lesions in patients with multiple actinic	Efudix cream	Efudex cream 1.5% Carac 0.5% (Dermik)—drug incorporated into microsphere

Type of preparation and general comments	UK preparation	USA
keratoses is tedious or impossible. For such cases 1–5% cream containing 5-fluorouracil is useful. It should be applied twice daily for 2–3 weeks. Patients should be warned about the inevitable inflammation and soreness which appears after a few days. Lesions on the scalp and face do better than those on the arms and hands		
Minoxidil May be used as a possible treatment for early male-pattern alopecia. The response is slow, and only a small minority of patients will obtain a dense regrowth even after 12 months. Hair regained will fall out when treatment stops—warn patients about this	Regaine liquid 2 or 5%—only on private prescription	Rogaine 2% solution Rogaine 5% solution for men
Capsaicin A topical analgesic useful for the treatment of post-herpetic neuralgia. Apply up to 3–4 times daily after lesions have healed. May take 2–4 weeks to relieve pain	Axsain cream (0.075%)	Zostrix cream (0.025%) Capzasin HP cream (0.075%) Axsain cream (0.075%)
Lithium succinate A topical anti-inflammatory used in seborrhoeic dermatitis	Efalith ointment	
Lidocaine/prilocaine A local anaesthetic for topical use. Applied on skin as a thick layer of cream under an occlusive dressing or on adult genital mucosa with no occlusive dressing. Read manufacturer's instructions for times of applicaion	Lidocaine and prilocaine (EMLA cream)	Lidocaine 4% (ELA-Max) Lindocaine 2.5%/Prilocaine 2.5% (Emla cream)

Systemic medication

We list here only preparations we use commonly for our patients with skin disease. **The doses given are the usual oral doses for adults**. We occasionally use some of these drugs for uses not approved by federal regulatory agencies. We have included some, but not all, of the side effects and interactions; these are more fully covered in the *British National Formulary* (BNF) (UK) and *Physician's Desk Reference* (PDR) (USA). Physicians prescribing these drugs should read about them there, in more detail, and specifically check the dosages before treating their patients. If possible, systemic medication should be avoided in pregnant women.

Main dermatological uses and usual adult doses	Adverse effects	Interactions	Other remarks
Antibacterials			
Cefalexin and Cefuroxime Cephalosporins not inactivated by penicillinase. For Gram-positive and -negative infections resistant to penicillin and erythromycin (Cefalexin 250–500 mg four times daily; Cefuroxine 250 mg twice daily)	Gut upsets Candidiasis Rarely, erythema multiforme or toxic epidermal necrolysis Transient hepatotoxicity Rarely nephrotoxic	Probenecid reduces excretion	Not usually indicated as first-line or blind therapy Ten per cent of penicillin allergic patients will react to this
Ciprofloxacin A 4-quinolone used for Gram-negative infections, especially pseudomonas, and Gram-positive infections. First choice for skin infections in the immunosuppressed if the causative organism is not yet known (500 mg twice daily)	Gut upsets Occasionally hepatotoxic and nephrotoxic Haemolysis in those deficient in glucose-6-phosphate dehydrogenase	Antacids reduce absorption Enhances effects of warfarin and theophylline	Crystalluria if fluid intake is inadequate Care if renal impairment Avoid in pregnancy, breast feeding, children and epileptics
Co-amoxiclav (Augmentin) A broad-spectrum penicillin combined with clavulanic acid: use if organisms resistant to both	Gut upsets Candidiasis Rashes, especially in infectious mononucleosis	As for other penicillins	Use with care in hepatic or renal failure, pregnancy, and breast feeding

Main dermatological uses and usual adult doses	Adverse effects	Interactions	Other remarks
erythromycin and flucloxacillin. Also for Gram-negative folliculitis (375 mg three times daily)			Avoid in those allergic to penicillin
Erythromycin 1 Acne vulgaris (250–500 mg twice daily) 2 Gram-positive infections, particularly staphylococcal and streptococcal. Useful with penicillin allergy (250–500 mg four times daily)	Gut upsets Rashes Cholestatic hepatitis if treatment prolonged (reversible and most common with estolate salt)	Increased risk of toxicity if given with theophylline or carbamezapine Potentiates effects of warfarin, ergotamine, cyclosporin A, disopyramide, carbamazepine, terfenadine, astemizole, theophylline, cisapride and digoxin	Avoid estolate in liver disease Care when hepatic dysfunction Excreted in human milk
Flucloxacillin Dicloxacillin and Cloxacillin Penicillins used for infections with penicillinase-forming staphylococci (250–500 mg four times daily)	Gut upsets Morbilliform eruptions Arthralgia Anaphylaxis	Probenecid increases blood level Reduces excretion of methotrexate	Accumulate in renal failure Atopics may be at increased risk of hypersensitivity reactions
Metronidazole 1 Anaerobic infections (400 mg three times daily) 2 Stubborn rosacea (200 mg twice daily) 3 Trichomoniasis (200 mg three times daily for 7 days)	Gut upsets Metallic taste Candidiasis Ataxia and sensory neuropathy Seizures	Potentiates effects of warfarin, phenytoin and lithium Drugs that induce liver enzymes (e.g. rifampicin, barbiturates, griseofulvin, phenytoin, carbamazepine, and smoking) increase destruction of metronidazole in liver and necessitate higher dosage May have disulfiram-like effect with alcohol (headaches, flushing, vomiting, abdominal pain)	Use lower dose in presence of liver disease Neurotoxicity more likely if central nervous system disease Carcinogenic and mutagenic in some non-human models
Minocycline A tetracycline used for acne and rosacea (50 mg daily or	Gut upsets Dizziness and vertigo	May impair absorption of oral contraceptives	Avoid in pregnancy and in children under 12 years

Continued p. 342

Main dermatological uses and usual adult doses	Adverse effects	Interactions	Other remarks
twice daily, or 100 mg daily in a modified release preparation)	Candidiasis Deposition in bones and teeth of fetus and children Deposition in skin and mucous membranes causes blue-grey pigmentation Benign intracranial hypertension Lupus erythematosus-like syndrome with hepatitis	May potentiate effect of warfarin	
Tetracycline and oxytetracycline Acne and rosacea (250–500 mg twice daily)	Gut upsets Candidiasis Rashes Deposition in bones and teeth of fetus and children Rare phototoxic reactions Benign intracranial hypertension	Absorption impaired when taken with food, antacids and iron Many impair absorption of oral contraceptives May potentiate effect of warfarin	Avoid in pregnancy and in children under 12 years Should not be used if renal insufficiency
Penicillin V (phenoxymethylpenicillin) 1 For infections with Gram-positive cocci (250–500 mg four times daily) 2 Prophylaxis of erysipelas (250 mg daily)	Gut upsets Morbilliform rashes Urticaria Arthralgia Anaphylaxis	Blood level increased by probenecid Reduces excretion of methotrexate	Accumulates in renal failure Atopics at increased risk of hypersensitivity reactions

Antifungals

Terbinafine
Dermatophyte infections when systemic treatment appropriate (as a result of site, severity or extent)
 	
Has replaced griseofulvin as first-choice systemic and fungal agent. Unlike itraconazole and fluconazole its action does not involve cytochrome P-450 dependent enzymes in the liver
Dose: 250 mg daily
  Tinea pedis: 2–6 weeks
  Tinea corporis: 4 weeks
  Tinea unguium: 12 weeks
	Gut upsets
	Headache
	Rashes—including toxic epidermal necrolysis
	Taste disturbance
	Rarely liver toxicity
		Plasma concentration reduced by rifampicin
		Plasma concentration increased by cimetidine
			Avoid in hepatic and renal impairment and when breast feeding
			Not for use in pregnancy
			Not yet recommended for children

Main dermatological uses and usual adult doses	Adverse effects	Interactions	Other remarks
Griseofulvin Has largely been superseded by newer antifungals Dermatophyte infections of skin, nails, and hair. Not for *Candida* or pityriasis versicolor (500 mg microsize daily)	Gut upsets Headaches, rashes, photosensitivity	Induces microsomal liver enzymes and so may increase elimination of drugs such as warfarin and phenobarbital	Not for use in pregnancy, liver failure, porphyria or systemic lupus erythematosus Men should not father children within 6 months of taking it Absorbed better when taken with fatty foods
Fluconazole 1 Candidiasis *Acute/recurrent vaginal* (single dose of 150 mg) *Mucosal (not vaginal) conditions* (50 mg daily) Oropharyngeal: 7–14 days Oesophagus: 14–30 days *Systemic candidiasis*—see manufacturer's instructions 2 Second-line treatment in some systemic mycoses, e.g. cryptococcal infections 3 Dermatophyte infections (except of nails) and pityriasis versicolor (50 mg daily for 2–6 weeks)	Gut upsets Rarely rashes Angioedema/anaphylaxis Liver toxicity May be worse in AIDS patients	Hydrochlorothiazide increases plasma concentration Rifampicin reduces plasma concentration Potentiates effects of warfarin, cyclosporin A and phenytoin May potentiate effects of sulphonylureas leading to hypoglycaemia May inhibit metabolism of astemizole causing serious dysrhythmias	Avoid in pregnancy Hepatic and renal impairment Use in children only if imperative and no alternative Avoid in children under 1 year and when breast feeding
Itraconazole 1 Candidiasis *Vulvovaginal* (200 mg twice daily) for 1 day *Oropharyngeal* (100 mg daily) for 15 days 2 Pityriasis versicolor (200 mg daily) for 7 days 3 Dermatophyte infections (100 mg daily) Tinea pedis and manuum for 30 days Tinea corporis for 15 days Tinea of nails—an intermittent regimen can be used (200 mg twice daily for 1 week per month, continued for three or four cycles)	Gut upsets Headache	Antacids reduce absorption Rifampicin and phenytoin reduce plasma concentration May potentiate effects of warfarin May increase plasma levels of digoxin and cyclosporin Inhibits metabolism of astemizole: this may lead to serious dysrhythmias	Avoid in hepatic impairment Avoid in children, in pregnancy and when breast feeding

Continued p. 344

Main dermatological uses and usual adult doses	Adverse effects	Interactions	Other remarks
Ketoconazole Widespread pityriasis versicolor (200 mg daily for 14 days or 400 mg each morning for 3 days)	As with fluconazole but greater incidence of liver toxicity	Same as fluconazole	Seldom used in UK. Monitor liver function continually if used for longer than 14 days. Chosen because of its cheapness
Nystatin 1 Recurrent vulval and perineal candidiasis 2 Persistent gastrointestinal candidiasis in immunosuppressed patients (500 000 units three times daily)	Unpleasant taste Gut upsets		Not absorbed and when given by mouth acts only on bowel yeasts

Antivirals

Aciclovir, famciclovir and valaciclovir (for dosages see specialist literature) Famciclovir and valaciclovir have the advantage that they need be taken only two or three time a day 1 Severe herpes simplex infections—primary or recurrent 2 Severe herpes zoster infections—use may reduce incidence of post-herpetic neuralgia 3 Prophylaxis for recurrent herpes simplex especially in the immunocompromised, to treat eczema herpeticum and to treat chickenpox in the immunocompromised	Rapid gut upsets, transient rise in urea and creatinine in 10% of patients after intravenous use Raised liver enzymes Reversible neurological reactions Decreases in haematological indices	Excretion may be delayed by probenicid Lethargy when intravenous aciclovir given with zidovudine	Adequate hydration of patient should be maintained Risk in pregnancy unknown Reduce dose in renal impairment No effect on virus in latent phase Must be given early in acute infections

Antihistamines

All those listed here are H_1-blockers though some dermatologists combine these with H_2-blockers in recalcitrant urticaria

Non-sedative

Used for urticaria and type I hypersensitivity reactions

Main dermatological uses and usual adult doses	Adverse effects	Interactions	Other remarks
Loratadine and desloratadine (Loratadine, 10 mg daily; desloratadine, 5 mg daily)		Not reported	Avoid in pregnancy and lactation
Cetirizine and levocetirizine (Cetirizine, 10 mg daily; levocetirizine, 5 mg daily)	Rarely sedate	Levocetirizine—delayed clearance with theophylline	Use half the usual dose when renal impairment
Fexofenadine (a metabolite of terfenadine) 60–180 mg daily			

Sedative

| Urticaria, type I hypersensitivity including intravenous use in anaphylaxis (p. 312). Also used as antipruritic agents in atopic eczema, lichen planus | Sedation (promethazine > trimeprazine (alimemazine) > hydroxyzine > chlorphenamine = diphenhydramine = cyproheptadine) Anticholinergic effects:
• dry mouth
• blurred vision
• urinary retention
• tachycardia
• glaucoma | Potentiate effect of alcohol and central nervous system depressants Potentiate effect of other anticholinergic drugs | Increased rate of elimination in children Sedation may be useful in an excited itchy patient Warn of risk of drowsiness when driving or operating dangerous machinery |

Chlorpheniramine
(4 mg three or four times daily)

Diphenhydramine
(25–30 mg four times daily)

Hydroxyzine
(10–50 mg four times daily)

Cyproheptadine
(4 mg four times daily)

Promethazine
(10–25 mg daily to three times daily)

Trimeprazine
(2.5–10 mg once or twice daily)

Continued p. 346

Main dermatological uses and usual adult doses	Adverse effects	Interactions	Other remarks
Anti-androgens			
Cyproterone acetate and ethinylestradiol (UK: Dianette; USA: not available) 1 Acne vulgaris, unresponsive to systemic antibiotics, in women only 2 Idiopathic hirsutism, one tablet (cyproterone acetate 2 mg, ethinylestradiol 35 mg) daily for 21 days, starting on fifth day of menstrual cycle and repeated after a 7-day interval. Treat for 6 months at least	As for combined oral contraceptives	Should not be given with other oral contraceptives	Contraindicated in pregnancy. Cyproterone acetate is an anti-androgen and if given to pregnant women may feminize a male fetus. For women of childbearing age, therefore, it must be given combined with a contraceptive (the ethinylestradiol component) Also contraindicated in liver disease, disorders of lipid metabolism, and with past or present endometrial carcinomas Not for use in males or children
Drospirenone and ethinyloestadiol (USA: Yasmin; UK: not available)	Hyperkalaemia	NSAIDS and ACE inhibitors increase risk of hyperkalaemia Increases shelf life of digoxin	Contraindicated if abnormal renal or hepatic function Drospirenone is an analogue of spironolactone. Avoid in pregnancy. May feminize male fetus
Spironolactone 25–50 mg daily for idiopathic hirsutism Used in USA	Hyperkalaemia		Avoid in pregnancy. Causes gynaecomastia Avoid if renal or hepatic impairment
Immunosuppressants			
Azathioprine For autoimmune conditions, e.g. systemic lupus erythematosus, pemphigus and bullous pemphigoid— often used to spare dose of systemic steroids (1–2.5 mg/kg daily). We strongly	Gut upsets Bone marrow suppression, usually leucopenia or thrombocytopenia Hepatotoxicity, pancreatitis Predisposes to infections, including warts	Increased toxicity if given with allopurinol	See comment about the need to check for thiopurine methyltransferase levels (in first column)

Main dermatological uses and usual adult doses	Adverse effects	Interactions	Other remarks
recommend checking thiopurine methyltransferase levels before starting treatment with azathioprine as homozygotes for the low-activity allele have a high risk of bone marrow suppression			Weekly blood checks are necessary for the first 8 weeks of treatment and thereafter at intervals of not longer than 3 months Reduce dosage if severe renal impairment Avoid in pregnancy Possible increased risk of lymphomas
Cyclosporin 1 Severe psoriasis when conventional treatment is ineffective or inappropriate 2 Short-term (max. 8 weeks) treatment of severe atopic dermatitis when conventional treatment ineffective or inappropriate (2.5 mg/kg daily in two divided doses). See p. 61 for guidance in use	Hepatic and renal impairment Hypertension Gut upset Hypertrichosis Gum hyperplasia Tremor Hyperkalaemia Occasionally facial oedema, fluid retention and convulsions Hypercholesterolaemia Hypomagnesia	(See *BNF* and *PDR* for fuller details) (Use with tacrolimus specifically contraindicated) 1 Drugs that may increase nephrotoxicity • Antibiotics (aminoglycosides, co-trimoxazole) • Non-steroidal anti-inflammatory drugs • Melphalan 2 Drugs that may increase cyclosporin blood level (by cytochrome P-450 inhibition) • Antibiotics (erythromycin, amphotericin B, cephalosporins, doxycycline, aciclovir) • Hormones (corticosteroids, sex hormones) • Diuretics (frusemide/furosamide thiazides) • Other (warfarin, H_2 antihistamines, calcium channel blockers, ACE inhibitors) 3 Drugs that may decrease cyclosporin levels (by cytochrome P-450 induction)	Contraindicated if abnormal renal function, hypertension not under control and concomitant premalignant or malignant conditions Monitor renal function and blood pressure as indicated on p. 61

Continued p. 348

Main dermatological uses and usual adult doses	Adverse effects	Interactions	Other remarks
		• Anticonvulsants (phenytoin, phenobarbital, carbamazepine, sodium valproate) • Antibiotics (isoniazide, rifampicin)	
Methotrexate Severe psoriasis unresponsive to local treatment (initially, 2.5 mg test dose and observe for 1 *week*, then 5–15 mg *once* a *week* orally or intramuscularly)	Gut upsets Stomatitis Bone marrow depression Liver or kidney dysfunction	Aspirin, probenecid, thiazide diuretics and some non-steroidal anti-inflammatory drugs delay excretion and increase toxicity Anti-epileptics, co-trimoxazole, and pyrimethamine increase antifolate effect Toxicity increased by cyclosporin and acitretin	Full blood count and liver function tests before starting treatment, and then weekly until therapy is stabilized. Thereafter test every 2–3 months. Avoid in pregnancy Reduce dose if renal or hepatic impairment Folinic acid given concomitantly prevents bone marrow depression Reduced fertility in males Many insist on a liver biopsy before treatment and periodically thereafter as this is the best way of detecting hepatic fibrosis Elderly may be more sensitive to the drug

Corticosteroids

Prednisone and prednisolone

Acute and severe allergic reactions, severe erythema multiforme, connective tissue disorders, pemphigus, pemphigoid and vasculitis (5–80 mg daily or on alternate days) Withdrawal should be gradual for patients who have received systemic corticosteroids for more than 3 weeks or those who have taken high doses	Impaired glucose tolerance Redistribution of fat (centripetal) Muscle wasting, proximal myopathy Osteoporosis and vertebral collapse Aseptic necrosis of head of femur Growth retardation in children Peptic ulceration Euphoria, psychosis or depression Cataract formation	Liver enzyme inducers (e.g. phenytoin, griseofulvin; rifampicin) reduce effect of corticosteroids Carbenoxolone and most diuretics increase potassium loss as a result of corticosteroids Corticosteroids reduce effect of many antihypertensive agents Corticostroids will interact with drugs that affect glucose metabolism	1 Before long-term treatment screen: • Chest X-ray • Blood pressure • Weight • Glycosuria • Electrolytes • Consider the need for a bone scan • Tuberculin skin test (USA) • Past history of peptic ulcer, cataracts/glaucoma, and affective psychosis

Main dermatological uses and usual adult doses	Adverse effects	Interactions	Other remarks
	Precipitation of glaucoma Increase in blood pressure Sodium and water retention Potassium loss Skin atrophy and capillary fragility Spread of infection Iatrogenic Cushing's syndrome		2 During treatment check blood passure, weight, glycosuria, and electrolytes regularly. Patients should carry a steroid treatment card or wear a labelled bracelet. Always bear in mind the possibility of masked infections and perforations 3 Long-term treatment has to be tapered off slowly to avoid adrenal insufficiency 4 Do not use for psoriasis or long-term for atopic eczema 5 Consider the need for adjunctive treatment for osteoporosis

Retinoids

Acitretin Severe psoriasis, resistant to other forms of treatment (may be used with PUVA, p. 59), palmoplantar pustulosis, severe ichthyoses, Darier's disease, pityriasis rubra pilaris (0.2–1.0 mg/kg daily) Acitretin is not recommended for children except under exceptional circumstances	1 *Mucocutaneous* (common) Rough, scaly, dry-appearing skin and mucous membranes Chafing Atrophy of skin and nails Diffuse thinning of scalp and body hair Curly hair Exuberant granulation tissue (especially toe nail folds) Disease flare-up Photosensitivity 2 *Systemic* Teratogenesis Diffuse interstitial skeletal hyperostosis Arthralgia, myalgia and headache Benign intracranial hypertension 3 *Laboratory abnormalities* Haematology: ↓ White blood cells ↑ Erythrocyte sedimentation rate	Avoid concomitant high doses of vitamin A Possible antagonism to anticoagulant effect of warfarin Increases plasma concentration of methotrexate Increases hepatotoxicity of methotrexate	All women of childbearing age must use effective oral contraception for 1 month before treatment, during treatment and for at least 2 years after treatment (see specialist literature for details) Patients should sign a consent form indicating that they know about the danger of teratogenicity Should not donate blood during or for 1 year after stopping the treatment (teratogenic risk) Regular screening should be carried out to exclude: 1 Abnormalities of liver function 2 Hyperlipidaemia

Continued p. 350

Main dermatological uses and usual adult doses	Adverse effects	Interactions	Other remarks
	Liver function tests: ↓ Bilirubin ↑ AST/ALT ↑ Alkaline phosphatase (abnormal in 20% of patients) Serum lipids: ↑ Cholesterol ↑ Triglycerides ↓ High-density lipoprotein (abnormal in 50% of patients)		3 Disseminated interstitial skeletal hyperostosis Avoid if renal or hepatic impairment
Isotretinoin (13 *cis*-retinoic acid) Severe acne vulgaris, unresponsive to systemic antibiotics (0.5–1.0 mg/kg daily for 16 weeks) (p. 154)	*See* Acitretin	*See* Acitretin	Females of childbearing age must take effective contraception for 1 month before treatment is started, during treatment, and for 3 months after treatment is stopped; check pregnancy test (s) before starting treatment and monthly. Females should sign a consent form which states the dangers of teratogenicity (see p. 154 for USA recommendations) Before starting a course of isotretinoin, patients and their doctors should know about the risk of the appearance or worsening of depression. The drug should be stopped immediately if there is any concern on this score (see p. 155). Avoid in renal or hepatic impairment Blood tests as for acitretin

Main dermatological uses and usual adult doses	Adverse effects	Interactions	Other remarks
Drugs acting on the central nervous system (CNS)			
Amitriptyline 1 Depression secondary to skin disease 2 Post-herpetic neuralgia (50–100 mg at night; start with 10–25 mg in the elderly)	Sedation, anticholinergic effects, cardiac dysrhythmias Confusion in the elderly Postural hypotension Jaundice Neutropenia May precipitate seizures in epileptics	Potentially lethal CNS stimulation with monoamine oxidase inhibitors Increases effects of other CNS depressants and anticholinergics Metabolism may be inhibited by cimetidine	Avoid in the presence of heart disease or hypertension Use small doses at first to avoid confusion in the elderly Warn about effects on skills such as driving
Doxepin Antidepressant with sedative properties sometimes used for antipruritic effect 10–50 mg at bedtime or twice daily	See amitriptyline	See amitriptyline	Avoid in breastfeeding
Diazepam Anxiety—often associated with skin disease (2 mg three times daily)	Sedation Impaired skills (e.g. driving) or ataxia Dependence (withdrawal may lead to sleeplessness, anxiety, tremors)	Potentiates effects of other CNS depressants including alcohol Breakdown inhibited by cimetidine and propranolol Liver enzyme inducers (e.g. phenytoin, griseofulvin, rifampicin) increase elimination	Use for short spells only (to avoid addiction) Avoid in pregnancy and breast feeding Use with care in presence of liver, kidney or respiratory diseases, and in the elderly
Miscellaneous			
Adrenaline (epinephrine) injection Emergency treatment for acute anaphylaxis 0.5 mg (0.5 ml of 1 in 1000 solution given as a slow subcutaneous or, rarely, intramuscular injection. May be repeated after 10 min if necessary) An Epipen is a convenient way in which patients can carry adrenaline with them for self-injection if needed	Tachycardia Cardiac dysrhythmias Anxiety Tremor Headache Hypertension Hyperglycaemia Hypokalaemia	If given with some β-blockers may lead to severe hypertension	Do not confuse the different strengths Give *slowly*, subcutaneously or intramuscularly, but *not* intravenously, except in cardiac arrest

Continued p. 352

Main dermatological uses and usual adult doses	Adverse effects	Interactions	Other remarks
Dapsone Leprosy, dermatitis herpetiformis, vasculitis, pyoderma gangrenosum (50–150 mg daily)	Haemolytic anaemia Methaemoglobinaemia Headaches Lethargy Hepatitis Peripheral neuropathy Exfoliative dermatitis Toxic epidermal necrolysis Agranulocytosis Aplastic anaemia Hypoalbuminaemia	Reduced excretion and increased side effects if given with probenecid	Regular blood checks necessary (weekly for first month, then every 2 weeks until 3 months, then monthly until 6 months and then 6-monthly) Not felt to be teratogenic, but should not be given during pregnancy and lactation if possible. For dermatitis herpetiformis, a gluten-free diet is preferable at these times Avoid in patients with glucose 6-phosphate dehydrogenase deficiency (screen for this, especially in USA)
Hydroxychloroquine Systemic and discoid lupus erythematosus, polymorphic light eruption: 200–400 mg daily, maintaining level at lowest effective dose. Must not exceed 6.5 mg/kg body weight/day (based on the ideal/lean body weight and not on the actual weight of the patient)	Retinopathy which may cause permanent blindness Corneal deposits Headaches Gut upsets, pruritus and rashes Worsening of psoriasis Vivid dreams	Should not be taken at the same time as other antimalarial drugs May raise plasma digoxin levels Potential neuromuscular toxicity if taken with gentamycin, kanamycin, or tobramycin Bioavailability decreased if given with antacids	In the UK, before treatment, patients should be asked about their visual acuity (not corrected with glasses). If it is impaired, or eye disease is present, assessment by an optometrist is advised and any abnormality should be referred to an ophthalmologist. The visual acuity of each eye should be recorded using a standard reading chart. In the USA all patients should have a pre-treatment ophthalmological assessment

Main dermatological uses and usual adult doses	Adverse effects	Interactions	Other remarks
			During treatment, patients should be asked annually about visual symptoms and their visual acuity should be monitored using the standard reading chart. Discontinue drug if any change occurs Reduce dose with poor renal or liver function Best avoided in the elderly and children Do not give automatic repeat prescriptions Prefer intermittent short courses to continuous treatment if possible
8-Methoxypsoralen (methoxsalen) Used usually with UVA as PUVA therapy (p. 59) Severe psoriasis, vitiligo, localized pustular psoriasis, cutaneous T-cell lymphoma; rarely, lichen planus, atopic dermatitis Tablets: 0.6–0.8 mg/kg body weight taken as a single dose 1–2 h before exposure to UVA Liquid (Ultra Capsules) (USA): 0.3 mg/kg body weight taken 1 h before exposure to UVA	Nausea Itching Photoxicity Catracts Lentigines Ageing changes of skin Hyperpigmentation Cutaneous neoplasms	Avoid other photosensitizers (Chapter 16)	The following should checked before treatment: • Skin. Examine for premalignant lesions and skin cancer • Eyes. Check for cataracts. Fundoscopic examination of retina. Visual acuity • Blood. Full blood count, liver and renal function tests and antinuclear factor test • Urine analysis Eyes should be protected with appropriate lenses for 24 h after taking the drug Protective goggles must be worn during radiation If feasible, shield face and genitalia during treatment

Continued p. 354

Main dermatological uses and usual adult doses	Adverse effects	Interactions	Other remarks
			Patients must protect skin against additional sun exposure after ingestion
			Monitor eyes for development of cataracts
			Try to avoid maintenance treatment, more than 250 treatments and a cumulative dose of more than 1000 joules/cm^2 (skin cancer risk)

Index

abnormal pigments 244
abscesses 31
acantholysis 109
acanthosis nigricans 283
aciclovir 344
acitretin (etretinate) 60, 349
acne 148–56
  androgen-secreting tumours 152
  apocrine 161
  cause 148–50
  congenital adrenal hyperplasia 151
  conglobate 150
  course 152
  differential diagnosis 152
  drug-induced 150, 151
  excoriated 151
  exogenous 151
  fulminans 151
  infantile 149, 150, 151
  investigations 152
  late onset 151
  mechanical 149
  polycystic ovarian syndrome 150, 151
  presentation 150–2
  prevalence 148
  treatment 152–6, 336
  tropical 150, 151
  virilization 149–50
  vulgaris 148–9
acne excorée 298
acneiform drug eruptions 311
acquired ichthyosis 43
acquired immunodeficiency syndrome 211–13
  course 211
  management 212–13
  pathogenesis 211
  skin changes 211–12
acral lentiginous melanoma 269, 272
acrochordon 256
acrocyanosis 132
actinic cheilitis 239
actinic keratoses 239, 263–5
  complications 264
  differential diagnosis 264
  histology 264
  investigations 264
  presentation 264
  treatment 264–5

actinic prurigo 239
actinic reticuloid 237–8
actinomycosis 223
acute dermatitis 111
acute febrile neutrophilic dermatosis 284
adapalene 153
Addison's disease 251
adhesion molecules 22
adrenaline 351
age-dependent prevalence of skin disorders 3
ageing of skin 239–41
AIDS *see* acquired immunodeficiency syndrome
alimemazine 345
alkaptonuria 291
allergens 77–9
allergic drug reactions 308
allergic (hypersensitivity) vasculitis 103–4, 310
alopecia 164
  androgenetic 166–7
  areata 64, 164–6
    cause 164
    course 164–5
    differential diagnosis 165
    exclamation mark hairs 164–5
    investigations 165
    nails in 176
    presentation 164
    treatment 165–6
  localized 164–8
  scarring 168
  totalis 165
  traction 167–8
  trichotillomania 167
  universalis 165
aluminium chloride 153
amelanotic melanoma 204
amitriptyline 350
amyloidosis 289
anagen 163
anaphylactoid purpura 103–4
anchoring fibrils 15
anchoring filaments 15
androgenetic alopecia 166–7
aneurin deficiency 287
angioedema 31
  hereditary 98, 99

angiokeratoma 185
angiokeratoma corporis diffusum 291
anhidrosis 160–1
annular lesions 32
anthrax, cutaneous 195–6
anti-androgens 346
antibacterials
  reactions to 308
  systemic 340–4
  topical 334
antibodies 21
anticonvulsants, reactions to 309
antifungals
  systemic 342–4
  topical 334–5
antigens 21
antihistamines 344–5
antiperspirants 331
antiphospholipid syndrome 134
antipruritics 330–1
antiretroviral drugs, reactions to 309
antivirals
  systemic 344
  topical 335
aphthous ulcers 182–3
apocrine acne 161
apocrine sweat glands 161
arcuate lesions 32
arrector pili muscles 17
arteries *see* blood vessel disorders
arthropods 224–31
  bed bugs (Hemiptera) 225
  insect bites 224, 225
  lice infestations (pediculosis) 226–7
  myiasis 225–6
  papular urticaria 224–5
  scabies 227–31
Arthus reaction 25
ash leaf macules 303
askamycin 86
asteatotic eczema 90–1
atherosclerosis 137, 140
athlete's foot 214–15
atopic dermatitis 74, 81–7
atopic eczema 81–7
  complications 84–5
  diagnostic criteria 83–4
  inheritance 82
  investigations 85

atopic eczema (*cont.*)
  presentation and course 82–3
  treatment 85–7
atopic palms 72
atrophy 32
atypical mole syndrome 259–60
augmentin 340–1
Auspitz's sign 51
autoimmune urticaria 96
autosomal dominant epidermolysis
    bullosa 117
autosomal recessive dystrophic
    epidermolysis bullosa 117
azathioprine 346
azelaic acid 153

B-cell lymphoma 281–2
Bacillus anthracis 196
bacterial infections 189–201
  erythrasma 189
  pitted keratolysis 189
  spirochaetal 193–5
    Lyme disease 195
    syphilis 193–5
    yaws 195
  staphylococcal 190–2
    carbuncle 192
    ecthyma 190–1
    furunculosis 191–2
    impetigo 190
    scalded skin syndrome 192
    toxic shock syndrome 192
  streptococcal 192–3
    cat-scratch disease 193
    cellulitis 193
    erysipelas 192–3
    erysipeloid 193
    necrotizing fasciitis 193
  trichomycosis axillaris 189
Bacteroides spp. 144, 161
balanitis 185
Balsam of Peru allergy 78
bamboo deformity 43
barrier preparations 329–30
basal cell carcinoma 265–7
  cause 265
  cicatricial (morphoeic) 267
  clinical course 266
  cystic 267
  differential diagnosis 267
  histology 267
  nodulo-ulcerative 266
  pigmented 267
  presentation 265–6
  superficial (multicentric) 267
  treatment 267
basal cell papilloma *see* seborrhoeic
    keratosis
basal layer 8
bath additives 328
bathing 319
Bazex syndrome 283
Bazin's disease 197
Beau's lines 175, 176
Becker's naevi 172

bed bugs (Hemiptera) 225
Behçet's disease 130, 182
benzocaine allergy 78
berloque dermatitis 252
bilateral acoustic neurofibromatosis
    302
black hairy tongue 180
black rubber mix allergy 78
blackheads 151
Blastomyces dermatitidis 222
blastomycosis 222
blood vessel disorders
  arteries 135–8
    arterial emboli 137
    atherosclerosis 137
    polyarteritis nodosa 104–6, 130,
      136
    pressure sores 137–8
    Raynaud's phenomenon 126,
      127, 135–6
    temporal arteritis 136–7
  small blood vessels 132–5
    acrocyanosis 132
    antiphospholipid syndrome 134
    erythema 133
    erythema ab igne 135
    erythrocyanosis 132
    erythromelalgia 132–3
    flushing 135
    livedo reticularis 133–4
    perniosis (chilblains) 132
    spider naevi 133
    telangiectases 133
  veins 138–47
    deep vein thrombosis 138
    gravitational syndrome 139–45
    purpura 145–7
    thrombophlebitis 138
    venous hypertension 139–45
    venous leg ulceration 139–45
blood vessels 17
blue naevi 259
body image 295
body lice 226–7
boils 191–2
Borrelia burgdorferi 195
botulinum toxin 160
Bowen's disease 187–8, 263
budesonide allergy 78
bullae 31
bullous disorders 107–18
  acquired epidermolysis bullosa 113
  acute dermatitis 111
  bullous impetigo 110
  cicatricial pemphigoid 112–13
  dermatitis herpetiformis 113–14
  diabetes and renal disease 114–15
  drug-related 310
  epidermolysis bullosa 116–17
  erythema multiforme 115
  immunological origin 107–10
  linear IgA bullous disease 113
  lupus erythematosus 115
  miliaria crystallina 110
  pemphigoid 15, 108, 111–12

pemphigoid gestationis 112
pemphigus 9, 25, 107–10, 108–9
pompholyx 89–90, 111
porphyria cutanea tarda 114
scalded skin syndrome 110
subcorneal pustular dermatosis
    110–11
toxic epidermal necrolysis 115–16
transient acantholytic dermatosis
    111
viral infections 111
bullous ichthyosiform erythroderma 43
bullous impetigo 110
bullous pemphigoid 24
bullous pemphigoid antigens 15
burrows 32
Buruli ulcers 200
butterfly sign 291
button-hole sign 301

cadherins 22, 23
café-au-lait patches 33, 301
calcipotriol 56–7
callosities 46–7
camouflaging preparations 330
Campbell de Morgan spots (cherry
    angiomas) 277
Candida albicans 92, 181, 218
Candida intertrigo 218
candidiasis 218–21
  chronic mucocutaneous 219
  genital 187, 219
  oral 181, 218
  systemic 220
capillary cavernous haemangioma
    276–7
capsaicin 339
carba mix allergy 78
carbuncle 192
carcinoma 239
cat-scratch disease 193
catagen 163
categories of skin disorders 1
causes of skin disorders 1
cefuroxime 340
cell cohesion 11
cell cycle 9
cell-mediated immune reactions 26–8
  elicitation/challenge phase 27–8
  sensitization phase 26–7
cellular adhesion molecules 22
cellulitis 193
central nervous system, drugs acting
    on 350
cetirizine 345
cetosteryl alcohol allergy 78
chemical-induced hyperpigmentation
    252
cherry angioma 277
chickenpox 206
chilblains 132
chloasma 251, 311
chlorocresol allergy 78
chlorphenamine 345
cholinergic urticaria 95, 99

chondrodermatitis modularis helicis 262
chrome allergy 77
chronic actinic dermatitis 237–8
cicatricial pemphigoid 112–13
ciprofloxacin 340
circinate lesions 32
clean ulcers 143–4
cleansing agents 329
cloxacillin 341
co-amoxiclav 340–1
coal tar preparations 58
cobalt allergy 77
Coccidioides immitis 222
coccidioidomycosis 222
cold urticaria 95, 99
collagen 16
collodion baby 42–3
colony stimulating factors 12
colophony allergy 78
comedones 32
compound melanocytic naevi 258
compression bandages 142
condyloma acuminata 185, 203
    treatment 205, 335
condyloma lata 204
connective tissue disorders 119–31
    Behçet's syndrome 130
    CREST syndrome 128
    dermatomyositis 125–6
    eosinophilic fasciitis 128–9
    lichen sclerosus 128
    lupus erythematosus 69, 115, 119–25
    mixed 129–30
    morphoea 129
    panniculitis 130–1
    polyarteritis nodosa 130
    Reiter's syndrome 130
    relapsing polychondritis 130
    rheumatoid arthritis 130
    systemic sclerosis 126–30
contact dermatitis
    allergic 80–1
        allergens 80
        cause 80
        investigations 81
        presentation and clinical course 80
        treatment 81
    genital 187
    irritant 76–80
        cause 76
        complications 77
        course 76–7
        differential diagnosis 77
        investigations 77
        treatment 77, 80
contact stomatitis 182
contact urticaria 96–7
corns 46–7
corticosteroids 348
    topical 57–8
cosmetic allergy 72, 77–8
cosmetic camouflage 153

Cowden's syndrome 183
crabs 227
creams 318
CREST syndrome 128
Crohn's disease 292
Cronkhite–Canada syndrome 250
crusts 32
cryoglobulinaemia 145–6
cryotherapy 324
curettage 323
currant bun appearance 255
Cushing's syndrome 251
cutaneous ageing 239–41
cutaneous horn 264
cutaneous lymphatics 17
cutaneous T-cell lymphoma 55
cutis marmorata 133
cutis rhomboidalis nuchae 240
cyclosporin 60–1, 346–7
cyproterone acetate 346
cytokines 11, 12, 21–2
cytology 35

dapsone 351
Darier's disease 44–5
De Sanctis–Cacchione syndrome 304
death 5
deep vein thrombosis 138
delayed pressure urticaria 95–6
Demodex folliculorum 156, 211
dendritic cells 18–19
depigmenting agents 330
depilatories 331
depression 5
dermabrasion 155–6
dermal papillae 7
dermatitis *see* eczema *and individual types of dermatitis*
dermatitis artefacta 295–7
dermatitis herpetiformis 108, 113–14
dermatofibroma 277
dermatofibrosarcoma protuberans 282
dermatological delusional disease 295
dermatological pathomimicry 296
dermatomyositis 120, 125–6
    complications 126
    course 125–6
    differential diagnosis 126
    and internal malignancy 283
    investigations 126
    presentation 125
    treatment 126
dermatophyte infections *see* ringworm
dermatoscopy 33–4
dermatoses of poverty 1
dermatosis papulosa nigra 255
dermis 7, 15–18
    blood vessels 17
    cells of 16
    cutaneous lymphatics 17
    fibres of 16–17
    ground substance 17
    muscles 17

nerves 17–18
    in psoriasis 50
dermo-epidermal junction 15
dermographism 95, 96, 99
desmocollins 9
desmogleins 9
desmoplakins 9
desquamation 11
desquamative gingivitis 179
diabetes 115
diabetes mellitus 284–5, 291
diabetic cheiropathy 285
diabetic dermopathy 285
diabetic sclerodactyly 285
diagnosis of skin disorders 29–40
    assessment 34
    examination 29–33
    history 29
    laboratory tests 39
    side-room and office tests 35–9
    tools and techniques 33–4
diascopy 33
diazepam 350
diet, in acne 155
diffuse cutaneous mastocytosis 279
diffuse hair loss 168–9
diphenhydramine 345
disability 4–5
discoid eczema 54–5
discoid lesions 32
discoid lupus erythematosus 69
discoid (nummular) eczema 89
discomfort 4
disfigurement 4
dithranol 58
Dowling–Meara epidermolysis bullosa 116
doxycycline 154
drug allergy 78–9
drug eruptions 307–13
    acneiform eruptions 311
    allergic 308
    allergic vasculitis 310
    bullous eruptions 310
    course 312
    differential diagnosis 312
    eczema 310
    erythema multiforme 310
    exfoliative dermatitis 310
    fixed 310–11
    hair loss 311
    hypertrichosis 311
    lichenoid 311
    mechanisms 307–8
    non-allergic 307–8
    photosensitivity 312
    pigmentation 311–12
    presentation 308–9
        antibiotics 308
        anticonvulsants 309
        antiretroviral drugs 309
        gold 309
        oral contraceptives 309
        penicillamine 308–9
        steroids 309

drug eruptions (cont.)
 purpura 310
 toxic epidermal necrolysis 311
 toxic (reactive) erythema 309
 treatment 312–13
 urticaria 310
 xerosis 312
dusting powders 318
dyshidrotic eczema see pompholyx
dysmorphophobia 295
dystrophic epidermolysis bullosa 117

ecchymosis 32
eccrine sweat glands 158–61
 generalized hyperhidrosis 159
 hypohidrosis and anhidrosis 160–1
 local hyperhidrosis 159–60
ecthyma 190–1
eczema 70–93
 acute 72, 75
 allergic contact dermatitis 80–1
 asteatotic 90–1
 atopic 74, 81–7
 causes 71
 chronic 72, 75–6
 classification of 70–1
 clinical appearance 72
 complications 73
 differential diagnosis 73–4
 discoid 89
 drug-related 310
 gravitational (stasis) 90
 histology 71–2
 investigations 74
 irritant contact dermatitis 76–80
 juvenile plantar dermatosis 91–2
 localized neurodermatitis 91
 nails in 175
 napkin dermatitis 92–3
 occupational dermatitis 81
 pompholyx 89–90
 seborrhoeic 87–9
 subacute 75
 terminology 70
 treatment 75–6
Ehlers–Danlos syndrome 16, 305–6
elastic fibres 17
electrosurgery 323–4
emboli 137
emollients 328
endocrine hyperpigmentation 251
eosinophilic fasciitis 128–9
ephelides see freckles
epidermal appendages 15
epidermal barrier 11
epidermal melanin unit 12
epidermal ridges 7
epidermis 7–15
epidermoid cysts 261
epidermolysis bullosa 116–17
 acquired 113
 autosomal dominant 117
 autosomal recessive dystrophic
  117
 dystrophic 117

junctional 117
 nails in 178
 simple 116–17
epidermolytic hyperkeratosis 43
Epidermophyton floccosum 215
epidermopoiesis 11–12
epiluminescence microscopy 33–4
epoxy resin allergy 78
erosions 32
erysipelas 192–3
erysipeloid 193
Erysipelothrix insidiosa 193
erythema 30, 133
erythema ab igne 135
erythema gyratum repens 283
erythema induratum 197
erythema infectiosum 214
erythema migrans 133, 195, 196
erythema multiforme 99–101
 bullous 115
 cause 99–100
 complications 100–1
 course 100
 differential diagnosis 101
 drug-related 310
 investigations 101
 presentation 100
 treatment 101
erythema nodosum 101–2
 and sarcoidosis 285
erythema nuchae 275
erythrasma 187, 189
erythrocyanosis 132
erythroderma 69
erythrodermic psoriasis 53–4
erythrohepatic (erythropoietic)
  protoporphyria 287
erythromelalgia 132–3
erythromycin 154, 341
ethinylestradiol 346
ethylenediamine dihydrochloride
  allergy 78
exclamation-mark hairs 164, 165
excoriations 32
exfoliatin 192
exfoliative dermatitis 69
 drug-related 310

Fabry's disease 291
fexofenadine 345
fibroblasts 16
fiddler's neck 149
fifth disease 214
figurate erythema 133
filariasis 231–2
finasteride 167
fissured tongue 180
fissures 32
fixed drug eruptions 310–11
flaps and grafts 323
fluconazole 343
5-fluorouracil 338–9
flushing 135
follicular mucinosis 289
folliculitis 211

Fordyce spots 183, 185
formaldehyde allergy 78
Fox–Fordyce disease 161
freckles 249
 differential diagnosis 260
frostbite 136
fungal infections 35, 214–23
 actinomycosis 223
 blastomycosis 222
 candidiasis see candidiasis
 coccidioidomycosis 222
 histoplasmosis 222
 mycetoma (Madura foot) 223
 pityriasis versicolor 221–2
 ringworm 214–18
  cause 214
  complications 216–17
  differential diagnosis 217
  investigations 217
  presentation and course 214–16
  treatment 217–18
 sporotrichosis 222–3
furred tongue 180
furunculosis 191–2

gangrene 136
gap junctions 9
gels 318
gene deletions 300–1
genetic disorders 300–6
 Ehlers–Danlos syndrome 16,
  305–6
 incontinentia pigmenti 305
 neurofibromatosis 301–2
 non-Mendelian genetics 300–1
 pseudoxanthoma elasticum 306
 tuberous sclerosis 302–4
 xeroderma pigmentosum 304–5
genitals 184–8
 benign problems 185–7
  dermatoses 187
  lichen sclerosus 185–6
  vulval and scrotal pruritus 186–7
  vulvovaginitis 185
 squamous cell carcinoma 187–8
geographic tongue 180
germinative layer 8
Gianotti–Crosti syndrome 213
gingival hyperplasia 309
gingivitis, desquamative 179
glomus tumours 178, 277
glossodynia 180
gold, reactions to 309
gonococcal septicaemia 196
Gottron's papules 125
graft-vs-host disease 286
granular cell layer 8
granuloma annulare 204
 and diabetes mellitus 284–5
gravitational (stasis) eczema 90
gravitational syndrome 139–45
griseofulvin 218, 343
groin, tinea infection 215, 216
Grover's disease 111
growth factors 11

guttate psoriasis 51, 52, 59
gyrate lesions 32

HAART therapy 213
haemangioma 276–7
  Campbell de Morgan spots (cherry
    angiomas) 277
  capillary cavernous (strawberry
    naevus) 276–7
  differential diagnosis 260
haematoma 32
hair 15, 162–72
  classification 162–3
  hair cycle 163–4
  lanugo 162
  terminal 163
  vellus 162
  white 248
  loss *see* alopecia; hair loss
hair cosmetics 172
hair follicles 8
hair loss
  diffuse 168–9
  drug-related 311
  patchy 168
  see also alopecia
hair-pulling 167, 298
hairy leukoplakia 180, 213
half-and-half nail 286
halo naevus 260
hand, foot and mouth disease 214
hands, tinea infection 215
haptens 21
harlequin fetus 43
head lice 226
heat stroke 160
heat urticaria 95
hemidesmosomes 15
Hemiptera 225
Hendersonula 217
Henoch–Schönlein purpura 103
hereditary angioedema 98, 99
herpangina 213
herpes simplex 208–9
herpes zoster 206–8
herpetic glossitis 180
hidradenitis suppurativa 152, 191
hirsutism 170–1
histiocytoma 277
histocompatibility antigens 22
Histoplasma capsulatum 222
histoplasmosis 222
hives *see* urticaria
Hodgkin's disease 281
Homan's sign 138
homing molecules 27
horny envelope 10
horny layer 10
humoral cytotoxic reactions 24–5
hydroxychloroquine 351–2
hydroxyzine 345
hyperhidrosis
  generalized 159
  local 159–60
hyperkeratotic warts 47

hypermelanosis 248–52
  chemicals causing 252
  chloasma 251
  Cronkhite-Canada syndrome 250
  endocrine hyperpigmentation 251
  freckles 249
  lentigo 249–50
  LEOPARD syndrome 250–1
  melanotic macule of lip 249, 250
  nutritional hyperpigmentation
    251–2
  Peutz–Jeghers syndrome 250
  poikiloderma 252
  porphyria 251
  postinflammatory 252
hypersensitivity reactions 23–8
  type I 23–4
  type II 24–5
  type III 25–6
  type IV 26–8
hypersensitivity urticaria 96, 99
hypertrichosis 170, 172
  drug-related 311
hypertrichosis lanuginosa, acquired
  283
hypodermis 7
hypohidrosis 160–1
hypohidrotic ectodermal dysplasia
  160, 169
hypopigmentation 244–8
  hypopituitarism 246
  oculocutaneous albinism 244–6
  phenylketonuria 246
  piebaldism 246
  postinflammatory depigmentation
    248
  vitiligo 246–7
  white hair 248
hypopituitarism 246
hypotrichosis *see* hair loss

IBIDS 43
ice-pick scars 156
ichthyoses 41–3
ichthyosiform erythroderma 43
ichthyosis
  acquired 283
  vulgaris 41–2
imidazolidinyl urea allergy 78
immediate hypersensitivity reactions
  23–4
immune complex-mediated reactions
  25–6
immune system of skin 18
  cellular components 18–21
  molecular components 21–3
immunoglobulin 21, 23
immunoglobulin E 74
immunoglobulin superfamily 22
immunosuppressants 346–8
impact of skin disorders 3–5
impetigo 190
  bullous 110
incontinentia pigmenti 305
infected ulcers 144

infections 189–223
  bacterial 189–201
  fungal 214–23
  viral 201–14
infective ulcers 141
infestations 224–32
  arthropods 224–31
  parasitic worms 231–2
inoculation tuberculosis 196–7
insect bites 224, 225
integrins 22, 23
interdigitating cells 18
interleukins 12
internal malignancy 283–4, 291
intertrigo 187
intradermal melanocytic naevi 259
intraepidermal carcinoma *see* Bowen's
  disease
iron deficiency 287, 291
isotretinoin 153, 154–5, 349–50
itching *see* pruritus
itraconazole 218, 343

jock itch 187
junctional epidermolysis bullosa 117
junctional melanocytic naevi 258
juvenile mastocytosis 279
juvenile plantar dermatosis 91–2

Kallmann's syndrome 42
Kaposi's sarcoma 211, 212, 279
Kasabach–Merritt syndrome 276
kathon allergy 78
Kawasaki's disease 213
keloid 278
keratinization 9, 10–11
keratinization disorders 41–7
  callosities and corns 46–7
  ichthyoses 41–3
  keratoderma of palms and soles
    45–6
  keratosis follicularis 44–5
  keratosis pilaris 44
  knuckle pads 46
keratinocytes 9–10, 18
  and wound healing 19
keratinosomes 10
keratins 11
keratoacanthoma 262–3
  cause 262
  clinical features 262
  differential diagnosis 262
  histology 262–3
  treatment 263
keratoderma
  blenorrhagicum 130
  climactericum 46
  of palms and soles 45–6
keratohyalin 10
keratolytics 331
keratosis follicularis 44–5
keratosis pilaris 44
kerion 216
ketoconazole 344
killer cells 21

Klippel–Trenaunay syndrome 275
knuckle pads 46
Köbner effect 50, 65, 202
koilonychia 175, 176
Koplik's spots 214
kwashiorkor 287

L cells 20–1
lamellar granules 10
lamellar ichthyosis 43
lamina densa 8, 15
lamina lucida 15
laminins 15
Langerhans cells 12, 13, 14, 18, 20
lanugo hairs 162
larva migrans 232
laser therapy 156, 326–7
latex allergy 96–7
lathyrism 16
Leishmania donovani 201
Leishmania tropica 201
leishmaniasis 201
lentigines 249–50
  differential diagnosis 260
lentigo maligna melanoma 269, 271
LEOPARD syndrome 1, 250–1
leprosy 197–200
  cause 197
  differential diagnosis 199
  epidemiology 197
  investigations 200
  presentation 197–9
  treatment 200
Leser–Trélat sign 255
leucocytoclastic vasculitis 103–4
leukaemia 281
lice 226–7
  body lice 226–7
  head lice 226
  pubic lice 227
  treatment 335
lichen planus 64–7
  cause 64
  complications 66
  course 66
  differential diagnosis 66
  genital 185
  investigations 66
  mouth 179–81
  nails in 66, 175–6
  presentation 64–6
  treatment 66
lichen sclerosus 129
  vulval 185–6
lichen simplex 91, 298
lichenification 32
lichenoid drug eruptions 311
lidocaine/prilocaine 339
light reactions 233–41
  actinic cheilitis 239
  actinic keratoses 239
  actinic prurigo 239
  carcinoma 239
  chronic actinic dermatitis (actinic
    reticuloid) 237–8

cutaneous ageing 239–41
lupus erythematosus 239
photoallergy 236–7
phototoxicity 235–6
polymorphic light eruption 238–9
porphyria cutanea tarda 239
solar urticaria 239
sunburn 234–5
linear epidermal naevus 257
linear IgA bullous disease 113
lipodermatosclerosis 139
lipoma 278
lithium succinate 339
livedo reticularis 105, 133–4
liver disease 285–6, 291
liver spots 250
local anaesthetics 37
localized neurodermatitis *see* lichen
    simplex
loratadine 345
lotions 318
lupus erythematosus 69, 115,
    119–25
  bullous 115
  discoid 69, 120, 121, 123–5
    course 123
    differential diagnosis 123–4
    investigations 124
    presentation 123
    treatment 124–5
  light reactions 239
  subacute 120, 122–3
    complications 123
    course 123
    differential diagnosis 123
    investigations 123
    presentation 122–3
    treatment 123
  systemic 119–22
    cause 119
    complications 119, 121
    course 119
    differential diagnosis 121
    investigations 121–2
    presentation 119
    treatment 122
lupus pernio 285
lupus vulgaris 196
Lyell's disease 115–16
Lyme disease 195
lymph vessel disorders 147
lymphangioma 277
lymphangitis 147
lymphocytes 16
lymphoedema 147
lymphoma
  cutaneous T-cell 280–1
  extracutaneous 281–2
    B-cell lymphoma 281–2
    Hodgkin's disease 281
    leukaemia 281

macroglossia 180
macules 30, 31
Madura foot 223

magnifying lens 33
malabsorption 286, 287
male pattern baldness 166–7
  see also alopecia
malignant melanoma 268–74
  acral lentiginous 269, 272
  amelanotic 204
  cause 269
  clinical features 269–70
  differential diagnosis 260, 273
  incidence 268–9
  lentigo maligna 269, 271
  metastatic 270
  microstaging 272–3
  nodular 269, 272
  prognosis 273
  subungual 270
  superficial spreading 269, 271
  totally amelanotic 270
  treatment 273–4
malignant ulcers 142
malnutrition 286, 287
mast cells 16, 21
mastocytoma 279
mastocytosis 279
measles 214
median rhomboid glossitis 180
Meissner corpuscles 18
melanocytes 12, 13
melanocytic naevi 257–61
  atypical mole syndrome 259–60
  blue naevi 259
  cause and evolution 257
  complications 260–1
  compound 258
  congenital 257–8
  differential diagnosis 260
  histology 260
  intradermal 259
  junctional 258
  Mongolian spots 259
  presentation 257–60
  Spitz naevi 259
  treatment 261
melanogenesis 12, 242–3
  control of 243
melanoma *see* malignant melanoma
melanosomes 12, 13
melanotic macule of lip 249, 250
membrane attack complex 24
Menkes' syndrome 169
mercapto-mix allergy 78
Merkel cells 12, 13, 14
methotrexate 60, 347–8
8-methoxypsoralen 352–3
metronidazole 341
Microsporum audouini 217
Microsporum canis 217
milia 261
miliaria 160
  crystallina 110, 161
  profunda 161
  rubra 161
minocycline 154, 341–2
minoxidil 339

mixed connective tissue disorder 120, 129–30
Mohs' surgery 323
molluscum contagiosum 204, 209–10
Mongolian spots 259
monilethrix 169
morphoea 121, 129
mosaicism 300
mouth 179–84
  aphthae 182–3
  bullous diseases 182
  candidiasis 181, 218
  contact stomatitis 182
  Cowden's syndrome 183
  lichen planus 179–81
  neurofibroma 183
  Peutz–Jeghers syndrome 183
  pregnancy tumours 183
  pseudoxanthoma elasticum 183
  squamous cell carcinoma 184
  telangiectasia 183
  ulcers 182
  venous lakes 183
mouth washes 333
mucinoses 289
mucocutaneous lymph node syndrome 213
Muir–Torre syndrome 284
mycetoma 223
mycobacterial infections 196–201
  leishmaniasis 201
  leprosy 197–200
  Mycobacterium marinum 200, 201
  Mycobacterium ulcerans 200–1
  tuberculosis 196–7
Mycobacterium bovis 196
Mycobacterium leprae 102, 197
Mycobacterium marinum 200, 201
Mycobacterium tuberculosis 196
Mycobacterium ulcerans 200–1
mycosis fungoides 280–1
myiasis 225–6
myxoedema 289
  pretibial 289
myxoid cysts 178

nail bed 173
nails 15, 172–9
  alopecia areata 176
  Beau's lines 175, 176
  biting 174
  clubbing 175
  colour changes 175
  connective tissue disorders 175
  Darier's disease 45
  dermatomyositis 125
  dermatophyte infection 176, 177–8
  eczema 175
  en raquette 174, 179
  epidermolysis bullosa 178
  glomus tumours 178, 277
  habit tic nail dystrophy 174
  half-and-half 286
  koilonychia 175, 176
  lamellar splitting 174

lichen planus 66, 175–6
  myxoid cysts 178
  nail-patella syndrome 178
  onychogryphosis 173, 174
  onycholysis 52, 53, 173, 174
  pachyonychia congenita 174, 178
  paronychia 176
    acute 177
    chronic 177
  peri-ungual fibroma 178, 303
  peri-ungual warts 178
  psoriasis 52, 53, 175
  pterygium 176
  splinter haemorrhages 173
  structure 173
  subungual exostosis 174, 178
  subungual haematoma 173
  in systemic disease 174–5
  telangiectatic capillaries 176
  tinea infection 215
  trauma 173–4
  tumours 178
  white 286
  yellow nail syndrome 178–9
napkin dermatitis 92–3
napkin psoriasis 53
natural killer cells 21
necrobiosis lipoidica 284
necrolytic migratory erythema 283
necrotizing fasciitis 193
Nelson's syndrome 251
neomycin allergy 78
nerves 17–18
Netherton's syndrome 43, 169
nettle rash *see* urticaria
neurodermatitis 91, 187
neurofibroma 278
neurofibromatosis 33, 301–2
neurological disease 291–2
neuroma 278
neurotic excoriations 297, 298
niacin deficiency 287
nickel allergy 77
Nikolsky test 111
nociceptors 18
nodular melanoma 269, 272
nodules 32
nummular lesions 32
nutritional hyperpigmentation 251–2
nystatin 344

occlusive therapy 319
occupational dermatitis 81
oculocutaneous albinism 244–6
  cause 244–5
  complications 245
  differential diagnosis 245
  investigations 245
  presentation and course 245
  treatment 246
Odland bodies 10
ointments 318
onchocerciasis 231
onychogryphosis 173, 174
onycholysis 52, 53, 173, 174

oral contraceptives, reactions to 309
orf 210–11
osteogenesis imperfecta 16
otitis externa
  AIDS 212
  preparations for 334
oxerutins 145
oxypentifylline 144
oxytetracycline 154, 342

Paccinian corpuscles 18
pachydermoperiostosis 284
pachyonychia congenita 174, 178
Paget's disease
  genital 185
  of the nipple 274–5
palmar erythema 133
panniculitic ulcers 142
panniculitis 130–1
papilloma 32
papular urticaria 224–5
papules 30
  surface contours 33
parabens-mix allergy 78
paraphenylene allergy 78
parapsoriasis 67–9
parasitic worms 231–2
  filariasis 231–2
  larva migrans 232
  onchocerciasis 231
  swimmer's itch 232
  threadworms 232
parasitosis, delusions of 295, 296
paratertiary butylphenol allergy 78
Parkes Weber syndrome 275
paronychia 176, 219
  acute 177
  chronic 177
pastes 318
patch testing 35–6
  contact dermatitis 77
  eczema 74
pearly penile papules 185
peau d'orange 282
pediculosis *see* lice
Pediculus humanus 226
Pediculus humanus capitis 226
Pediculus humanus corporis 226
pegs 7
pemphigoid 15, 108, 111–12
  cicatricial 112–13, 182
  gestationis 112
  mouth 182
pemphigoid gestationis 112, 293
pemphigus 9, 25, 108–9
  mouth 182
penicillamine, reactions to 308–9
penicillin V 342
percutaneous absorption 315
perforating disorders 286
perfume allergy 77
peri-ungual fibroma 178, 303
peri-ungual warts 178
perinosis 132
petechiae 30, 32

Peutz–Jeghers syndrome 1, 183
  hyperpigmentation in 250
pharmacological urticaria 96
phenylketonuria 246, 289–91
photoallergy 236–7
photochemotherapy 59–60
photodermatitis 236
photodynamic therapy 325–6
photopatch testing 74
photosensitivity 312
phototherapy 325–6
phototoxicity 235–6
Phthirus pubis 226
piebaldism 246
pigmentation 32
  drug-related 311–12
  liver disease 286
  renal disease 286
pigmentation disorders 242–52
  decreased melanin pigmentation
    244–8
    hypopituitarism 245
    oculocutaneous albinism
      244–6
    phenylketonuria 245
    piebaldism 245
    postinflammatory
      depigmentation 248
    vitiligo 245–7
    white hair 248
  genetics 243
  increased pigmentation
    (hypermelanosis) 248–52
    chemicals causing 252
    chloasma 251
    Cronkhite–Canada syndrome
      250
    endocrine hyperpigmentation
      251
    freckles 249
    lentigo 249–50
    LEOPARD syndrome 250–1
    melanotic macule of lip 249
    nutritional hyperpigmentation
      251–2
    Peutz–Jeghers syndrome 250
    poikiloderma 252
    porphyria 251
    postinflammatory 252
  melanogenesis 242–3
  normal skin colour 242–3
pilar cysts 261
pimicrolimus 86
pinworms 232
pitted keratolysis 189
pityriasis alba 248
pityriasis lichenoides 69
pityriasis rosea 55, 63–4
pityriasis rubra pilaris 67
pityriasis versicolor 221–2
Pityrosporum orbiculare 221
plant allergy 78
plantar corns 204
plaques 30
plucked chicken appearance 306

poikiloderma 32, 252
poikiloderma vasculare atrophicans
  280
polyarteritis nodosa 104–6, 130,
  136
polycystic ovarian syndrome 150,
  151, 152
polycythaemia 291
polymorphic light eruption 238–9
pompholyx 89–90, 111
porphyria 286–9
  acute intermittent 288
  congenital erythropoietic 287
  cutaneous hepatic *see* porphyria
    cutanea tarda
  erythrohepatic (erythropoietic)
    protoporphyria 287
  hyperpigmentation in 251
  variegate 288–9
porphyria cutanea tarda 115, 239,
  287–8
port-wine stains 4, 275, 276
postinflammatory depigmentation
  248
postinflammatory hyperpigmentation
  252
potassium hydroxide 35
prayer sign 285
prednisolone 348
prednisone 348
pregnancy 293
  dermatoses 293
  hyperpigmentation in 251
pregnancy tumours 183
premycotic eruption 67–9
preservative allergy 78
preservatives 318–20
pressure sores 137–8
prevalence of skin disorders 1–3
prick testing 36–7
  atopic eczema 85
  eczema 74
prickle cell layer 8, 9
primin allergy 78
profilaggrin 10
promethazine 345
properdin 24
Propionibacterium acnes 149
prurigo nodularis 298
prurigo of pregnancy 293
pruritic urticarial papules and plaques
  of pregnancy 293
pruritus 18, 291–2
  genital 186–7
  internal malignancy 283, 291
  liver disease 285, 291
  renal disease 286, 291
pseudofolliculitis barbae 152
Pseudomonas aeruginosa 144
Pseudomonas pyocyanea 174
pseudoporphyria 115, 289
  see also porphyria
pseudoxanthoma elasticum 183,
  306
psoralens 236, 252

psoriasis 3, 48–62
  and alopecia 168
  cause and pathogenesis 48–50
    altered epidermal maturation
      49
    epidermal cell kinetics 49
    genetics 48–9
    inflammation 49–50
  complications 54
  differential diagnosis 54–5
  eruptive/unstable 59
  genital 185
  histology 51
  investigations 55
  nails in 52, 53, 175
  precipitation factors 50–1
  presentation 51–4
    erythrodermic psoriasis 53,
      54
    flexures 52, 53
    guttate 51, 52, 59
    localized pustular psoriasis 53,
      54
    nails 52
    napkin psoriasis 53
    palms and soles 53
    plaque pattern 51
    scalp 52, 59
  treatment 55–62, 336–8
    calcipotriol 56–7
    coal tar preparations 58
    corticosteroids 57–8
    cyclosporin 61
    dithranol 58
    methotrexate 61–2
    photochemotherapy 59–60
    retinoids 57, 61
    tacalcitol 57
    ultraviolet radiation 58–9
    vitamin D analogues 56
psoriatic arthropathy 54
psychological reaction to skin disease
  294–9
  body image 295
  dermatitis artefacta 295–8
  dermatological delusional disease
    295
  emotional factors triggering
    dermatoses 299
pterygium 176
pubic lice 227
punch biopsy 38
purpura 30, 32, 145–7
  drug-related 310
pustular psoriasis 53, 54
pustules 30, 31
pyoderma gangrenosum 142,
  292–3
pyogenic folliculitis 152
pyogenic granuloma 277
pyridoxine deficiency 287

quaternium 15 allergy 78
Queyrat's erythroplasia 187, 188
quinoline mix allergy 78

radioallergosorbent test *see* RAST
     test
radiotherapy 324–5
RAST test 74
     urticaria 99
Raynaud's phenomenon 126, 127,
     135–6
reactive erythema 94–102
     erythema multiforme 99–101
     erythema nodosum 101–2
     urticaria 94–9
Refsum's syndrome 43
Reiter's syndrome 130, 220
relapsing polychondritis 130
renal disease 115, 286, 291
renal failure 251
reticulate lesions 32
reticulin 17
retiform lesions 32
retinoids 349–50
     local 57
retinol deficiency 287
rheumatoid arthritis 130
rhinophyma 157
riboflavine deficiency 287
ringworm 214–18
     cause 214
     complications 216–17
     differential diagnosis 217
     investigations 217
     presentation and course 214–16
     scalp 168, 216
     treatment 217–18
     see also tinea
Rochalimaea henselae 193
rodent ulcer *see* basal cell carcinoma
rosacea 152, 156–8
     cause and histopathology 156
     clinical course and complications
          156
     differential diagnosis 157
     treatment 157–8, 336
rubber allergy 78
rubella 214
Rud's syndrome 43

sailor's skin 240
salmon patches 275
salt-split technique 113
sarcoidosis 285, 286
Sarcoptes scabiei 227
satyr's tuft 171
saucerization excision 322–3
scabies 227–31
     cause 227–8
     complications 229–30
     course 229
     detection of 35
     differential diagnosis 230
     epidemiology 228
     investigations 230
     presentation 228–9
     treatment 230–1, 335
scalded skin syndrome 110, 192
scales 32

scalp
     metastases 282
     psoriasis 52, 59
     ringworm 168, 216
scalpel biopsy 37–8
scar sarcoidosis 285
scars 32
scleromyxoedema 289
Scopulariopsis 217
scrofuloderma 197
scurvy 287
sebaceous cysts 261
sebaceous gland disorders 15,
          148–58
     acne 148–56
     rosacea 156–8
sebaceous naevi 265
seborrhoeic eczema 55, 87–9
     AIDS 211, 212
     cause 88–9
     complications 89
     genital 187
     investigations 89
     presentation and course 87–8
     treatment 89
seborrhoeic keratosis 255–6
     cause 255
     clinical course 255
     differential diagnosis 255, 260
     investigations 256
     presentation 255
     treatment 256
seborrhoeic warts *see* seborrhoeic
          keratosis
selectins 22, 23
sesquiterpene allergy 78
Sézary cells 281
shampoos 329
shave excision 322
shower gels 328
sinus 32
skin biopsy 37–8, 321
skin failure 5
skin function and structure 7–28
skin surface microscopy 33–4
skin tags 256
smooth tongue 180
solar elastosis 240
solar urticaria 95, 99, 239
spider naevi 133
     and liver disease 286
spinous cell layer 9–10
Spitz naevi 259
sporotrichosis 222–3
Sporotrichum schencki 222
sprays 318
squamous cell carcinoma 267–8
     cause 268
     clinical presentation and course
          268
     genitals 187–8
     histology 268
     mouth 184
     treatment 268
squamous cell papilloma 254–5

stanozolol 144
Staphylococcus aureus 76, 110, 161,
          190, 192
Staphylococcus epidermidis 189
steroids 331–2
     combinations 332–3
     reactions to 309
     topical, pharmacology 316
Stevens–Johnson syndrome 100
stork bites 275
strawberry naevus 276–7
strawberry tongue 213
Streptococcus milleri 161
striae 32
Sturge–Weber syndrome 1, 275
subcorneal pustular dermatosis
          110–11
subungual exostosis 174, 178
subungual haematoma 173
subungual melanoma 270
sulphur 153
sunblocks 330
sunburn 234–5
sunscreens 330
superantigens 21
superficial spreading melanoma 269,
          271
suppurative hidradenitis 161
surgery 321–4
     curettage 323
     electrosurgery 323–4
     excision 321–3
     flaps and grafts 323
     microscopically controlled excision
          323
     skin biopsy 37–8, 321
sweat gland disorders 158–61
     apocrine sweat glands 161
     eccrine sweat glands 158–61
          generalized hyperhidrosis 159
          hypohidrosis and anhidrosis
               160–1
          local hyperhidrosis 159–60
sweat glands 15
     apocrine 161
     eccrine 158–61
     see also sweat gland disorders
Sweet's syndrome 284
swimmer's itch 232
syphilis 193–5
     cause 193
     clinical course 194
     differential diagnosis 194–5
     investigations 195
     presentation 194
     secondary 55
     treatment 195
systemic sclerosis 120, 126–30
     complications 127
     course 127
     differential diagnosis 127
     investigations 127
     presentation 126–7
     treatment 127–8
systemic therapy 320, 340–53

T lymphocytes 19–20
T-cell gene receptor rearrangements 19–20
T-cell receptor rearrangements 19–20
T-cytotoxic cells 19
T-helper/inducer cells 19
tacalcitol 57
talon noir 273
tazarotene 57, 153
telangiectasia 32, 127, 133, 134, 158
  mouth 183
telogen 163
telogen effluvium 168–9
temporal arteritis 136–7
terbinafine 218, 342
terminal hairs 163
tetracycline 154, 342
thiuram-mix allergy 78
threadworms 232
thrombophlebitis 138
  and internal malignancy 283
thrombotic ulcers 141
thrush *see* candidiasis
thyroid disease 291
tic nail dystrophy 174
tinea capitis 216
tinea corporis 216
tinea cruris 187
tinea incognito 217
tinea pedis 214–15
tinea unguium 55
tinker's tartan 135
tixocortol pivalate allergy 78
tongue, problems of 180
tonofibrils 10
tonofilaments 9–10
topical immune mediators 334
topical treatment 315–20, 328–39
  active ingredients 315
  percutaneous absorption 315
  preservatives 318–20
  vehicles (bases) 315–18
toxic epidermal necrolysis 115–16,
    192, 311
toxic (reactive) erythema 309
toxic shock syndrome 192
toxic sock syndrome 92
traction alopecia 167–8
transient acantholytic dermatosis
    111
treatment 314–20
  cryotherapy 324
  laser therapy 156, 326–7
  phototherapy 325–6
  radiotherapy 324–5
  surgery 321–4
    curettage 323
    electrosurgery 323
    excision 321–3
    flaps and grafts 323
    microscopicall controlled
        excision 323
    skin biopsy 321
  systemic therapy 320
  therapeutic options 314–15

topical treatment 315–20
  active ingredients 315
  methods of application 319–20
  percutaneous absorption 315
  preservatives 318
  vehicles (bases) 315–18
Treponema pallidum 193, 195
trichomycosis axillaris 189
Trichophyton mentagrophytes 215
Trichophyton rubrum 214
Trichophyton schoenleini 216
Trichophyton tonsurans 217
trichorrhexis nodosa 169
trichothiodystrophy 43
trichotillomania 167, 298
trimeprazine 345
trimethoprim 154
tuberculides 197
tuberculosis 196–7
tuberous sclerosis 302–4
tumours 32, 253–82
  dermis 275–82
    benign 275
    Campbell de Morgan spots 277
    capillary cavernous
        haemangioma (strawberry
        naevus) 276, 277
    combined vascular
        malformations of limbs 275
    cutaneous metastases 282
    dermatofibroma 278
    dermatofibrosarcoma
        protuberans 282
    developmental abnormalities of
        blood vessels 275
    extracutaneous lymphoma
        281–2
    glomus tumours 277
    haemangioma 276–7
    Kaposi's sarcoma 211, 212,
        279–80
    keloid 278
    lipoma 278–9
    lymphangioma 277–8
    lymphoma and leukaemia 280–2
    malformations 275
    malignant 279–80
    mastocytosis 279
    mycosis fungoides 280–1
    neurofibroma 278
    neuroma 278
    port-wine stains 275, 276
    pyogenic granuloma 277
    salmon patches (stork bites) 275
  epidermis and appendages 254–75
    actinic keratoses 263–5
    basal cell carcinoma 265–7
    benign 254–62
    chondrodermatitis nodularis
        helicis 262
    epidermoid and pilar cysts 261
    intraepidermal carcinoma
        (Bowen's disease) 263
    keratoacanthoma 262–3
    linear epidermal naevus 257

    malignant 265–75
    malignant melanoma 268–74
    melanocytic naevi 257–61
    milia 261
    Paget's disease of the nipple
        274–5
    premalignant 262–5
    sebaceous naevi 265
    seborrhoeic keratosis 255–6
    skin tags (acrochordon) 256
    squamous cell carcinoma 267–8
    squamous cell papilloma 254–5
    viral warts 254
    prevention 253–4
tylosis 45, 46
Tzanck smear 35

ulcerative colitis 64
ulcers 32
ultraviolet B radiation therapy 58–9,
    155
urticaria 22, 94–9
  autoimmune 96
  cause 94–5
  cholinergic 95
  classification 95
  cold 95
  complications 97
  contact 96–7
  course 97
  delayed pressure 95–6
  dermographism 95, 96
  differential diagnosis 97–8
  drug-related 310
  heat 95
  hypersensitivity 96
  investigations 98–9
  papular 224–5
  pharmacological 96
  presentation 97
  solar 95, 99, 239
  treatment 99
urticaria pigmentosa 279
urticarial vasculitis 103

vagabond's disease 226
varicella 206
vasculitis 102–6, 140–1
  leucocytoclastic 103–4
  polyarteritis nodosa 104–6
  Wegener's granulomatosis 106
vehicles (bases) 315–18
veiled cells 18
veins *see* blood vessel disorders
vellus hairs 162
venous hypertension 139–45
  cause 139
  clinical features 139
  complications 139–40
  differential diagnosis 140–2
  investigations 142
  treatment 142
    local therapy 143–4
    oral treatment 144–5
    physical measures 142–3

venous lakes 183
venous ulcers 139–45
 treatment 338
vesicles 30, 31
viral infections 201–14
 acquired immunodeficiency
   syndrome 211–13
 erythema infectiosum (fifth disease)
   214
 Gianotti-Crosti syndrome 213
 hand, foot and mouth disease
   214
 herpangina 213
 herpes simplex 208–9
 herpes zoster 206–8
 measles 214
 molluscum contagiosum
   209–10
 mucocutaneous lymph node
   syndrome (Kawasaki's
   disease) 213
 orf 210–11
 rubella 214
 varicella (chickenpox) 206
 viral warts 201–5
viral warts 254
vitamin A deficiency 287
vitamin B$_1$ deficiency 287
vitamin B$_2$ deficiency 287
vitamin B$_6$ deficiency 287

vitamin B$_7$ deficiency 287
vitamin C deficiency 287
vitamin D analogues 56
vitamin D, synthesis 12
vitiligo 64, 246–8
 causes and types 246
 clinical course 246
 differential diagnosis 246–7
 treatment 247–8
Von Recklinghausen's
   neurofibromatosis 301,
   302
vulvovaginitis 185

warts 201–5, 254
 anogenital *see* condyloma
   acuminata
 cause 201–2
 common 202
 complications 204
 course 203–4
 differential diagnosis 204
 facial 203, 205
 hyperkeratotic 47
 mosaic 203
 penile 203
 peri-ungual 178
 plane 203, 205
 plantar 202, 203, 204–5
 presentation 202–3

seborrhoeic *see* seborrhoeic
   keratosis
 treatment 204–5, 335
Weber–Cockayne epidermolysis
   bullosa 116
Wegener's granulomatosis 106
wet wrap dressings 75, 319
wheals 30, 31
white hair 248
white nails 286
Wickham's striae 65
wood alcohol allergy 78
Wood's light 33, 217
wound healing 19

X-linked ichthyosis 11
X-linked recessive ichthyosis 42
xanthelasma 289, 290
xanthoma 289
 eruptive 290
 generalized plane 290
 and liver disease 286
 plane 290
 tuberous 290
xeroderma pigmentosum 304–5
xerosis 312

yaws 195
yellow nail syndrome 178–9

zinc sulphate 144

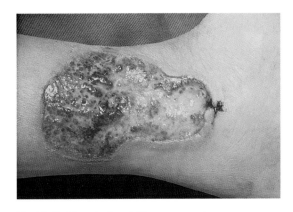

Fig. 11.10 Chronic ulcer failing to respond to treatment. Biopsy, taken from rolled edge, excluded malignant change.

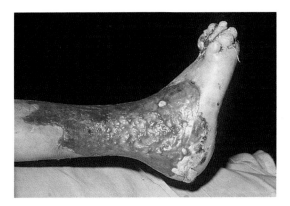

Fig. 11.11 Large, shallow and recalcitrant ulcer complicating rheumatoid arthritis.

Table 11.7 Causes of leg ulceration.

Venous hypertension	See Table 11.6
Arterial disease	Atherosclerosis
	Buerger's disease
	Giant cell arteritis
	Polyarteritis nodosa
	Systemic sclerosis
Small vessel disease	Diabetes mellitus
	Systemic lupus erythematosus
	Rheumatoid arthritis
	Systemic sclerosis
	Allergic vasculitis
Abnormalities of blood	Immune complex disease
	Sickle cell anaemia
	Cryoglobulinaemia
Neuropathy	Diabetes mellitus
	Leprosy
	Syphilis
	Syringomyelia
	Peripheral neuropathy
Infection	'Tropical ulcer'
	Tuberculosis
	Deep fungal infections
Tumour	Squamous cell carcinoma
	Malignant melanoma
	Kaposi's sarcoma
	Basal cell carcinoma
Trauma	Injury
	Artefact
	Iatrogenic

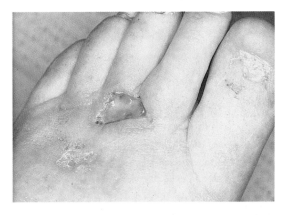

Fig. 11.12 This ulcer on the foot was not caused by venous insufficiency but cryoglobulins were detected.

The involvement of larger vessels is heralded by painful nodules that may ulcerate. The intractable deep sharply demarcated ulcers of rheumatoid arthritis are caused by an underlying vasculitis (Fig. 11.11).

Thrombotic ulcers. Skin infarction (Fig. 11.12), leading to ulceration, may be caused by embolism or by the increased coagulability of polycythaemia or cryoglobulinaemia.

Infective ulcers. Infection is now a rare cause of leg ulcers in the UK but ulcers caused by tuberculosis, leprosy, atypical mycobacteria, diphtheria and deep fungal infections, such as sporotrichosis or chromoblastomycosis, are still seen in the tropics.

Panniculitic ulcers. These may appear at odd sites, such as the thighs, buttocks or backs of the calves. The most common types of panniculitis that ulcerate are lupus panniculitis, pancreatic panniculitis and erythema induratum (p. 130).

Malignant ulcers. Those caused by a squamous cell carcinoma (p. 267) are the most common, but both malignant melanomas (p. 268) and basal cell carcinomas (p. 265) can present as flat lesions, which expand, crust and ulcerate. Furthermore, squamous cell carcinoma can arise in any longstanding ulcer, whatever its cause.

Pyoderma gangrenosum (p. 292). These large and rapidly spreading ulcers may be circular or polycyclic, and have a blue, indurated, undermined or pustular margin. Pyoderma gangrenosum may complicate rheumatoid arthritis, Crohn's disease, ulcerative colitis or blood dyscrasias.

Investigations

Most chronic leg ulcers are venous, but other causes should be considered if the signs are atypical. In patients with venous ulcers, a search for contributory factors, such as obesity, peripheral artery disease, cardiac failure or arthritis, is always worthwhile. Investigations should include the following.

- Urine test for sugar.
- Full blood count to detect anaemia, which will delay healing.
- Swabbing for pathogens (see Bacterial superinfection above).
- Venography, colour flow duplex scanning and the measurement of ambulatory venous pressure help to detect surgically remediable causes of venous incompetence.
- Doppler ultrasound may help to assess arterial circulation when atherosclerosis is likely. It seldom helps if the dorsalis pedis or posterior tibial pulses can easily be felt. If the maximal systolic ankle pressure divided by the systolic brachial pressure ('ankle brachial pressure index') is greater than 0.8, the ulcer is unlikely to be caused by arterial disease.
- Cardiac evaluation for congestive failure.

Treatment

Venous ulcers will not heal if the leg remains swollen and the patient chair-bound. Pressure bandages take priority over other measures but not for atherosclerotic ulcers with an already precarious arterial supply. A common error is to use local treatment that is too elaborate. As a last resort, admission to hospital for elevation and intensive treatment may be needed, but the results are not encouraging; patients may stay in the ward for many months only to have their apparently well-healed ulcers break down rapidly when they go home.

The list of therapies is extensive. They can be divided into the following categories: physical, local, oral and surgical.

Physical measures

Compression bandages and stockings

Compression bandaging, with the compression graduated so that it is greatest at the ankle and least at the top of the bandage, is vital for most venous ulcers; it reduces oedema and aids venous return. The bandages are applied over the ulcer dressing, from the forefoot to just below the knee. Self-adhesive bandages (e.g. Secure Forte and Coban) are convenient and have largely replaced elasticated bandages. Bandages stay on for 2–7 days at a time and are left on at night. One four-layer compression bandaging system includes a layer of orthopaedic wool (Velband), a standard crepe, an elasticated bandage (e.g. Elset and Litepress) and an elasticated cohesive bandage (e.g. Secure Forte and Coban): it requires changing only once a week and is very effective. The combined four layers give a 40-mmHg compression at the ankle. Once an ulcer has healed, a graduated compression stocking (e.g. Duomed, Medi Strumpf, or Venosan 2502/2003 (UK) or Jobst or Teds (USA)) from toes to knee (or preferably thigh), should be prescribed, preferably at pressures of at least 35 mmHg. A foam or felt pad may be worn under the stockings to protect vulnerable areas against minor trauma. The stocking should be put on before rising from bed. Care must be taken with all forms of compression to ensure that the arterial supply is satisfactory and not compromised.